Dandy
(1886-1946)

Grashey
(1876-1950)

Sweet
(1860-1926)

Law
(1875-1947)

Caldwell
(1870-1918)

Béclère, A.
(1856-1939)

Graham
(1883-1957)

Scholten B. Jones

MERRILL'S ATLAS OF

RADIOGRAPHIC POSITIONING & PROCEDURES

FOURTEENTH EDITION | VOLUME THREE

MERRILL'S ATLAS OF

RADIOGRAPHIC POSITIONING & PROCEDURES

Bruce W. Long, MS, RT(R)(CV), FASRT, FAEIRS
Director and Associate Professor
Radiologic Imaging and Sciences Programs
Indiana University School of Medicine
Indianapolis, Indiana

Jeannean Hall Rollins, MRC, BSRT(R)(CV)
Associate Professor
Medical Imaging and Radiation Sciences Department
Arkansas State University
Jonesboro, Arkansas

Barbara J. Smith, MS, RT(R)(QM), FASRT, FAEIRS
Instructor, Radiologic Technology
Medical Imaging Department
Portland Community College
Portland, Oregon

ELSEVIER

ELSEVIER

3251 Riverport Lane
St. Louis, Missouri 63043

MERRILL'S ATLAS OF RADIOGRAPHIC POSITIONING
AND PROCEDURES, FOURTEENTH EDITION

ISBN: 978-0-323-56768-8 (vol 1)
ISBN: 978-0-323-56767-1 (vol 2)
ISBN: 978-0-323-56766-4 (vol 3)
ISBN: 978-0-323-56667-4 (set)

Notices

Practitioners and researchers must always rely on their own experience and knowledge in evaluating and using any information, methods, compounds or experiments described herein. Because of rapid advances in the medical sciences, in particular, independent verification of diagnoses and drug dosages should be made. To the fullest extent of the law, no responsibility is assumed by Elsevier, authors, editors or contributors for any injury and/or damage to persons or property as a matter of products liability, negligence or otherwise, or from any use or operation of any methods, products, instructions, or ideas contained in the material herein.

Previous editions copyrighted 2016, 2012, 2007, 2003, 1999, 1995, 1991, 1986, 1982, 1975, 1967, 1959, and 1949.

International Standard Book Number: 978-0-323-56667-4

Executive Content Strategist: Sonya Seigafuse
Director, Content Development: Laurie Gower
Content Development Specialist: Betsy McCormac
Publishing Services Manager: Julie Eddy
Book Production Specialist: Clay S. Broeker
Design Direction: Brian Salisbury

Printed in the United States of America

Last digit is the print number: 9 8 7 6 5 4

PREVIOUS AUTHORS

Vinita Merrill
1905-1977

Vinita Merrill was born in Oklahoma in 1905 and died in New York City in 1977. Vinita began compilation of *Merrill's* in 1936, while she worked as Technical Director and Chief Technologist in the Department of Radiology and Instructor in the School of Radiography at the New York Hospital. In 1949, while employed as Director of the Educational Department of Picker X-Ray Corporation, she wrote the first edition of the *Atlas of Roentgenographic Positions.* She completed three more editions from 1959 to 1975. Seventy-four years later, Vinita's work lives on in the fourteenth edition of *Merrill's Atlas of Radiographic Positioning & Procedures.*

Philip W. Ballinger, PhD, RT(R), FASRT, FAEIRS, became the author of *Merrill's Atlas* in its fifth edition, which published in 1982. He served as author through the tenth edition, helping to launch successful careers for thousands of students who have learned radiographic positioning from *Merrill's.* Phil currently serves as Professor Emeritus in Radiologic Sciences and Therapy, Division of the School of Health and Rehabilitation Sciences, at The Ohio State University. In 1995, he retired after a 25-year career as Radiography Program Director and, after ably guiding *Merrill's Atlas* through six editions, he retired as *Merrill's* author. Phil continues to be involved in professional activities such as speaking engagements at state, national, and international meetings.

Eugene D. Frank, MA, RT(R), FASRT, FAEIRS, began working with Phil Ballinger on the eighth edition of *Merrill's Atlas* in 1995. He became the coauthor in its ninth, 50th-anniversary edition, published in 1999. He served as lead author for the eleventh and twelfth editions and mentored three coauthors. Gene retired from the Mayo Clinic/Foundation in Rochester, Minnesota in 2001 after 31 years of employment. He was Associate Professor of Radiology in the College of Medicine and Director of the Radiography Program. He also served as Director of the Radiography Program at Riverland Community College, Austin, Minnesota, for 6 years before fully retiring in 2007. He is a Fellow of the ASRT and AEIRS. In addition to *Merrill's*, he is the coauthor of two radiography textbooks, *Quality Control in Diagnostic Imaging* and *Radiography Essentials for Limited Practice.* He now works in hospice through Christian Hospice Care and helps design and equip x-ray departments in underdeveloped countries.

THE MERRILL'S TEAM

Bruce W. Long, MS, RT(R)(CV), FASRT, FAEIRS, is Director and Associate Professor of the Indiana University Radiologic and Imaging Sciences Programs, where he has taught for 33 years. A Life Member of the Indiana Society of Radiologic Technologists, he frequently presents at state and national professional meetings. His publication activities include 28 articles in national professional journals and two books, *Orthopaedic Radiography* and *Radiography Essentials for Limited Practice,* in addition to being coauthor of the *Atlas.* The fourteenth edition is Bruce's fourth on the Merrill's team and second as lead author.

Jeannean Hall Rollins, MRC, BSRT(R)(CV), is an Associate Professor in the Medical Imaging and Radiation Sciences department at Arkansas State University, where she has taught for 27 years. She presents regularly at national meetings. Her publication activities include articles, book reviews, and chapter contributions. Jeannean's first contribution to *Merrill's Atlas* was on the tenth edition as coauthor of the trauma radiography chapter. The fourteenth edition is Jeannean's fourth on the Merrill's team and second as a coauthor. Her previous role was writing the workbook, *Mosby's Radiography Online,* and the Instructor Resources that accompany *Merrill's Atlas.*

Barbara J. Smith, MS, RT(R)(QM), FASRT, FAEIRS, is an instructor in the Radiologic Technology program at Portland Community College, where she has taught for 34 years. The Oregon Society of Radiologic Technologists inducted her as a Life Member in 2003. She presents at state, regional, national, and international meetings, is a trustee with the American Registry of Radiologic Technologists (ARRT), and is involved in professional activities at these levels. Her publication activities include articles, book reviews, and chapter contributions. As coauthor, her primary role on the Merrill's team is working with the contributing authors and editing Volume 3. The fourteenth edition is Barb's fourth on the Merrill's team.

Tammy Curtis, PhD, RT(R)(CT)(CHES), is an associate professor at Northwestern State University, where she has taught for 18 years. She presents at the state, regional, and national levels and is involved in professional activities at the state and national levels. Her publication activities include articles, book reviews, and book contributions. Previously, Tammy served on the advisory board and submitted several projects to the *Atlas.* In particular, for the twelfth edition, Tammy submitted an updated photo of the original author, Vinita Merrill, which she discovered after a 3-year search of historical records. Her primary role on the Merrill's team is to update the workbook and work with the coauthors of the textbook to review content for all three volumes. The fourteenth edition is Tammy's second on the Merrill's team.

ADVISORY BOARD

This edition of *Merrill's Atlas* benefits from the expertise of a special advisory board. The following board members have provided professional input and advice and have helped the authors make decisions about *Atlas* content throughout the preparation of the fourteenth edition:

Kimberly Cross, MSRS, RT(R)(CT)
Clinical Coordinator and Assistant Program
   Director
Emory University Medical Imaging Program
Emory Department of Radiology and Imaging
   Sciences
Atlanta, Georgia

Parsha Y. Hobson, MPA, RT(R)
Professor, Program Director, and Chairperson
Radiography, Public Health, Health Sciences,
   and Health Information
Passaic County Community College
Paterson, New Jersey

Robin J. Jones, MS, RT(R)
Associate Professor and Clinical Coordinator
Radiologic Sciences Program
Indiana University Northwest
Gary, Indiana

James G. Murrell, MSRS, RT(R)(M)(QM)
(CT), CRT(R)(F), FAEIRS
Dean of Imaging Sciences and Radiologic
   Technology Program Director
Brightwood College
Los Angeles, California

Christine Preachuk, RT(R), CAE
Clinical Educator, Health Sciences Centre,
   Winnipeg Regional Health Authority
Clinical Faculty Member, Medical Radiologic
   Technology Program, Red River College
Winnipeg, Manitoba, Canada

Marilyn J. Lewis Thompson, MBA,
RT(R)(M)
Clinical Coordinator
Saint Luke's School of Radiologic
   Technology at Saint Luke's Hospital of
   Kansas City
Saint Luke's College of Health Sciences
Kansas City, Missouri

CHAPTER CONTENT EXPERTS

Valerie F. Andolina, RT(R)(M)
Mammography Technologist
Radiology
Lee Health
Fort Myers, Florida

Leila Bussman-Yeakel, MEd, RT(R)(T)
Program Director and Assistant Professor
Radiation Therapy Program
Mayo Clinic School of Health Sciences
Rochester, Minnesota

Derek Carver, MEd, RT(R)(MR)
Manager of Education and Training
Department of Radiology
Boston Children's Hospital
Boston, Massachusetts

Rex T. Christensen, MHA, RT(R)(MR)(CT), CIIP, MRSO
Associate Professor and MRI Program Director
School of Radiologic Sciences
Weber State University
Ogden, Utah

Cheryl DuBose, EdD, RT(R)(MR)(CT)(QM), MRSO
Department Chair
Medical Imaging and Radiation Sciences
Arkansas State University
Jonesboro, Arkansas

Angela Franceschi, MEd, CCLS
Certified Child Life Specialist
Radiology
Boston Children's Hospital
Boston, Massachusetts

Steven G. Hayes Jr., MSRS, RT(R)
Radiology Supervisor
IU Health
Methodist Hospital
Indianapolis, Indiana

Tracy Iversen, RT(R)(M)(QM)
Rapid City, South Dakota

Nancy M. Johnson, MEd, RT(R)(CV)(CT)(QM), FASRT
Dean, Professional and Technical Education
Academic Affairs
GateWay Community College
Phoenix, Arizona

Raymond J. Johnson, BS, CNMT, PET
Certified Nuclear Medicine Technologist/ Certified PET Technologist
Radiology/Nuclear Medicine
John Peter Smith Health Network
Fort Worth, Texas

Lois J. Layne, MSHA, RT(R)(CV)
Privacy Specialist
Centralized Privacy
Covenant Health
Knoxville, Tennessee

Cheryl Morgan-Duncan, MAS, RT(R)(M)
Instructor
Radiography Program
Passaic County Community College
Staff Mammographer
Mammography
St Joseph's Regional Medical Center
Paterson, New Jersey

Susanna L. Ovel, RT, RDMS, RVT
Senior Sonographer
Medical Imaging
Sutter Medical Foundation
Sacramento, California

Paula Pate-Schloder, MS, RT(R)(CV)(CT)(VI), FAEIRS
Department Chair
Medical Imaging
Misericordia University
Dallas, Pennsylvania

Lynette Petrie, MEd, RT(R)(CV)
Vascular and Interventional Radiologic Technologist
New Hanover Regional Medical Center
Wilmington, North Carolina

Bartram J. Pierce, BS, RT(R)(MR), MRSO
MRI Safety Officer/MR Technologist II
Radiology—MRI
The Corvallis Clinic, PC
Corvallis, Oregon
Adjunct Professor
Medical Imaging
Portland Community College
Portland, Oregon

Jessica L. Saunders, RT(R)(M)
Senior Technologist
Mammography
Elizabeth Wende Breast Care
Rochester, New York

Raymond Thies, BS, RT(R)
Radiologic Technologist II
Radiology
Boston Children's Hospital
Boston, Massachusetts

Sharon R. Wartenbee, RTR, BD, CBDT, FASRT
Senior DXA Technologist
Avera Medical Group
McGreevy Clinic
Sioux Falls, South Dakota

Gayle K. Wright, BS, RTR, CT, MR
Instructor, Radiography
Instructor, Program Coordinator—CT and MRI
Medical Imaging
Portland Community College
Portland, Oregon

PREFACE

Welcome to the fourteenth edition of *Merrill's Atlas of Radiographic Positioning & Procedures*. This edition continues the tradition of excellence begun in 1949, when Vinita Merrill wrote the first edition of what has become a classic text. Over the past 70 years, *Merrill's Atlas* has provided a strong foundation in anatomy and positioning for thousands of students around the world who have gone on to successful careers as imaging technologists. *Merrill's Atlas* is also a mainstay for everyday reference in imaging departments all over the world. As the coauthors of the fourteenth edition, we are honored to follow in Vinita Merrill's footsteps.

Learning and Perfecting Positioning Skills

Merrill's Atlas has an established tradition of helping students learn and perfect their positioning skills. After covering preliminary steps in radiography, radiation protection, and terminology in the introductory chapters, the first two volumes of the *Atlas* teach anatomy and positioning in separate chapters for each bone group or organ system. The student learns to position the patient properly so that the resulting radiograph provides the information the physician needs to correctly diagnose the patient's problem. The *Atlas* presents this information for commonly requested projections as well as for those less commonly requested, making it the only reference of its kind in the world.

The third volume provides basic information about a variety of special imaging modalities, such as mobile and surgical imaging, pediatrics, geriatrics, computed tomography (CT), vascular radiology, magnetic resonance imaging (MRI), sonography, nuclear medicine technology, bone densitometry, and radiation therapy.

Merrill's Atlas is not only a comprehensive resource to help students learn but also an indispensable reference as they move into the clinical environment and ultimately into practice as imaging professionals.

New to This Edition

Since the first edition of *Merrill's Atlas* in 1949, many changes have occurred. This new edition incorporates many significant changes designed not only to reflect the technologic progress and advancements in the profession but also to meet the needs of today's radiography students. The major changes in this edition are highlighted as follows.

ORGANIZATION

The fourteenth edition of the *Atlas* has been completely reorganized to emphasize all procedures listed in the Content Specifications for the ARRT Radiography Examination and in the ASRT Radiography Curriculum and to better reflect the order in which the majority of educators teach radiographic positioning and procedures. Most notably, the thoracic viscera and abdomen chapters are now the first two positioning and procedures chapters. Outdated chapters were removed, while still relevant materials were moved to appropriate chapters and updated to current practice. Selected chapter titles and anatomic terms have been updated to ensure consistency with the ARRT Content Specifications and the ASRT Curriculum Guide.

NEW PATIENT PHOTOGRAPHY

All patient positioning photographs have been replaced in Chapter 7. Additional new patient positioning photographs have been strategically added to better reflect current practice. The new photographs show positioning detail to a greater extent and in some cases from a more realistic perspective. In addition, the equipment in these photos is more modern, and computed radiography plates and occasionally direct digital detectors are used. The use of electronic central ray angle indicators enables a better understanding of where the central ray should enter the patient.

NEW IMAGES

Updated digital images were added to selected chapters, including Chapters 11, 12, 15, and 17. Many MRI images in the sectional anatomy chapter (24) were replaced by images with improved contrast.

IMAGE RECEPTORS AND COLLIMATION

Descriptions and sizes of image receptors on each projection page have been updated to include only those used in current practice. Greater emphasis has been placed on collimation size and field light coverage. This is increasingly important as many imaging departments use only a single, large IR size. A constant reminder has been added to properly place a radiographic marker in the exposure field.

REVISED IMAGE EVALUATION CRITERIA

All image evaluation criteria have been revised and reorganized to improve the student's ability to learn what constitutes a quality image. In addition, the criteria are presented in a way that improves the ability to correct positioning errors.

SIGNIFICANT VOLUME 1 CHAPTER UPDATES

Radiographic compensating filter material has been moved to Chapter 1 to place it with the rest of the general concepts material. Appropriate soft tissue neck material from the deleted anterior part of the neck chapter was moved to the thoracic viscera chapter (3) and updated to reflect current practice. Appropriate long bone measurement material from the deleted long bone measurement chapter was moved to the lower extremity chapter (7) and updated to reflect current practice. Scoliosis radiography material was updated in the vertebral column chapter (9) to reflect current practice.

SIGNIFICANT VOLUME 2 CHAPTER UPDATES

New projections have been added to the trauma chapter (12) to ensure complete coverage of procedures tested by the ARRT. In chapter 15, the modified barium swallow (swallowing dysfunction study) and other contrast media procedures of the GI tract have been updated to reflect current practice. Outdated procedures have been removed from the urinary system and venipuncture chapter (16), while sonography images of urinary anatomy have been added, as has the latest information on the relationships between radiographic contrast media administration and BUN, creatinine, and GFR. The chapter on the reproductive system (17) has been updated to include sonography of the male reproductive system.

SIGNIFICANT VOLUME 3 CHAPTER UPDATES

The vascular, cardiac, and interventional radiography chapter (27) has been significantly updated, especially with regard to ancillary equipment and interventional procedures, to reflect current practice. The nuclear medicine chapter (29) has been reorganized, and radiopharmaceuticals material has been updated.

Learning Aids for the Student
POCKET GUIDE TO RADIOGRAPHY

The new edition of *Merrill's Pocket Guide to Radiography* complements the revision of *Merrill's Atlas*. Instructions for positioning the patient and the body part for all of the essential projections are presented in a complete yet concise manner. Tabs are included to help the user locate the beginning of each section. Space is provided for the user to write in specifics of department techniques.

RADIOGRAPHIC POSITIONING AND PROCEDURES WORKBOOK

The new edition of this workbook features extensive review and self-assessment exercises that supplement the first 25 chapters in *Merrill's Atlas* in one convenient volume. To complement the textbook, similar content was merged and rearranged to better reflect the order in which the majority of students learn radiographic positioning and procedures. Chapters were removed to coincide with changes in the *Atlas*. Relevant material was updated to current practice and integrated into appropriate chapters. Terminology was updated to match the Content Specifications for the ARRT Radiography Examination, the ASRT Radiography Curriculum, and the evolution of digital imaging. The features of the previous editions, including anatomy labeling exercises, positioning exercises, and self-tests, are still available. However, this edition features more image evaluations to give students additional opportunities to evaluate radiographs for proper positioning and more positioning questions to complement the workbook's strong anatomy review. The comprehensive multiple-choice tests at the end of each chapter help students assess their comprehension of the whole chapter. New exercises in this edition focus on improved understanding of essential projections and the need for appropriate collimated field sizes for digital imaging. Additionally, review and assessment exercises in this edition have been expanded for the chapters on pediatrics, geriatrics, vascular and interventional radiography, sectional anatomy, and computed tomography in Volume 3. Exercises in these chapters help students learn the theory and concepts of these special techniques with greater ease. Answers to the workbook questions are found on the Evolve website.

Teaching Aids for the Instructor
EVOLVE INSTRUCTOR ELECTRONIC RESOURCES

This comprehensive resource provides valuable tools such as lesson plans, PowerPoint slides, and an electronic test bank for teaching an anatomy and positioning class. The test bank includes more than 1500 questions, each coded by category and level of difficulty. Four exams are already compiled in the test bank to be used "as is" at the instructor's discretion. The instructor also has the option of building new tests as often as desired by pulling questions from the ExamView pool or using a combination of questions from the test bank and questions that the instructor adds.

Evolve may be used to publish the class syllabus, outlines, and lecture notes; set up "virtual office hours" and e-mail communication; share important dates and information through the online class Calendar; and encourage student participation through Chat Rooms and Discussion Boards. Evolve allows instructors to post exams and manage their grade books online. For more information, visit *www.evolve.elsevier.com* or contact an Elsevier sales representative.

MOSBY'S RADIOGRAPHY ONLINE

Mosby's Radiography Online: Merrill's Atlas of Radiographic Positioning & Procedures is a well-developed online course companion for the textbook and workbook. This online course includes animations with narrated interactive activities and exercises, as well as multiple-choice assessments that can be tailored to meet the learning objectives of your program or course. The addition of this online course to your teaching resources offers greater learning opportunities while accommodating diverse learning styles and circumstances. This unique program promotes problem-based learning with the goal of developing critical thinking skills that will be needed in the clinical setting.

EVOLVE—ONLINE COURSE MANAGEMENT

Evolve is an interactive learning environment designed to work in coordination with *Merrill's Atlas*. Instructors may use Evolve to provide an Internet-based course component that reinforces and expands on the concepts delivered in class.

We hope you will find this edition of *Merrill's Atlas of Radiographic Positioning & Procedures* the best ever. Input from generations of readers has helped to keep the *Atlas* strong through 13 editions, and we welcome your comments and suggestions. We are constantly striving to build on Vinita Merrill's work, and we trust that she would be proud and pleased to know that the work she began 70 years ago is still so appreciated and valued by the imaging sciences community.

Bruce W. Long
Jeannean Hall Rollins
Barbara J. Smith
Tammy Curtis

ACKNOWLEDGMENTS

In preparing for the fourteenth edition, our advisory board continually provided professional expertise and aid in the decision making on the revision of this edition. The advisory board members are listed on p. vii. We are most grateful for their input and contributions to this edition of the *Atlas*.

Contributors

The group of radiography professionals listed below contributed to this edition of the *Atlas* and made many insightful suggestions. We are most appreciative of their willingness to lend their expertise.

We would like to extend special recognition and appreciation to Chris Brown, BS, RT(R); radiography student Madison Kolthoff; and the imaging professionals at Eskenazi Health in Indianapolis, Indiana, for their assistance with on-site photography for scoliosis and long bone measurement radiography. We would also like to thank Sally Powell, RT(R), imaging supervisor at Riley Hospital for Children, and student radiographer Madeline Pfister for their assistance with on-site photography for scoliosis radiography.

We would like to extend special recognition and appreciation to the imaging professionals and Gena Morris, RT(R), RDMS, PACS administrator at NEA Baptist Hospital in Jonesboro, Arkansas, for their time, effort, and expertise during this revision process. Additionally, we would also like to thank the imaging professionals and Mitzi Pierce, MSHS, RT(R)(M), radiology educator at St. Bernard's Medical Center in Jonesboro, Arkansas.

We would like to extend special recognition and appreciation to April Apple, RT(R), Senior Staff Technologist, Duke University Medical Center, for providing a new and more accurate image for the West Point method of the shoulder.

Finally, our deepest appreciation to our faith, family, and colleagues, whose support and encouragement remain an indispensable part of this work.

CONTENTS

20
MOBILE RADIOGRAPHY

STEVEN G. HAYES JR.

Principles of Mobile Radiography

Mobile radiography using transportable radiographic equipment allows imaging services to be brought to the patient. In contrast to the large stationary machines found in radiography rooms, compact mobile radiography units can produce diagnostic images in virtually any location (Fig. 20.1). Mobile radiography is commonly performed in patients' rooms, emergency departments, intensive care units, surgery, recovery rooms, and nursery and neonatal units. Some machines are designed for transport by automobile or van to extended-care facilities or other off-site locations requiring radiographic imaging services.

Mobile radiography was first used by the military for treating battlefield injuries during World War I. Small portable units were designed to be carried by soldiers and set up in field locations. Although mobile equipment is no longer "carried" to the patient, the term *portable* has persisted and is often used in reference to mobile procedures.

This chapter focuses on the most common projections performed with mobile radiography machines. The basic principles of mobile radiography are described and helpful hints are provided for successful completion of the examinations.

An understanding of common projections enables the radiographer to perform most mobile examinations ordered by the physician.

Mobile X-Ray Machines

Mobile x-ray machines are not as sophisticated as the larger stationary machines in the radiology department. Although mobile units are capable of producing images of most body parts, they vary in their exposure controls and power sources (or generators).

A typical mobile x-ray machine has controls for setting kilovolt (peak) (kVp) and milliampere-seconds (mAs). The mAs control automatically adjusts milliamperage (mA) and time to preset values. Maximum settings differ among manufacturers, but mAs typically range from 0.04 to 320 and kVp from 40 to 130. The total power of the unit ranges from 15 to 25 kilowatts (kW), which is adequate for most mobile projections. By comparison, the power of a stationary radiography unit can reach 150 kW (150 kVp, 1000 mA) or more.

Some mobile x-ray machines have preset anatomic programs (APRs) similar to stationary units. The APRs use exposure techniques with predetermined values based on the selected examination. The radiographer can adjust these settings as needed to compensate for differences in the size or condition of a patient. The much wider dynamic range available with CR or DR and the ability to manipulate the final image with computer software can provide images of proper density.

Some mobile units have direct digital capability, where the image is acquired immediately on the unit. These machines have a flat-panel detector, similar to those found in a DR table bucky. The detector either is connected to the portable unit by a tethered cord or communicates through wireless technology (Fig. 20.2).

Technical Considerations

Mobile radiography presents the radiographer with challenges different from those associated with performing examinations with stationary equipment in the radiology department. Although the positioning of the patient and placement of the central ray are essentially the same, three important technical matters must be clearly understood to perform optimal mobile examinations: the *grid,* the *anode heel effect*, and the *source-to-image receptor distance (SID)*. In addition, exposure technique charts must be available (Fig. 20.3).

Fig. 20.1 Radiographer moving a battery-operated mobile radiography machine to a patient's room.

GRID

The phosphor used in CR imaging plates is very sensitive to the image degradation effects of scattered radiation. Therefore, in performing portable radiography with CR imaging plates, it is important to use a grid.

For optimal imaging, a grid must be level, centered to the central ray, and correctly used at the recommended focal distance, or radius. When a grid is placed on an unstable surface such as the mattress of a bed, the weight of the patient can cause the grid to tilt "off level." If a longitudinal grid tilts transversely, the central ray forms an angle across the long axis. Image density is then lost as a result of grid "cutoff" (Fig. 20.4). If the grid tilts longitudinally, the central ray angles through the long axis. In this case, grid cutoff is avoided, but the image may be distorted or elongated.

A grid positioned under a patient can be difficult to center. If the central ray is directed to a point transversely off the midline of a grid more than 1 to $1\frac{1}{2}$ inches (2.5 to 3.8 cm), a cutoff effect similar to that produced by an off-level grid results. The central ray can be centered longitudinally to any point along the midline of a grid without cutoff. Depending on the procedure, beam-restriction problems may occur. If this happens, a portion of the image is "collimated off," or patient exposure is excessive because of an oversized exposure field.

Fig. 20.2 (A) The machine on the left is an analog mobile unit, and the other two are digital units. Notice that the two digital mobile units have computer screens. (B) Mobile digital screen with a chest image.

MOBILE RADIOGRAPHIC TECHNIQUE CHART

AMX—4   40-inch SID   CR IP   8:1 grid

Part	Projection	Position	cm—kVp	mAs	Grid
Chest	AP	Supine/upright	21—120	3.2	Yes
	AP	Lateral decubitus	21—85	6.25	Yes
Abdomen	AP	Supine	23—74	25	Yes
	AP	Lateral decubitus	23—74	32	Yes
Pelvis	AP	Supine	23—74	32	Yes
Femur (distal)	AP	Supine	15—70	10	Yes
	Lateral	Dorsal decubitus	15—70	10	Yes
C-spine	Lateral	Dorsal decubitus	10—62	20	Yes
NEONATAL					
Chest/abdomen	AP	Supine	7—64	0.8	No
	Lateral	Dorsal decubitus	10—72	1	No

Fig. 20.3 Sample radiographic technique chart showing manual technical factors used for the 10 common mobile projections described in this chapter. The kVp and mAs factors are for the specific centimeter measurements indicated. Factors vary depending on the actual centimeter measurement.

Fig. 20.4 Mobile radiograph of proximal femur and hip, showing comminuted fracture of left acetabulum. (A) Poor-quality radiograph resulted when grid was transversely tilted far enough to produce significant grid cutoff. (B) Excellent-quality repeat radiograph on the same patient, performed with grid accurately positioned perpendicular to central ray.

Fig. 20.5 The directions of the grid lines are marked on the front of the grid as either transverse *(short dimension)* or longitudinal *(long dimension)*. Focal ranges are clearly identified for proper use.

Grids used for mobile radiography are often of the focused type. However, some radiology departments continue to use the older, parallel-type grids. All focused grids have a recommended focal range, or radius, that varies with the grid ratio. Projections taken at distances greater or less than the recommended focal range can produce cutoff in which image density is reduced on lateral margins. Grids with a lower ratio have a greater focal range, but they are less efficient for cleaning up scatter radiation. The radiographer must be aware of the *exact* focal range for the grid used. Most focused grids used for mobile radiography have a ratio of 6:1 or 8:1 and a focal range of about 36 to 44 inches (91 to 112 cm). This focal range allows mobile examinations to be performed efficiently. Inverting a focused grid causes a pronounced cutoff effect similar to that produced by improper distance.

Today most grids are mounted on a protective frame, and the IR is easily inserted behind the grid (Fig. 20.5). The direction of the grid lines is usually marked to indicate if it is transverse (short dimension) or longitudinal (long dimension). The examinations described in this chapter present methods of ensuring proper grid and IR placement for projections that require a grid.

ANODE HEEL EFFECT

Another consideration in mobile radiography is the *anode heel effect*. The heel effect causes a decrease of image density under the anode side of the x-ray tube. The heel effect is more pronounced with the following:
- Short SID
- Larger field sizes
- Small anode angles

Short SIDs and large field sizes are common in mobile radiography; here the radiographer has control of the anode-cathode axis of the x-ray tube relative to the body part. Correct placement of the anode-cathode axis with regard to the anatomy is essential. In performing a mobile examination, the radiographer may not always be able to orient the anode-cathode axis of the tube to the desired position because of limited space and maneuverability in the room. For optimal mobile radiography, the anode and cathode sides of the x-ray tube should be clearly marked to indicate where the high-tension cables enter the x-ray tube, and the radiographer should use the heel effect maximally (Table 20.1).

SOURCE-TO-IMAGE RECEPTOR DISTANCE

The SID should be maintained at 40 inches (102 cm) for most mobile examinations. A standardized distance for all patients and projections helps to ensure consistency in imaging. Longer SIDs—40 to 48 inches (102 to 122 cm)—require increased mAs to compensate for the additional distance. The mA limitations of a mobile unit necessitate longer exposure times when the SID exceeds 40 inches (102 cm). Despite the longer exposure time, a radiograph with motion artifacts may result if the SID is greater than 40 inches (102 cm). In addition, motion artifacts may occur in the radiographs of critically ill adult patients and infants or small children who require chest and abdominal examinations but may be unable to hold their breath.

RADIOGRAPHIC TECHNIQUE CHARTS

A radiographic technique chart should be available for use with every mobile machine. The chart should display, in an organized manner, the standardized technical factors for all the radiographic projections done with the machine (see Fig. 20.3). A caliper should also be available; this device is used to measure the thickness of body parts to ensure that accurate and consistent exposure factors are used. Measuring the patient also allows the radiographer to determine the optimal kVp level for all exposures (Fig. 20.6).

TABLE 20.1
Cathode placement for mobile projections

Part	Projection	Cathode placement
Chest	AP	Diaphragm
	AP—decubitus	Down side of chest
Abdomen	AP	Diaphragm
	AP—decubitus	Down side of abdomen
Pelvis	AP	Upper pelvis
Femur	AP	Proximal femur
	Lateral	Proximal femur
Cervical spine	Lateral	Over lower vertebrae (40-inch (102-cm) SID only)
Chest and abdomen in neonate	All	No designation[a]

[a]Not necessary because of small field size of the collimator.
Note: The cathode side of the beam has the greatest intensity.

Fig. 20.6 Radiographer measuring the thickest portion of the femur to determine the exact technical factors needed for the examination.

Radiation Safety

Radiation protection for the radiographer, others in the immediate area, and the patient is of paramount importance when mobile examinations are performed. *Mobile radiography produces some of the highest occupational radiation exposures for radiographers.* The radiographer should wear a lead apron and stand as far away from the patient, x-ray tube, and useful beam as the room and the exposure cable allow. The recommended *minimal* distance is 6 ft (2 m). For a horizontal (cross-table) x-ray beam or for an upright AP chest projection, the radiographer should stand at a right angle (90 degrees) to the primary beam and the object being radiographed. The least amount of scatter radiation occurs at this position (Fig. 20.7). Shielding and distance have a greater effect on exposure reduction, however, and should always be considered first.

The most effective means of radiation protection is *distance.* The radiographer should inform all persons in the immediate area that an x-ray exposure is about to occur so that they may leave to avoid exposure. Lead protection should be provided for any individuals who are unable to leave the room and for individuals who may have to hold a patient or IR.

Patients should be shielded as necessary with appropriate radiation protection devices for any of the following situations:

- X-ray examinations performed on children
- X-ray examinations performed on patients of reproductive age
- Any examination for which the patient requests protection
- Examinations in which the gonads lie in or near the useful beam
- Examinations in which shielding would not interfere with imaging of the anatomy that must be shown (Fig. 20.8)

In addition, the source-to-skin distance (SSD) cannot be less than 12 inches (30 cm), in accordance with federal safety regulations.[1]

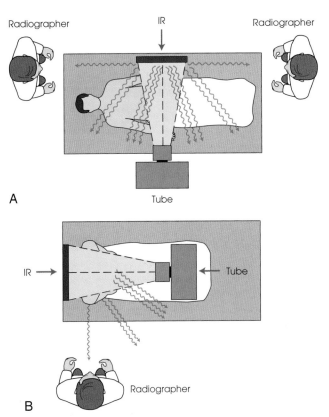

Fig. 20.7 Whenever possible, the radiographer should stand at least 6 feet (2 m) from the patient and useful beam. The lowest amount of scatter radiation occurs at a right angle (90 degrees) from the primary x-ray beam. (A) Note radiographer standing at either the head or the foot of the patient at a right angle to the x-ray beam for dorsal decubitus position lateral projection of the abdomen. (B) Radiographer standing at right angle to the x-ray beam for AP projection of the chest. *IR,* Image receptor.

Isolation Considerations

Two types of patients are often cared for in isolation units: (1) patients who have infectious microorganisms that could be spread to health care workers and visitors and (2) patients who need protection from potentially lethal microorganisms that may be carried by health care workers and visitors. Optimally, a radiographer entering an isolation room should have full knowledge of the patient's disease, the way in which it is transmitted, and the proper way to clean and disinfect equipment before and after use in the isolation unit. Because of the confidentiality of patient records, the radiographer may be unable to obtain information about a patient's specific disease. However, all patients must be treated with universal precautions.

If isolation is used to protect the patient from receiving microorganisms (reverse isolation), a different protocol may be required. Institutional policy regarding isolation procedures should be available and strictly followed.

In performing mobile procedures in an isolation unit, the radiographer should wear the required protective apparel for the specific situation: gown, cap, mask, shoe covers, and gloves. All of this apparel is not needed for every isolation patient. All persons entering a strict isolation unit wear a mask, a gown, and gloves, but only gloves are worn for drainage secretion precautions. Radiographers should always wash their hands with warm soapy water before putting on gloves. The x-ray machine is taken into the room and moved into position. The IR is placed into a clean protective cover. Pillowcases would not protect the IR or the patient if body fluids soaked through them. A clean, impermeable cover should be used in situations in which body fluids may come into contact with the IR. For examinations of patients in strict isolation, two radiographers may be required to maintain a safe barrier (see Chapter 1).

After finishing the examination, the radiographer should remove and dispose of the mask, cap, gown, shoe covers, and gloves according to institutional policies. All equipment that touched the patient or the patient's bed must be wiped with a disinfectant according to appropriate aseptic technique. The radiographer should wear new gloves, if necessary, while cleaning equipment. Handwashing is repeated before the radiographer leaves the room.

Fig. 20.8 Patient ready for mobile chest examination. Note lead shield placed over the patient's pelvis. This shield does not interfere with the examination.

Performing Mobile Examinations

INITIAL PROCEDURES

The radiographer should plan for the trip out of the radiology department. Ensuring that all of the necessary devices (e.g., IR, IR protective covers, grid, tape, caliper, markers, and positioning blocks) are transported with the mobile x-ray machine provides greater efficiency in performing examinations. Many mobile x-ray machines are equipped with storage areas for transporting IRs and supplies. If a battery-operated machine is used, the radiographer should check the machine to ensure that it is acceptably charged. An inadequately charged machine can interfere with performance and affect the quality of the radiograph.

Before entering the patient's room with the machine, the radiographer should follow several important steps (Box 20.1). The radiographer begins by checking that the correct patient is going to be examined. After confirming the identity of the patient, the radiographer enters, makes an introduction as a radiographer, and informs the patient about the x-ray examinations to be performed. While in the room, the radiographer observes any medical appliances—such as chest tube boxes, catheter bags, and intravenous (IV) poles—that may be positioned next to or hanging on the sides of the patient's bed. The radiographer should ask family members or visitors to step out of the room until the examination is finished. If necessary, the nursing staff should be alerted that assistance is required.

Communication and cooperation between the radiographer and nursing staff members are essential for proper patient care during mobile radiography. In addition, communication with the patient is *imperative,* even if the patient is or appears to be unconscious or unresponsive.

EXAMINATION

Chairs, stands, IV poles, wastebaskets, and other obstacles should be moved from the path of the mobile machine. Lighting should be adjusted if necessary. If the patient is to be examined in the supine position, the base of the mobile machine should be positioned toward the middle of the bed. If a seated patient position is used, the base of the machine should be toward the foot of the bed.

For lateral and decubitus radiographs, positioning the base of the mobile machine parallel to or directly perpendicular to the bed allows the greatest ease in positioning the x-ray tube. Room size can also influence the base position used.

The radiographer may sometimes have difficulty accurately aligning the x-ray tube parallel to the IR while standing at the side of the bed. When positioning the tube above the patient, the radiographer may have to check the x-ray tube and IR alignment from the foot of the bed to ensure that the tube is not tilted.

For all projections, the primary x-ray beam must be collimated no larger than the size of the IR. When the central ray is correctly centered to the IR, the light field coincides with or fits within the borders of the IR.

A routine and consistent system for labeling and separating exposed and unexposed IRs should be developed and maintained. It is easy to "double expose" IRs during mobile radiography, particularly if many examinations are performed at one time. Using DR imaging eliminates the chance of double exposure.

Most institutions require additional identification markers for mobile examinations. Typically the time of examination (especially for chest radiographs) and technical notes such as the position of the patient are indicated. A log may be maintained for each patient and kept in the patient's room. The log should contain the exposure factors used for the projections and other notes regarding the performance of the examination.

PATIENT CONSIDERATIONS

A brief but total assessment of the patient must be conducted before and during the examination. Some specific considerations to keep in mind are described in the following sections.

Assessment of the patient's condition

A thorough assessment of the patient's condition and room allows the radiographer to make necessary adaptations to ensure the best possible patient care and imaging outcome. The radiographer assesses the patient's level of alertness and respiration and determines the extent to which the patient is able to cooperate and the limitations that may affect the procedure. Some patients may be experiencing varying degrees of drowsiness because of their medications or medical condition. Many mobile examinations are performed in patients' rooms immediately after surgery; these patients may be under the influence of various anesthetics. It is always important to communicate with the patient even if he or she is not alert.

BOX 20.1

Preliminary steps for the radiographer before mobile radiography is performed

- Announce your presence to the nursing staff and ask for assistance if needed.
- Determine that the correct patient is in the room.
- Introduce yourself to the patient and family as a radiographer and explain the examination.
- Observe the medical equipment in the room and other apparatus and IV poles with fluids. Move the equipment if necessary.
- Ask family members and visitors to leave.[a]

[a]A family member may have to be present for the examination of a small child.

Patient mobility

The radiographer must never move a patient or part of the patient's body without assessing the patient's ability to move or tolerate movement. *Gentleness* and *caution* must prevail at all times. If unsure, the radiographer should always check with the nursing staff or physician. Many patients who undergo total joint replacement may be unable to move the affected joint for many days without assistance, but this may not be evident to the radiographer. Some patients may be able to indicate verbally their ability to move or their tolerance for movement. *The radiographer should never move a limb that has been operated on or is broken unless the nurse, the physician, or sometimes the patient grants permission.* Inappropriate movement of the patient by the radiographer during the examination may harm the patient.

Fractures

Patients can have various fractures and fracture types, ranging from one simple fracture to multiple fractures of many bones. A patient lying awake in a traction bed with a simple femoral fracture may be able to assist with a radiographic examination. Another patient may be unconscious and have multiple broken ribs, spinal fractures, or a severe closed head injury.

Few patients with multiple fractures are able to move or tolerate movement. The radiographer must be cautious, resourceful, and work in accordance with the patient's condition and pain tolerance. If a patient's trunk or limb must be raised into position for a projection, the radiographer should have ample assistance so that the part can be raised safely without causing harm or intense pain.

Interfering devices

Patients who are in intensive care units or orthopedic beds because of fractures may be attached to various devices, wires, and tubing. These objects may be in the direct path of the x-ray beam and consequently produce artifacts on the image. Experienced radiographers know which of these objects can be moved out of the x-ray beam. When devices such as fracture frames cannot be moved, it may be necessary to angle the central ray or adjust the IR to obtain the best radiograph possible. In many instances, the objects have to be radiographed along with the body part (Fig. 20.9). The radiographer must exercise caution in handling any of these devices and should never remove traction devices without the assistance of a physician.

Positioning and asepsis

During positioning, the patient often perceives the IR (with or without a grid) as cold, hard, and uncomfortable. Before the IR is put in place, the patient should be warned of possible discomfort and assured that the examination will be for as short a time as possible. The patient will appreciate the radiographer's concern and efficiency in completing the examination as quickly as possible.

If the surface of the IR inadvertently touches bare skin, it can stick, making positioning adjustments difficult. An imaging plate cover over the IR protects the patient's skin, helps keep the IR clean, and assists with infection control. IRs should be wiped off with a disinfectant for asepsis and infection control after each patient. *The skin of older patients may be thin and dry and can be torn by manipulation of the IR if care is not taken.*

The IR must be enclosed in an appropriate, impermeable barrier in any situation in which it may come in contact with blood, body fluids, and other potentially infectious material. A contaminated IR can be difficult and sometimes impossible to clean. Approved procedures for disposing of used barriers must be followed.

Fig. 20.9 (A) Mobile radiograph of chest. Note various objects in the image that could not be removed for the exposure. (B) Mobile radiograph of proximal femur and hip. Metal buckles could not be removed for the exposure.

AP PROJECTION[a]
Upright or supine

Image receptor: The IR should be 14 × 17 inches (35 × 43 cm) lengthwise or crosswise, depending on body habitus.

Position of patient
Depending on the condition of the patient, the projection should be performed with the patient in the upright position or to the greatest angle the patient can tolerate, whenever possible. Use the supine position for critically ill or injured patients.

---

[a]The nonmobile projection is described in Chapter 3.

Position of part
- Center the midsagittal plane to the IR.
- To include the entire chest, position the IR under the patient with the top about 2 inches (5 cm) above the relaxed shoulders. The exact distance depends on the size of the patient. When the patient is supine, the shoulders may move to a higher position relative to the lungs. Adjust accordingly.
- Make sure that the patient's shoulders are relaxed; then internally rotate the patient's arms to prevent scapular superimposition of the lung field if not contraindicated.
- Make sure that the patient's upper torso is not rotated or leaning toward one side (Fig. 20.10).
- *Shield gonads.*
- *Respiration*: Inspiration unless otherwise requested. If the patient is receiving respiratory assistance, carefully watch the patient's chest to determine the inspiratory phase for the exposure.

Central ray
- Perpendicular to the long axis of the sternum and the center of the IR. The central ray should enter about 3 inches (7.6 cm) below the jugular notch at the level of T7.

Collimation
- Adjust to at least 14 × 17 inches (35 × 43 cm) on the collimator, less for smaller patients.

Exposure considerations
- A grid must be used for all mobile chest examinations if the exposure technique is more than 90 kVp. (Review the manufacturer's protocol for the exact kVp levels for the unit being used.) When a crosswise-positioned longitudinal grid is used, the central ray must be perpendicular to the grid to prevent grid cutoff.

Fig. 20.10 Mobile AP chest: partially upright.

Structures shown

This projection shows the anatomy of the thorax, including the heart, trachea, diaphragmatic domes, and, most importantly, the entire lung fields, including vascular markings (Fig. 20.11).

EVALUATION CRITERIA

The following should be clearly shown:

- Evidence of proper collimation
- No motion; well-defined (not blurred) diaphragmatic domes and lung fields
- Lung fields in their entirety, including costophrenic angles
- Pleural markings
- Ribs and thoracic intervertebral disk spaces faintly visible through heart shadow
- No rotation, with medial portion of clavicles and lateral border of ribs equidistant from vertebral column
- Radiograph markers as appropriate (R or L marker, and any to indicate how the patient is positioned; that is, supine, sitting upright, etc.).

NOTE: To ensure the proper angle from the x-ray tube to the IR, the radiographer can double-check the shadow of the shoulders from the field light projected onto the IR. If the shadow of the shoulders is thrown far above the upper edge of the IR, the angle of the tube must be corrected.

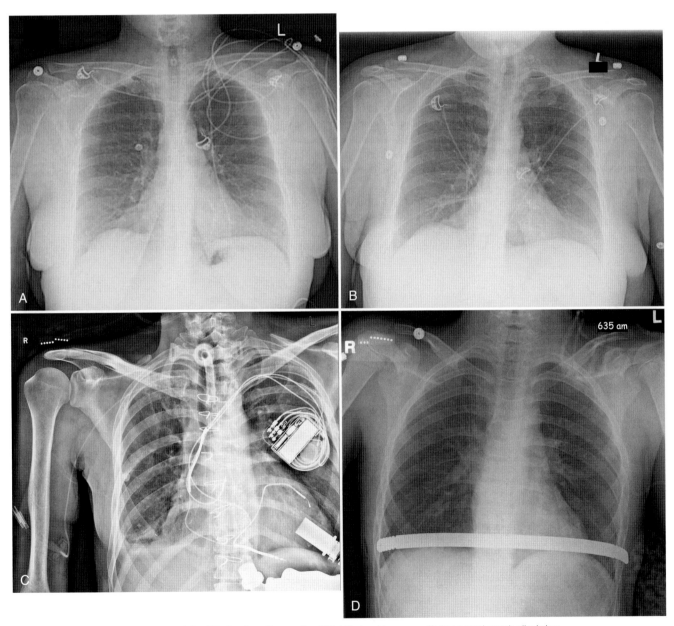

Fig. 20.11 Mobile AP chest radiographs. (A) AP chest image with incorrect cephalic tube angle resulting in an apical lordotic image in which the ribs appear boxy, the clavicles are projected too high, and the heart has a distorted silhouette. A tangle of lead wire is seen over the upper left chest. (B) Repeat image with the correct angle, central ray perpendicular to the long axis of the sternum. The radiographer has also positioned the lead wires appropriately. (C) Mobile PICC placement image to visualize the PICC line from entrance to tip. Also seen are the tracheostomy, pacemaker, sternal wires, and ventricular assist device. (D) Adolescent postoperative patient with strut placed for pectus excavatum repair. Ice pack is seen in the lower right corner of the image.

AP OR PA PROJECTION[b]

Right or left lateral decubitus position

> **Image receptor:** The IR should be a 14 × 17 inches (35 × 43 cm) with a lengthwise grid.

Position of patient

- Place the patient in the lateral recumbent position.
- Flex the patient's knees to provide stabilization, if possible.
- Place a firm support under the patient to elevate the body 2 to 3 inches (5 to 8 cm) and prevent the patient from sinking into the mattress.
- Raise both of the patient's arms up and away from the chest region, preferably above the head. An arm lying on the patient's side can imitate a region of free air.
- Make sure that the patient cannot roll off the bed.

[b]The nonmobile projection is described in Chapter 3.

Position of part

- Position the patient for the AP projection whenever possible. It is much easier to position an ill patient (particularly the arms) for an AP.
- Adjust the patient to ensure a lateral position. The coronal plane passing through the shoulders and hips should be vertical.
- Place the IR behind the patient and below the support so that the lower margin of the chest is visible.
- Adjust the grid so that it extends approximately 2 inches (5 cm) above the shoulders. The IR should be supported in position and not leaning against the patient to avoid distortion (Fig. 20.12).
- *Shield gonads.*
- *Respiration*: Inspiration unless otherwise requested.

Central ray

- Horizontal and perpendicular to the center of the IR, entering the patient at a level of 3 inches (7.6 cm) below the jugular notch.

Collimation

- Adjust to 14 × 17 inches (35 × 43 cm) on the collimator.

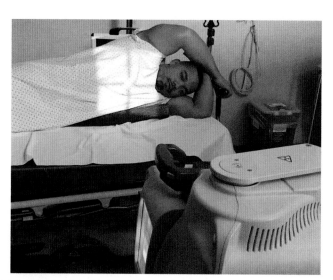

Fig. 20.12 Mobile AP chest: left lateral decubitus position. Note gray pad placed under the chest to elevate it. The block is necessary to ensure that the left side of chest is included on the image.

Structures shown

This projection shows the anatomy of the thorax, including the entire lung fields and any air or fluid levels that may be present (Fig. 20.13).

EVALUATION CRITERIA

The following should be clearly shown:
- Evidence of proper collimation
- No motion
- No rotation
- Affected side in its entirety (upper lung for free air and lower lung for fluid)
- Patient's arms out of region of interest
- Radiographic markers as appropriate

NOTE: Fluid levels in the pleural cavity are best visualized with the affected side down, which also prevents mediastinal overlapping. Air levels are best visualized with the unaffected side down. The patient should be in position for at least 5 minutes before the exposure is made to allow air to rise and fluid levels to settle.

Fig. 20.13 Mobile AP chest radiographs performed in lateral decubitus positions in critically ill patients. (A) Left lateral decubitus position. The patient has a large right pleural effusion *(arrow)* and no left effusion. The complete left side of thorax is visualized because of elevation on a block. (B) Right lateral decubitus position. The patient has a right pleural effusion *(arrows)*, cardiomegaly, and mild pulmonary vascular congestion. The complete right side of thorax is visualized because of elevation on a block.

AP PROJECTION[c]

Image receptor: The IR should be a 14 × 17 inches (35 × 43 cm) with a lengthwise grid.

Position of patient

- If necessary, adjust the patient's bed to achieve a horizontal bed position.
- Place the patient in a supine position.

Position of part

- Position the grid under the patient to show the abdominal anatomy from the pubic symphysis to the upper abdominal region.
- Keep the grid from tipping side to side by placing it in the center of the bed and stabilizing it with blankets or towels if necessary.
- Use the patient's draw sheet to roll the patient; this makes it easier to shift the patient from side to side during positioning of the IR and provides a barrier between the patient's skin and the grid.
- Center the midsagittal plane of the patient to the midline of the grid.

[c]The nonmobile projection is described in Chapter 4.

- Center the grid to the level of the iliac crests. If the emphasis is on the upper abdomen, center the grid 2 inches (5 cm) above the iliac crests or high enough to include the diaphragm.
- Adjust the patient's shoulders and pelvis to lie in the same plane (Fig. 20.14).
- Move the patient's arms out of the region of the abdomen.
- *Shield gonads.* This may not be possible in a female patient.
- *Respiration*: Expiration.

Central ray

- Perpendicular to the center of the grid along the midsagittal plane and at the level of the iliac crests or the 10th rib laterally.

Collimation

- Adjust to 14 × 17 inches (35 × 43 cm) on the collimator.

Structures shown

This projection shows the following: the inferior margin of the liver; the spleen, kidneys, and psoas muscles; calcifications; and evidence of tumor masses. If the image includes the upper abdomen and diaphragm, the size and shape of the liver may be seen (Fig. 20.15).

EVALUATION CRITERIA

The following should be clearly shown:
- Evidence of proper collimation
- No motion
- Outlines of the abdominal viscera
- Abdominal region, including pubic symphysis or diaphragm (both may be seen on some patients)
- Vertebral column in center of image
- Psoas muscles, lower margin of liver, and kidney margins
- No rotation
- Symmetric appearance of vertebral column and iliac wings
- Radiographic markers as appropriate

NOTE: Hypersthenic patients may require two separate projections using a crosswise grid. One grid is positioned for the upper abdomen and the other for the lower abdomen.

Fig. 20.14 Mobile AP of the abdomen.

Fig. 20.15 Mobile AP abdominal radiographs. (A) Abdomen without pathology. The entire abdomen is seen in this patient. (B) Because of this patient's large body habitus, two crosswise (landscape) images of the abdomen were necessary to include all abdominal structures. Counting of vertebral bodies ensures adequate overlap. Note the large amount of free air, indicative of a perforated bowel. (C) Mobile AP abdominal image of a pediatric patient. Ingested jewelry bead is seen in the fundus of the stomach.

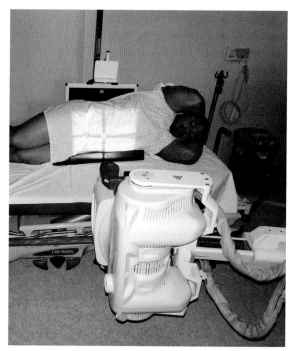

Fig. 20.16 Mobile AP abdomen: left lateral decubitus position. Note black blocks placed under the abdomen to level the abdomen and keep the patient from sinking into the mattress.

AP OR PA PROJECTION[d]

Left lateral decubitus position

> **Image receptor:** The IR should be a 14 × 17 inches (35 × 43 cm) with a lengthwise grid.

Position of patient
- Place the patient in the left lateral recumbent position unless requested otherwise.
- Flex the patient's knees slightly to provide stabilization.
- If necessary, place a firm support under the patient to elevate the body and keep the patient from sinking into the mattress.
- Raise both of the patient's arms away from the abdominal region if possible. The right arm lying on the side of the abdomen may imitate a region of free air.
- Make sure that the patient cannot fall out of bed.

Position of part
- Use the PA or AP projection, depending on the room layout.
- Adjust the patient to ensure a true lateral position. The coronal plane passing through the shoulders and hips should be vertical.
- Place the grid vertically in front of the patient for a PA projection and behind the patient for an AP projection. The grid should be supported in position and not leaned against the patient; this position prevents grid cutoff.
- Position the grid so that its center is 2 inches (5 cm) above the iliac crests to ensure that the diaphragm is included. The pubic symphysis and lower abdomen do not have to be visualized (Fig. 20.16).
- Before making the exposure, ensure that the patient has been in the lateral recumbent position for at least 5 minutes to allow air to rise and fluid levels to settle.
- *Shield gonads.*
- *Respiration*: Expiration.

---

[d]The nonmobile projection is described in Chapter 4.

Central ray

• Horizontal and perpendicular to the center of the grid, entering the patient along the midsagittal plane

Collimation

• Adjust to 14 × 17 inches (35 × 43 cm) on the collimator.

Structures shown

Air or fluid levels within the abdominal cavity are shown. These projections are especially helpful in assessing free air in the abdomen. The right border of the abdominal region must be visualized (Fig. 20.17).

EVALUATION CRITERIA

The following should be clearly shown:
- Evidence of proper collimation
- No motion
- Well-defined diaphragm and abdominal viscera
- Air or fluid levels if present
- Right and left abdominal wall and flank structures
- No rotation
- Symmetric appearance of vertebral column and iliac wings
- Radiographic markers as appropriate

NOTE: Hypersthenic patients may require two projections using a 14 × 17 inches (35 × 43 cm) grid positioned crosswise to visualize the entire abdominal area. A patient with a long torso may require two projections with the grid lengthwise to visualize the entire abdominal region.

Fig. 20.17 Mobile AP of the abdomen: left lateral decubitus position. Free intraperitoneal air is seen on the upper or right side of the abdomen *(arrow)*. The radiograph is slightly underexposed to show free air more easily.

AP PROJECTION[f]

Most mobile AP and lateral projections of the femur may be radiographs of the middle and distal femur taken while the patient is in traction. The femur cannot be moved, which presents a challenge to the radiographer.

Image receptor: The IR should be a 14 × 17 inches (35 × 43 cm) with a grid lengthwise.

Position of patient

- The patient is in the supine position.

[f]The nonmobile projection is described in Chapter 7.

Position of part

- Cautiously place the grid lengthwise under the patient's femur, with the distal edge of the grid low enough to include the fracture site, pathologic region, and knee joint.
- Elevate the grid with towels, blankets, or blocks under each side, if necessary, to ensure proper grid alignment with the x-ray tube.
- Center the grid to the midline of the affected femur.
- Ensure that the grid is placed parallel to the plane of the femoral condyles (Fig. 20.20).
- *Shield gonads.*
- *Respiration*: Suspended.

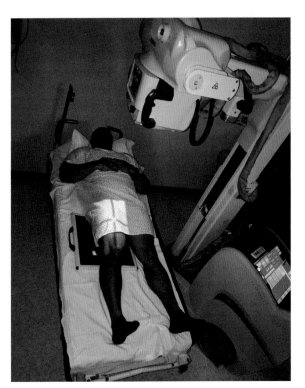

Fig. 20.20 Mobile of the AP femur.

Central ray

- Perpendicular to the long axis of the femur and centered to the grid.
- Make sure that the central ray and grid are aligned to prevent grid cutoff.

Collimation

- Adjust to top at ASIS for hip, bottom at tibial tuberosity for knee, 1 inch (2.5 cm) on side of the shadow of the femur, and 17 inches (43 cm) in length.

DIGITAL RADIOGRAPHY

The thickest portion of the femur (proximal area) must be carefully measured, and an appropriate kVp must be selected to penetrate this area. The computer cannot form an image of the anatomy in this area if penetration does not occur. A light area of the entire proximal femur would result. Positioning the cathode over the proximal femur would improve CR image quality.

Structures shown

The distal two-thirds of the femur, including the knee joint, are shown (Fig. 20.21).

EVALUATION CRITERIA

The following should be clearly shown:
- Evidence of proper collimation
- Most of femur, including knee joint
- No knee rotation
- Adequate penetration of proximal portion of femur
- Any orthopedic appliance, such as plate and screw fixation
- Radiographic markers as appropriate

NOTE: If the entire length of the femur must be visualized, an AP projection of the proximal femur can be performed by placing a 14 × 17 inches (35 × 43 cm) grid lengthwise under the proximal femur and hip. The top of the grid is placed at the level of the ASIS to ensure that the hip joint is included. The central ray is directed to the center of the grid and long axis of the femur (see Fig. 20.4).

Fig. 20.21 Mobile of the AP femur showing a fracture of the midshaft with femoral rod placement. The knee joint is included on the image.

Fig. 20.22 Mobile of the mediolateral left femur. An assistant wearing a lead apron holds and positions the right leg and femur and steadies the grid.

Fig. 20.23 Mobile lateromedial of the left femur. The grid is placed between the legs and steadied by the patient.

LATERAL PROJECTION[g]

Mediolateral or lateromedial projection

Dorsal decubitus position

It may not be possible to move the femur, which presents a challenge to the radiographer. The *mediolateral* projection is generally preferred because more of the proximal femur is demonstrated.

> **Image receptor:** The IR should be 14 × 17 inches (35 × 43 cm) with a grid lengthwise.

Position of patient

- The patient is in the supine position.

Position of part

- Determine whether a mediolateral or lateromedial projection is to be performed.

Mediolateral projection

- Visualize the optimal length of the patient's femur by placing the grid in a vertical position next to the lateral aspect of the femur.
- Place the distal edge of the grid low enough to include the patient's knee joint.
- Have the patient, if able, hold the upper corner of the grid for stabilization; otherwise support the grid firmly in position.
- Support the unaffected leg by using the patient's support (or a trapeze bar if present) or a support block.
- Elevate the unaffected leg until the femur is nearly vertical. An assistant may have to elevate and hold the leg of a critically ill patient. The assistant may also steady the grid and must wear a lead apron for protection (Fig. 20.22).

Lateromedial projection

- Place the grid next to the medial aspect of the affected femur (between the patient's legs) and make sure that the knee joint is included (Fig. 20.23).
- Make sure that the grid is placed *perpendicular* to the epicondylar plane.
- *Shield gonads.*
- *Respiration:* Suspended.

---

[g]The nonmobile projection is described in Chapter 7.

Central ray

- Perpendicular to the long axis of the femur, entering at its midpoint.
- Make sure that the central ray and grid are aligned to prevent grid cutoff; the central ray is centered to the femur and not to the center of the grid.

Collimation

- Adjust to top at ASIS for hip, bottom at the tibial tuberosity of the knee, 1 inch (2.5 cm) on the side of the shadow of the femur and 17 inches (43 cm) in length.

The thickest portion of the femur (proximal area) must be measured carefully, and an appropriate kVp must be selected to penetrate this area. The computer cannot form an image of any anatomy in this area if penetration does not occur. A light area of the entire proximal femur would result. Positioning the cathode over the proximal femur would improve CR image quality.

Structures shown

This projection shows the distal two-thirds of the femur, including the knee joint, without superimposition of the opposite thigh (Fig. 20.24).

The following should be clearly shown:
- Evidence of proper collimation
- Most of femur, including knee joint
- Patella in profile
- Superimposition of femoral condyles
- Opposite femur and soft tissue out of area of interest
- Adequate penetration of proximal portion of femur
- Orthopedic appliance if present
- Radiographic markers as appropriate

Fig. 20.24 Mobile of the lateral femur showing midshaft fractures and femoral rod placement. The knee joints are included on the image. (A) Mediolateral. (B) Lateromedial.

Fig. 20.25 Mobile of the lateral cervical spine.

LATERAL PROJECTION[h]
Right or left dorsal decubitus position

> **Image receptor:** The IR should be 10 × 12 inches (24 × 30 cm) with a grid lengthwise; imaging may be performed with a nongrid IR on smaller patients.

Position of patient
- Position the patient in the supine position with arms extended down along the sides of the body.
- Observe whether a cervical collar or another immobilization device is being used. *Do not remove the device without the consent from the physician or authorized personnel.*

Position of part
- Ensure that the upper torso, cervical spine, and head are not rotated.
- Place the grid lengthwise on the right or left side, parallel to the neck.
- Place the top of the grid approximately 1 inch (2.43 cm) above the external acoustic meatus (EAM) so that the grid is centered to C4 (upper thyroid cartilage).
- Raise the chin slightly. *If the patient has a new trauma, suspected fracture, or known fracture of the cervical region, check with the physician before elevating the chin. Improper movement of a patient's head can disrupt a fractured cervical spine.*
- Immobilize the grid in a vertical position. The grid can be immobilized in multiple ways if a holding device is unavailable. Another method is to place pillows or a cushion between the side rail of the bed and the IR, holding the IR next to the patient. Tape also works well in many instances (Fig. 20.25).
- Have the patient relax the shoulders and reach for the feet if possible.
- *Shield gonads.*
- *Respiration:* Full expiration to obtain maximum depression of the shoulders.

---

[h]The nonmobile projection is described in Chapter 9.

Central ray

- Horizontal and perpendicular to the center of the grid. This should place the central ray at the level of C4 (upper thyroid cartilage).
- Make sure that proper alignment of the central ray and grid is maintained to prevent grid cutoff.
- Because of the great object-to-image receptor distance (OID), SID of 60 to 72 inches (158 to 183 cm) is recommended. This also helps show C7.

Collimation

- Adjust top at top of ear attachment (TEA), bottom to jugular notch, and 1 inch (2.5 cm) on the sides of the neck.

DIGITAL RADIOGRAPHY

To ensure that the lower cervical vertebrae are fully penetrated, the kVp must be set to penetrate the C7 area.

Structures shown

This projection shows the seven cervical vertebrae, including the base of the skull and the soft tissues surrounding the neck (Fig. 20.26).

EVALUATION CRITERIA

The following should be clearly shown:
- Evidence of proper collimation
- All seven cervical vertebrae, including interspaces and spinous processes
- Neck extended when possible so that rami of mandible are not overlapping C1 or C2
- C4 in center of grid
- Radiographic markers as appropriate
- Superimposed posterior margins of each vertebral body

NOTE: It is essential that C6 and C7 be included on the image. To accomplish this, the radiographer should instruct the patient to relax the shoulders toward the feet as much as possible. If the examination involves pulling down on the patient's arms, the radiographer should exercise extreme caution and evaluate the patient's condition carefully to determine whether pulling of the arms can be tolerated. Fractures or injuries of the upper limbs, including the clavicles, must be considered. Applying a strong pull to the arms of a patient in a hurried or jerking manner can disrupt a fractured cervical spine. If the lateral projection does not adequately visualize the lower cervical region, the Twining method, sometimes referred to as the "swimmer's" position, which eliminates pulling of the arms, may be recommended for patients who have experienced trauma or have a known cervical fracture. One arm must be placed above the patient's head (the Twining method is described in Chapter 9).

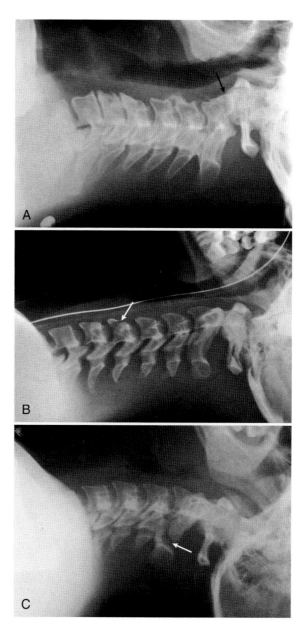

Fig. 20.26 Mobile of the lateral cervical spine obtained at the patient's bedside several weeks after trauma. (A) Entire cervical spine shows slight anterior subluxation of the dens on the body of C2 (arrow). (B) Entire cervical spine shows nearly vertical fracture through the body of C5 with slight displacement (arrow). (C) First five cervical vertebrae show vertical fractures through the posterior aspects of the C2 laminae (arrow) with 4-mm displacement of the fragments. Earlier radiographs showed that C6 and C7 were unaffected and did not need to be included in this follow-up radiograph.

Mobile Radiography

Fig. 20.27 (A) Side panel of the isolette being lowered to gain access to the IR tray. (B) IR being placed on a special tray for placement below the infant.

AP PROJECTION

The chest and abdomen combination described here is typically ordered for premature newborns who are in the neonatal intensive care unit. If a chest or abdomen projection is ordered separately, the radiographer should adjust the central ray and collimator accordingly.

> **Image receptor:** The IR should be 8 × 10 inches (20 × 24 cm) or 10 × 12 inches (24 × 30 cm).

Position of patient

Position the infant supine in the center of the IR. Some bassinets have a special tray to hold the IR. Positioning numbers along the tray permits accurate placement of the IR (Fig. 20.27). If the IR is directly under the infant, cover the IR with a soft warm blanket.

Fig. 20.28 Neonatal intensive care unit bassinet with a premature infant. Overhead heating unit *(arrow)* is moved out of the way to accommodate mobile x-ray machine tube head.

Position of part

- *Carefully* position the x-ray tube over the infant (Fig. 20.28).
- Make sure that the chest and abdomen are not rotated.
- Move the infant's arms away from the body or over the head and bring the legs down and away from the abdomen. The arms and legs may have to be held by a nurse, who should wear a lead apron.
- Leave the head of the infant rotated. (See note at the end of this section.)
- Adjust the collimators closely to the chest and abdomen (Fig. 20.29).
- *Shield gonads.*
- *Respiration:* Inspiration. Neonates have an extremely fast respiratory rate and cannot hold their breath. Make the best attempt possible to perform the exposure on full inspiration (Fig. 20.30).

Fig. 20.29 Mobile chest and abdomen radiograph of a neonate. Note the male gonadal shield. (In actual practice, the IR is covered with a soft warm blanket.)

Fig. 20.30 Radiographs on inspiration and expiration in a neonate. (A) Left side of chest is shown at full expiration. Note the lack of normal lung markings and the illusion of massive pulmonary disease. The diaphragm is not seen, and the heart appears enlarged. (B) Repeat radiograph of the same patient performed correctly at full inspiration. Diaphragm may be seen correctly at the level of the 10th posterior rib. The same technical factors were used for both exposures.

(Courtesy Department of Radiology, Rochester General Hospital, Rochester, NY. From Cullinan AM, Cullinan JE: *Producing quality radiographs*, ed 2, Philadelphia, 1994, Lippincott.)

Central ray

- Perpendicular to the midpoint of the chest and abdomen along the midsagittal plane.

Collimation

- Adjust top to 1 inch (2.5 cm) above shoulders, bottom at lower rib margins for chest or to pubic symphysis if chest and abdomen requested, and 1 inch (2.5 cm) on sides.

Structures shown

The anatomy of the entire chest and abdomen is shown (Fig. 20.31).

EVALUATION CRITERIA

The following should be clearly shown:
- Evidence of proper collimation
- Anatomy from apices to pubic symphysis in the thoracic and abdominal regions
- No motion
- No blurring of lungs, diaphragm, and abdominal structures
- No rotation of patient
- Radiographic markers as appropriate

NOTE: When performing an AP or lateral projection of the chest, the radiographer should keep the head and neck of the infant straight so that the anatomy in the upper chest and airway is accurately visualized. However, straightening the head of a neonate in the supine position can inadvertently advance an endotracheal tube too far into the trachea. It is sometimes more important to leave the head of an intubated neonatal patient rotated in the position in which the infant routinely lies to obtain accurate representation of the position of the endotracheal tube on the radiograph.

Fig. 20.31 Mobile AP chest and abdominal radiograph of a neonate. Exposure technique shows the anatomy of entire chest and abdomen. Note gonadal shield accurately positioned on this male infant (*arrow*).

LATERAL PROJECTION
Dorsal decubitus position

Image receptor: The IR should be 8 × 10 inches (20 × 24 cm) or 10 × 12 inches (24 × 30 cm). Most premature neonates cannot be turned on their sides or placed upright for a lateral projection.

Position of patient
- *Carefully* place the x-ray tube on the side of the bassinet.
- Position the infant supine on a radiolucent block covered with a soft warm blanket. If a radiolucent block is not readily available, an inverted box of tissues works well.

Position of part
- Ensure that the infant's chest and abdomen are centered to the IR and not rotated.
- Move the infant's arms above the head. The infant's arms may have to be held up by a nurse, who should wear a lead apron.
- Place the IR lengthwise and vertical beside the patient and immobilize it.
- Leave the head of the infant rotated. (See note on p. 28.)
- Adjust the collimators closely to the chest and abdomen (Fig. 20.32).
- *Shield gonads.*
- *Respiration:* Inspiration. Neonates have an extremely fast respiratory rate and cannot hold their breath. Make the best attempt possible to perform the exposure on full inspiration.

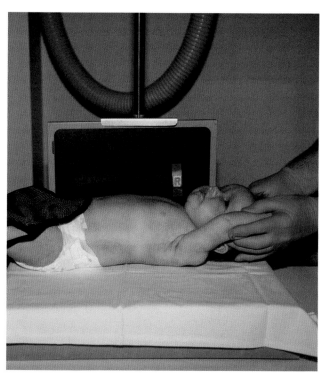

Fig. 20.32 Mobile lateral chest and abdominal radiograph of a neonate in dorsal decubitus position. The infant is positioned on a raised block with the IR below the block.

Central ray

- Horizontal and perpendicular to the midpoint of the chest and abdomen along the midcoronal plane

Collimation

- Adjust top to 1 inch (2.5 cm) above shoulders, bottom at lower rib margins for chest or to pubic symphysis if chest and abdomen requested, and 1 inch (2.5 cm) on sides.

Structures shown

This projection shows the anatomy of the entire chest and abdomen, with special attention to the costophrenic angles in the posterior chest. If present, air and fluid levels are visualized (Fig. 20.33).

EVALUATION CRITERIA

The following should be clearly shown:
- Evidence of proper collimation
- Anatomy of chest and abdomen from apices to pubic bone
- No motion
- No blurring of lungs, diaphragm, and abdominal structures
- No rotation of patient
- Air and fluid levels if present
- Radiographic markers as appropriate

References

1. National Council on Radiation Protection: *Report 102: medical x-ray, electron beam and gamma ray protection for energies up to 50 Mev*, Bethesda, MD, 1989.

Selected bibliography

Adler AM, Carlton RR: *Introduction to radiography and patient care*, ed 4, Philadelphia, 2007, Saunders.

Bontrager KL: *Textbook of radiographic positioning*, ed 7, St Louis, 2010, Mosby.

Bushong SC: *Radiologic science for technologists*, ed 9, St Louis, 2008, Mosby.

Ehrlich RA, McClosky ED: *Patient care in radiography*, ed 7, St Louis, 2009, Mosby.

Hall-Rollins J, Winters R: Mobile chest radiography: improving image quality, *Radiol Technol* 71:5, 2000.

Statkiewicz-Sherer MA, et al: *Radiation protection in medical radiography*, ed 6, St Louis, 2011, Mosby.

Tucker DM, et al: Scatter in computed radiography, *Radiology* 188:271, 1993.

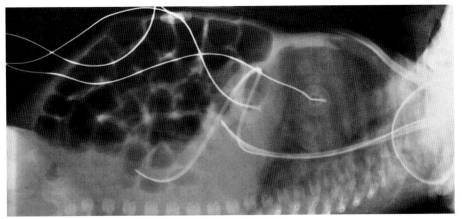

Fig. 20.33 Mobile lateral chest and abdominal radiograph of a neonate in dorsal decubitus position. Exposure technique shows the anatomy of the entire chest and abdomen.

21

SURGICAL RADIOGRAPHY

TRACY IVERSEN

Surgical radiology is a dynamic experience. The challenges a radiographer encounters in the surgical suite are unique. Knowing the machinery and its capabilities and limitations is most important; in that regard, the radiographer can enter any operating room (OR) case, whether routine or extraordinary, and, with good communication, be able to perform all tasks well. An understanding of common procedures and familiarity with equipment enables the radiographer to perform most mobile examinations ordered by the physician. Surgical radiography can be a challenging and exciting environment for the radiographer but can also be intimidating and stressful. Surgical radiology requires educated personnel familiar with specific equipment routinely used during common surgical procedures. It requires expertise in teamwork. Preparedness and familiarity with equipment are key. Standard health and safety protocols must be followed to avoid contamination and to ensure patient safety. These are the basics, and the pieces come together in surgical radiology in distinctive ways.

This chapter focuses on the most common procedures performed in the surgical area. The basic principles of mobile imaging are detailed, and helpful suggestions are provided for successful completion of the examinations. This chapter is not intended to cover every possible combination of examinations or situations that a radiographer may encounter; rather it provides an overview of the surgical setting and a summary of common examinations. The scope of radiologic examinations in a surgical setting is vast and may differ greatly among health care facilities (Box 21.1). The goals of this chapter are to (1) provide an overview of the surgical setting and explain the role of the radiographer as a vital member of the surgical team, (2) assist the radiographer in developing an understanding of the imaging equipment used in surgical situations, and (3) present common radiographic procedures performed in the OR. The radiographer should review the surgery department protocols because they vary from institution to institution.

Surgical Team

At no other time is a patient so well attended as during a surgical procedure. A surgeon, one or two assistants, a surgical technologist, an anesthesia provider, a circulating nurse, and various support staff surround the patient. These individuals, each with specific functions to perform, form the OR team. This team literally has the patient's life in its hands. The OR team has been described as a symphony orchestra, with each person an integral entity in unison and harmony with his or her colleagues for the successful accomplishment of the expected outcomes. The OR team is subdivided, according to the functions of its members, into sterile and nonsterile teams.

BOX 21.1

Scope of surgical radiography

Surgical fluoroscopic procedures
- Abdomen: cholangiogram
- Chest-line placement: bronchoscopy
- Cervical spine: anterior cervical discectomy and fusion
- Lumbar spine
- Hip: cannulated hip screws or hip pinning, decompression hip screw
- Femoral and tibial nailing
- Extremity fluoroscopy
- Humerus: shoulder in beach chair position
- Femoral/tibial arteriogram

Mobile surgical radiography procedures
- Localization examinations of cervical, thoracic, and lumbar spine
- Mobile extremity examinations in operating room

STERILE TEAM MEMBERS

Sterile team members scrub their hands and arms, don a sterile gown and gloves over proper surgical attire, and enter the sterile field. The sterile field is the area of the OR that immediately surrounds and is specially prepared for the patient. To establish a sterile field, all items necessary for the surgical procedure are sterilized. After this process, the scrubbed and sterile team members function within this limited area and handle only sterile items (Fig. 21.1). The sterile team consists of the following members:

- *Surgeon:* The surgeon is a licensed physician who is specially trained and qualified by knowledge and experience to perform surgical procedures. The surgeon's responsibilities include preoperative diagnosis and care, selection and performance of the surgical procedure, and postoperative management of care. The surgeon assumes full responsibility for all medical acts of judgment and for the management of the surgical patient.

- *Surgical assistant:* The first assistant is a qualified surgeon or resident in an accredited surgical educational program. The assistant should be capable of assuming responsibility for performing the procedure for the primary surgeon. Assistants help to maintain visibility of the surgical site, control bleeding, close wounds, and apply dressings. The assistant's role varies depending on the institution and with the type of procedure or surgical specialty.

- *Physician assistant:* The physician assistant is a nonphysician allied health practitioner who is qualified by academic and clinical training to perform designated procedures in the OR and in other areas of surgical patient care.

- *Scrub nurse:* The scrub nurse is a registered nurse (RN) who is specially trained to work with surgeons and the medical team in the OR.

- *Certified surgical technologist (CST):* The CST is responsible for maintaining the integrity, safety, and efficiency of the sterile field throughout the surgical procedure. The CST prepares and arranges instruments and supplies and assists the surgical procedure by providing the required sterile instruments and supplies. In some institutions, a licensed practical nurse (LPN) or RN may assume this role.

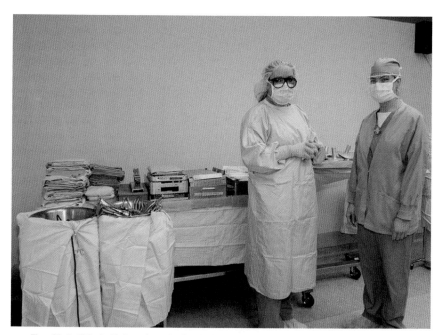

Fig. 21.1 OR staff showing sterile *(left)* and nonsterile *(right)* team members.

NONSTERILE TEAM MEMBERS

Nonsterile team members do not enter the sterile field; they function outside and around it. They assume responsibility for maintaining sterile techniques during the surgical procedure, but they handle supplies and equipment that are not considered sterile. Following the principles of aseptic technique, they keep the sterile team supplied, provide direct patient care, and respond to any requests that may arise during the surgical procedure.

- *Anesthesia provider:* The anesthesia provider is a physician (anesthesiologist) or certified RN anesthetist who specializes in administering anesthetics. Choosing and applying appropriate agents and suitable techniques of administration, monitoring physiologic functions, maintaining fluid and electrolyte balance, and performing blood replacements are essential responsibilities of the anesthesia provider during the surgical procedure.

- *Circulator:* The circulator is preferably an RN. The circulator monitors and coordinates all activities within the OR, provides supplies to the CST during the surgical procedure, and manages the care of the patient.
- *Radiographers:* The radiographer's role in the OR is to provide intraoperative imaging in a variety of examinations and with various types of equipment.
- *Others:* The OR team may also include biomedical technicians, monitoring technologists, and individuals who specialize in the equipment or monitoring devices necessary during the surgical procedure.

Proper Surgical Attire

Surgical attire protocols may change from institution to institution but should be available for review, understood, and followed by all staff members. Although small variances in protocol exist among institutions, there are common standards.

Large amounts of bacteria are present in the nose and mouth, on the skin, and on the attire of personnel who enter the restricted areas of the surgical setting. Proper facility design and surgical attire regulations are important ways of preventing transportation of microorganisms into surgical settings, where they may infect patients' open wounds. Infection control practices also involve personal measures, including personal fitness for work, skin disinfection (patient and personnel), preparation of personnel hands, surgical attire, and personal technique (surgical conscience).

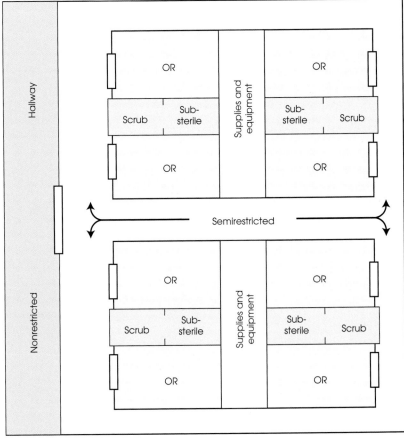

Fig. 21.2 OR suite layout showing restricted, nonrestricted, and semirestricted areas. ORs are "restricted."

Operating Room Attire

The OR should have specific written policies and procedures for proper attire to be worn within the semirestricted and restricted areas of the OR suite. The dress code should include aspects of personal hygiene important to environmental control. Protocol is strictly monitored so that everyone conforms to established policy.

Street clothes should never be worn within semirestricted or restricted areas of the surgical suite (Fig. 21.2). Clean, fresh attire should be donned at the beginning of each shift in the OR suite and as needed if the attire becomes wet or soiled. Blood-stained or soiled attire, including shoe covers, is unattractive and can also be a source of cross-infection or contamination. Soiled attire is not worn outside of the OR suite, and steps should be taken to remove soiled clothing immediately on exiting. OR attire should not be hung in a locker for wearing a second time. Underclothing should be clean and totally covered by the scrub suit (Fig. 21.3). Other aspects of proper attire include the following:

- *Protective eyewear:* Occupational Safety and Health Administration (OSHA) regulations require eyewear to be worn when contamination from blood or body fluids is possible.
- *Masks:* Masks should be worn at all times in the OR but are not necessary in all semirestricted areas.
- *Shoe covers:* Shoe covers should be worn when contamination from blood or body fluids can be reasonably anticipated. Shoe covers should be changed whenever they become torn, soiled, or wet and should be removed before leaving the surgical area.
- *Caps:* Caps should be worn to cover and contain hair at all times in the restricted and semirestricted areas of the OR suite. Hoods are also available to cover hair, such as facial hair, that cannot be contained by a cap and mask.
- *Gloves:* Gloves should be worn when contact with blood or body substances is anticipated.
- *Radiation badge and identification:* A radiation badge and proper identification should be worn at all times.

PERSONAL HYGIENE

A person with an acute infection, such as a cold, open cold sore, or sore throat, is known to be a carrier of transmittable conditions and should not be permitted within the OR suite. Daily body cleanliness and clean hair are also important because good personal hygiene helps to prevent transportation of microbial fallout that can cause open wound infections. Daily body cleanliness and clean, dandruff-free hair help prevent superficial wound infections.

Fig. 21.3 Properly attired radiographers with protective eyewear and additional headwear to cover facial hair or long hair.

Dance of the Operating Room

The concepts of sterile and aseptic technique date back to Hippocrates, who boiled wine and water to pour into open wounds in an attempt to prevent infection. Galen changed the technique a bit and began boiling the instruments instead, and shortly thereafter Semmelweis noted a dramatic decline in postoperative infection by having the staff wash their hands and change gowns between surgical procedures.

Maintaining the sterile field in an OR suite can be like a well-choreographed dance when the team works well together. Certain moves and rules must be followed. Proper adherence to aseptic technique eliminates or minimizes modes and sources of contamination. Basic principles must be observed during the surgical procedure to provide the patient with a well-defined margin of safety. Everyone who cares for patients must carry out effective hospital and OR infection control programs. Infection control involves a wide variety of concepts including methods of environmental sanitation and maintenance of facilities; cleanliness of the air and equipment in the OR suite; cleanliness of the skin and apparel of patients, surgeons, and personnel; sterility of surgical equipment; strict aseptic technique; and careful observance of procedural rules and regulations.

Up to 10,000 microbial particles can be shed from the skin per minute. Nonsterile team members should not reach over a sterile field. When working over the sterile field (e.g., performing a posteroanterior [PA] lumbar spine), the sterile field should be covered with a sterile drape to protect the field (Fig. 21.4). The technologist cannot move the radiographic equipment into position over the sterile field until after the sterile cover is in place. A sterile team member should fold over the sterile drape on itself, and then a nonsterile team member should carefully remove the covering drape, being careful not to compromise the sterile field. If a sterile field is compromised, the OR staff should be notified immediately.

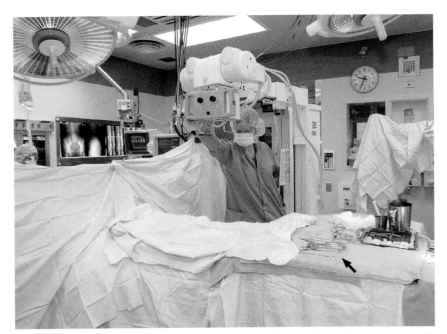

Fig. 21.4 Radiographer leaning over the sterile field while positioning the x-ray tube. The sterile incision site over which the radiographer works is properly covered to maintain a sterile field. Note the sterile instruments in the foreground (arrow). The radiographer should never move radiographic equipment over uncovered sterile instruments or an uncovered surgical site.

Communication is of utmost importance. As a result of the surgical sterile field, the radiographer is unable to help position the IR or the patient. Good, professional communication is essential while using sound, basic knowledge of anatomy and positioning. The radiographer may have to instruct the surgeon or resident on the proper position to visualize the desired portion of the anatomy best.

PROPER IR HANDLING IN THE STERILE FIELD

To maintain proper universal precautions, the radiographer must follow specific steps when handling an IR in the OR.

- *Surgical technologist (CST) taking the IR:* The CST holds a sterile IR cover open toward the radiographer. The radiographer should hold one end of the IR while placing the other end of the IR into the sterile IR cover. The CST grasps the IR and wraps the protective cover securely (Fig. 21.5).

Fig. 21.5 Radiographer and CST place wireless DR detector into the sterile drape.

- *Radiographer accepting the IR after exposure:* After the exposure has been made, the radiographer needs to retrieve the IR. The CST should carefully open the sterile drape, exposing the detector for the technologist to grasp (Fig. 21.6). The CST would then dispose of the drape. In the event of an urgent situation in which the CST needs to hand the IR over, the radiographer must be wearing gloves to accept a covered IR that has been in the sterile field or under an open incision. The protective cover is possibly contaminated with blood or body fluids and should be treated accordingly. The radiographer should grasp the IR, open the protective cover carefully away from himself or herself or others so as not to spread blood or body fluids, and then ask another nonsterile person to remove the IR from the cover. The radiographer should dispose of the sterile cover in a proper receptacle and remember to remove gloves before handling the IR or any other equipment because the gloves are now considered contaminated. If contamination of the IR occurs, the radiographer should use hospital-approved disinfectant for cleaning before leaving the OR (Box 21.2). Hand hygiene should be performed whenever entering or exiting the OR.

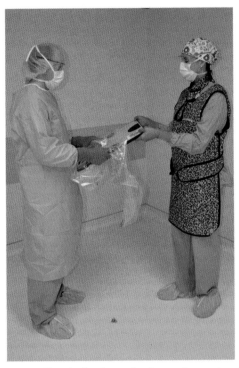

Fig. 21.6 CST correctly opens the sterile drape for the radiographer to remove the IR from the now-contaminated bag, being careful not to brush contaminants from bag onto self or others.

ENEMIES OF THE STERILE FIELD

Lengthy or complex procedures increase the chance of sterile field contamination. Physical limitations, such as crowding, poor lighting, and staffing levels, are also a consideration. The floor is always considered contaminated. The radiographer should not place IRs, lead aprons, and shields on the floor.

BOX 21.2

Principles of aseptic techniques

- Only sterile items are used within the sterile field.
- Only sterile persons handle sterile items or touch sterile areas.
- Nonsterile persons touch only nonsterile items or areas.
- Movement within or around a sterile field must not contaminate the sterile field.
- Items of doubtful sterility must be considered nonsterile.
- When a sterile barrier is permeated, it must be considered contaminated.
- Sterile gowns are considered sterile in front from the shoulder to the level of the sterile field and at the sleeves from the elbow to the cuff.
- Tables are sterile only at table level.
- Radiographers should not walk between two sterile fields if possible.
- Radiographers should avoid turning their backs toward the sterile field in compromised spaces.
- The radiographer should watch the front of clothing when it is necessary to be next to the patient.
- The radiographer must be aware of machinery close to the sterile field, including lead aprons hanging from the portable machine that may swing toward the sterile field.
- The lead apron needs to be secured if it is being worn next to the sterile field. The apron can easily slip forward when raising one's arms up to position the tube. A properly worn apron does not compromise the sterile field or jeopardize proper body mechanics.
- When positioning an IR under the OR table, the radiographer should not lift the sterile drapes above table level because this would compromise the sterile field.

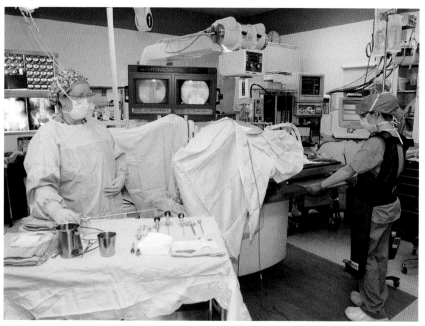

Fig. 21.7 In-room urologic radiographic equipment used for retrograde ureterograms.

Equipment

The radiographer must be well acquainted with the radiologic equipment. Some procedures may seldom occur. The radiographer should not fear a rare procedure if good communication and equipment knowledge are in place. IR holders enable the radiographer to perform cross-table projections on numerous cases and eliminate the unnecessary exposure of personnel who may volunteer to hold the IR. In mobile radiography, exposure times may increase for larger patients, and a holder eliminates the chance of motion from handheld situations.

Some OR suites, such as those used for stereotactic or urologic cases, have dedicated radiologic equipment (Fig. 21.7). Most radiographic examinations in the OR are performed with mobile equipment, however.

Mobile image machines are not as sophisticated as larger stationary machines in the radiology department. Mobile fluoroscopic units, often referred to as *C-arms* because of their shape (Fig. 21.8), are commonplace in the surgical suite. Mobile radiography is also widely used in the OR.

Good communication is imperative when providing safe and efficient imaging during a surgical case. It is important to establish a common language of terms between the surgeon and the technologist for C-arm operation (Fig. 21.9).

Fig. 21.8 (A) C-arm radiographic/fluoroscopic system used in the OR. (B) Mini-mobile C-arm used for extremity examinations in OR.

Cleaning of Equipment

The x-ray equipment should be cleaned after each surgical case. If possible, the radiographer should clean the mobile image machine, including the base, in the OR suite, especially when the equipment is obviously contaminated with blood or surgical scrub solution. Cleaning within the OR helps reduce the possibility of cross-contamination. The x-ray equip-ment must be cleaned with a hospital-approved cleaning solution. Cleaning solutions should not be sprayed in the OR suite during the surgical procedure. If cleaning is necessary during the surgical procedure, opening the cleaning container and pouring the solution on a rag for use prevents possible contamination from scattered spray. Gloves should always be worn during cleaning. The underside of the image machine should be checked to ensure contaminants that might have splashed up from the floor are removed. Cleaning the equipment after an isolation case is necessary to prevent the spread of contaminants. All equipment that is used less frequently should undergo a thorough cleaning at least once a week and just before being taken into the OR.

Fig. 21.9 (A) C-arm up or C-arm down movement. (B) When C-arm is positioned perpendicular to the patient C-arm in or C-arm out movement allows for medial to lateral movement without needing to move the patient. (C) C-arm *pan* movement allows scanning evenly along the long axis of a body part, for example, a femur during a femoral nailing. (D) C-arm *tilt* movement allows for angled images such as inlet or outlet images of the pelvis when the C-arm is positioned perpendicular to the patient. (E) C-arm *arc* movement allows for oblique projections such as Judet images of a fractured acetabulum when the C-arm is positioned perpendicular to the patient. (F) C-arm *pivot* allows limited pan-type movement without moving the base of the machine, while following contrast during an intraoperative cholangiogram, for example.

Radiation Exposure Considerations

Radiation protection for the radiographer, others in the immediate area, and the patient is of paramount importance when mobile fluoroscopic examinations are performed. The radiographer should wear a lead, or lead equivalent, apron and stand as far away from the patient, x-ray tube, and useful beam as the procedure, OR, and exposure cable allow. The most effective means of radiation protection is *distance*. The recommended *minimal* distance is 6 ft (2 m). When possible, the radiographer should stand at a right angle (90 degrees) to the primary beam and the object being radiographed. The least amount of scatter radiation occurs at this position. The greatest amount of scatter radiation occurs on the tube side of the fluoroscopic machine. It is recommended that the x-ray tube always be placed *under the patient* (Fig. 21.10). Because of the significant amount of exposure to the facial and neck region, the x-ray tube should never be placed above the patient unless absolutely necessary.

The OR may have signs posted outside the room warning of radiation in use, or "lead aprons required when entering this room." Lead or lead equivalent protection should be provided for individuals who are unable to leave the room.

The patient's gonads should be shielded with appropriate radiation protection devices during examinations in which shielding would not interfere with imaging of the anatomy that must be shown. When fluoroscopic equipment with the tube *under* the table is to be used, shielding should be placed under the patient. In addition, the source-to-skin distance (SSD) should not be less than 12 inches (29 cm).

Fluoroscopic Procedures for the Operating Room
OPERATIVE (IMMEDIATE) CHOLANGIOGRAPHY

Operative cholangiography, introduced by Mirizzi in 1932, is performed during biliary tract surgery. After the bile has been drained from the ducts, and in the absence of obstruction, this technique permits the major intrahepatic ducts and the extrahepatic ducts to be filled with contrast medium.

The value of operative cholangiography is such that it has become an integral part of biliary tract surgery. It is used to investigate the patency of the bile ducts and the functional status of the sphincter of the hepatopancreatic ampulla to reveal the presence of calculi that cannot be detected by palpation. Intraoperative cholangiography can also show such conditions as small intraluminal neoplasms and stricture or dilation of the ducts. When the pancreatic duct shares a common channel with the distal common bile duct before emptying into the duodenum, it is sometimes seen on operative cholangiograms because it has been partially filled by reflux.

After exposing, draining, and exploring the biliary tract, and frequently after excising the gallbladder, the surgeon injects the contrast medium. This solution is usually introduced into the common bile duct through a needle, small catheter, or (after cholecystectomy) an inlaying T tube. When the latter route is used, the procedure is referred to as *delayed operative* or *operative T-tube cholangiography.*

mR/hr
A >300
B 100-500
C 50-100
D 25-50
E 10-25
F <10

Fig. 21.10 Radiation safety with C-arm. In the *upper image*, less radiation reaches the facial and neck region when the x-ray tube is under the patient. This is the recommended position of the C-arm. In the *lower image*, there is a greater amount of radiation reaching the facial and neck regions.

(From Giese RA, Hunter DW: Personnel exposure during fluoroscopy. *Postgrad Radiol* 8:162, 1988.)

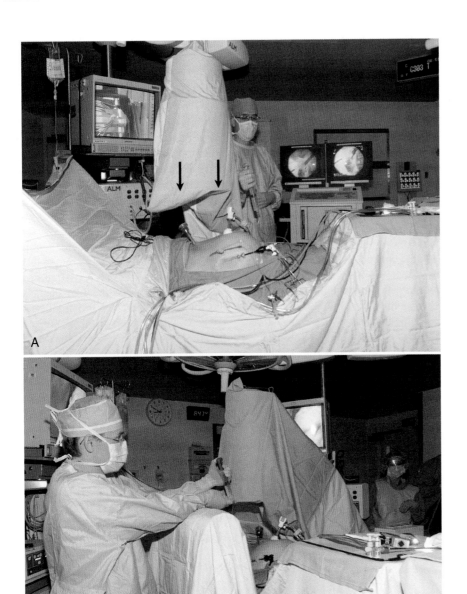

Position of patient

The patient is supine with the abdomen exposed. In laparoscopic cases, such as cholecystectomy, the abdomen is distended because air is injected into the abdominal cavity to allow adequate room for maneuvering of the camera and instruments. The radiographer should ensure no obstacles would impede the movement of the C-arm (Fig. 21.11).

NOTE: The CR comes from under the table, so appropriate shielding should be placed under the patient and placed so as not to obscure any pertinent anatomy.

Position of C-arm

Center the C-arm in the PA projection over the right side of the abdomen below the rib line. The patient may be tilted to the left or in the Trendelenburg position to aid in the flow of contrast medium to the complete biliary system. The C-arm should be tilted or canted until the PA projection is achieved. The C-arm may also have to be rotated to ensure that the spine does not obscure the biliary system. When the position is obtained, the surgeon injects contrast medium into the duct system under fluoroscopy. The radiographer should do the following:

- Provide radiation protection for all persons in the room.
- Remember that examination is optimal with suspended respiration.

Because of the length of time it may take for contrast medium to fill all ducts, respiration may be suspended at intervals throughout the examination.

Fig. 21.11 (A) C-arm in correct position for an abdominal cholangiogram. The assistant surgeon checks syringe for air bubbles before handing it to the surgeon for injection. The radiographer positioned fluoroscopic image intensifier (*arrows*) carefully to avoid hitting laparoscopic instruments protruding from the patient's abdomen. (B) Surgeon, standing behind a sterile draped lead shield, injecting contrast media for an operative cholangiogram.

Structures shown

This examination shows the biliary system full of contrast medium, including a portion of the cystic duct, the branches of the hepatic duct, the common bile duct, and often the pancreatic duct.

EVALUATION CRITERIA

- Biliary system should be completely filled with contrast medium (Fig. 21.12).
- No extravasation of contrast medium occurs at the injection site.
- Biliary system should not be obscured by any extraneous anatomy or instrumentation.
- Prompt emptying of contrast medium into the duodenum occurs.
- Proper radiographic technique is maintained.
- Sterile field is maintained.

A   B

Fig. 21.12 Images of anatomy visualized during a cholangiogram using fluoroscopy. (A) Intraoperative cholangiogram. (B) Intraoperative cholangiogram showing pancreatic duct *(arrow)*.

CHEST (LINE PLACEMENT, BRONCHOSCOPY)

Position of patient

The patient is supine with the arms secured at his or her sides. The radiographer should ensure there are no bars or supports in the table that would obscure the view of the chest. Allow room under the table for the C-arm to maneuver.

Position of C-arm

The C-arm should be covered with a sterile drape before entering the field. The C-arm enters the sterile field perpendicular to the patient and in position for a PA projection. If the surgeon prefers, the radiographer can reverse or invert the image to obtain anatomic position. Radiation protection should be provided for all persons in the room.

- *Line placement:* Find the point of insertion and follow the catheter to its end (Fig. 21.13). This examination is done to ensure there are no kinks in the catheter and to show it is in proper position. Numerous catheters may be used in the OR. They are usually inserted to deliver medicines to chronically ill patients.
- *Rigid and flexible bronchoscopy:* Bronchoscopy may be done to perform biopsies, place stents, or dilate the bronchi.

Structures shown

Structures shown include all anatomy of the chest cavity, including the heart, lung fields, and ribs, and any instrumentation that may be introduced during the procedure. These instruments may include catheters, guidewires, bronchoscopes, stent devices, dilation balloons, or biopsy instruments.

EVALUATION CRITERIA

- Pertinent parts of the chest are distinguished easily.
- Proper radiographic technique and contrast are maintained on the monitor.
- Image on the monitor is in true anatomic position or per the physician's preference.
- Sterile technique is maintained.

Fig. 21.13 Patient and C-arm in position for Hickman catheter placement. Introduction of catheter begins in the upper thorax and is completed with the catheter in the heart.

CERVICAL SPINE (ANTERIOR CERVICAL DISKECTOMY AND FUSION)

Position of patient

The patient is supine with the chin elevated and the neck in flexion. The patient's arms are at his or her sides.

Position of C-arm
PA projection

Cover the C-arm with sterile drape. Enter the sterile field perpendicular to the patient. Tilt the C-arm 15 degrees cephalad and center the beam over the cervical spine. Raise the C-arm to allow the surgeon to work if necessary. Ensure the spine is in the center of the monitor, and the top of spine and skull are at the top of the screen with no rotation.

Lateral projection

Rotate the C-arm under the table into lateral position with the beam parallel to the floor. Angle the C-arm either cephalad or caudal to obtain a true lateral view. Raise or lower the C-arm to bring the spine into the center of the field of view. Rotate the image on the monitor to the same plane as the patient with the spine parallel with the floor. Cases in which a PA projection is unnecessary may opt to have the C-arm positioned in "rainbow" fashion or arched over the patient (Fig. 21.14).
- Ensure there are no obstacles under the table that impede movement of the C-arm.
- The C-arm is often positioned before the patient is draped. In this case, the surgical team drapes the C-arm into the sterile field. Ensure that the C-arm can be moved out of the way without disturbing any instrumentation.

Structures shown

These positions show the affected area of the cervical spine and any hardware that may be introduced (Fig. 21.15). Because this surgery is most often performed to repair physiologic defects, abnormalities (e.g., osteophytes, degenerated disk spaces, subluxation) may be visible, especially in the lateral view.

EVALUATION CRITERIA

- Cervical spine and its affected part are in the center of the monitor to maintain proper radiographic technique.
- Image is rotated in the same plane as the patient.
- PA projection should show spinous processes in the center of spinous bodies.
- Lateral projection should show the bodies in profile and the interarticular facets aligned.
- Sterile field is maintained.

Fig. 21.14 C-arm placed in rainbow position for cervical procedures.

Fig. 21.15 Fluoroscopic image of cervical spine in lateral projection showing plate and screws used to fuse vertebrae.

LUMBAR SPINE
Position of patient

The patient is prone and positioned on chest rolls or a frame to flex the spine. His or her arms are placed on arm boards and located by the head of the table to bring them out of the field of view.

Position of C-arm
AP projection

Cover the C-arm with a sterile drape. The C-arm enters the field perpendicular to the patient. Center the beam in the AP projection over the affected area of the spine. Raise the C-arm to leave enough room between the IR and the patient so that the surgeon can work without being obstructed (Fig. 21.16). Ensure there is nothing in or under the table to impair the view of the spine.

Fig. 21.16 (A) C-arm correctly placed in rainbow position for lateral lumbar procedures. The rainbow position is used especially for larger patients in which the table size or size of the patient would not allow enough elevation of the C-arm to include the lumbar spine. (B) C-arm positioned under the table. (C) C-arm positioned for AP projection of lumbar spine.

Lateral projection

- Rotate the C-arm under the table into lateral position. Raise or lower the C-arm to bring the spine into the center of the monitor. The C-arm may need to be angled cephalad or caudal to obtain true lateral projection. Rotate the image on the monitor until the image is in same plane as the patient. The C-arm may be arched over the patient for the lateral projection, especially on hypersthenic patients, because rotating the C-arm under the table would not allow a great enough height to visualize the lumbar region.
- The surgical team members place sterile drapes over both ends of the C-arm when they drape the patient.

Structures shown

These projections show the affected area of the spine, which includes the bodies, disk spaces, spinous processes, lamina, pedicles, and facets. When the case is completed, there is hardware in the spine, such as rods, plates, and screws, to hold the spine in alignment. A bone graft or interbody fusion device may also exist in the disk space to fuse the bones together (Fig. 21.17).

Fluoroscopic Procedures for the Operating Room

Fig. 21.17 Fluoroscopic lateral projection image of lumbar spine with instrumentation.

Fig. 21.18 AP projection fluoroscopic images during laparoscopic lumbar fusion.

HIP (CANNULATED HIP SCREWS OR HIP PINNING)

Position of patient

The patient is supine with the legs abducted and the affected leg held in traction. The patient's arm on the affected side is crossed over the body to be kept out of the field of view.

- These procedures are often done using an isolation drape or "shower curtain." In these cases, it is not necessary to cover the C-arm with a sterile drape; however, a nonsterile bag over the tube is recommended to prevent povidone-iodine (Betadine) staining of the C-arm.

Position of C-arm

Position the C-arm between the patient's legs, and center the beam over the affected hip (Fig. 21.19). To obtain the lateral projection, rotate the C-arm under the leg and table to a lateral position (Fig. 21.20). Do not dislodge any instrumentation when rotating the C-arm.

Fig. 21.19 C-arm positioned for PA projection of the hip.

Fig. 21.20 C-arm properly positioned for lateral projection of the hip. After preliminary images are obtained, the hip is prepared for incision, and the C-arm is sterile draped.

- Before the procedure, the surgeon manipulates the leg under fluoroscopy to reduce the fracture (Fig. 21.21).
- The C-arm may have to be manipulated to achieve projections and may not be in true PA or lateral projection. Note the position of the C-arm on PA and lateral projections to return to this angle when necessary.
- When hardware is in the hip, rotate the C-arm under fluoroscopy to ensure that no hardware is in the hip joint space.

Fig. 21.21 PA projection of the hip with fracture of femoral neck.

Structures shown

This examination shows all parts of the proximal femur and hip joint, including the acetabular rim, femoral head and neck, and greater and lesser trochanters. Hardware may include cannulated screws or pins running parallel with the femoral neck used to reduce the fracture (Fig. 21.22).

EVALUATION CRITERIA

- Hip is centered on monitor and in correct plane.
- Lateral side of femur and acetabular rim must be visualized to determine a starting point and to ensure no hardware enters the joint.
- Lesser trochanter is visible in profile on PA projection. Greater trochanter lies behind the femoral neck and shaft in lateral view.
- Proper radiographic technique is maintained.
- Sterile field is maintained.
- Radiation protection is provided for the surgical team.

Fig. 21.22 PA projection (A) and lateral projection (B) fluoroscopic images of hip fracture reduction.

FEMUR NAIL

Position of patient and C-arm

During this procedure, a rod is inserted into the intramedullary (IM) canal to reduce a fracture of the shaft of the femur (Fig. 21.23). This rod or nail can be introduced either antegrade through the greater trochanter or retrograde through the popliteal notch.

Antegrade femoral nailing

During antegrade nailing, the patient is either supine or in the lateral position. In the supine position, the affected leg would most likely be in traction to help reduce the fracture. The legs would be abducted, and the unaffected leg would be flexed at the knee and hip and raised to allow the C-arm enough room to enter the sterile field. The patient's arm on the injured side is draped across the chest to keep it from obstructing the surgeon. The C-arm is positioned between the patient's legs, parallel to the unaffected leg, and cen-

tered over the hip. The C-arm may have to be rotated forward or backward to obtain a true PA projection. Rotate the C-arm under the table for a lateral projection.

With the patient in lateral position, the affected leg is extended forward to clear the opposite leg. The lateral position requires the radiographer to enter the sterile field and rotate the C-arm under the table to find a PA projection of the femur. Lateral projection is achieved with the tube starting in a true PA projection, rotating the C-arm forward 10 to 15 degrees, and tilting it 5 to 10 degrees cephalad.

Fig. 21.23 Image of midshaft femoral fracture with guide rod being inserted to align fracture.

Retrograde femoral nailing

During the retrograde femoral nailing, the patient is supine with the injured leg exposed and the knee flexed and supported with a bump. This position allows the surgeon access to the popliteal notch without injuring the patella.

The sterile field is entered with the C-arm perpendicular to the patient. The C-arm is tilted cephalad to account for the flexed knee and to find the PA projection. The C-arm is rotated under the table for lateral position (Fig. 21.24).

Method

- Instruments or hardware may protrude from the operative site. Be sure to avoid disturbing these instruments or hardware or allowing them to puncture a sterile drape.
- Center the C-arm over the fracture site during canal reaming to ensure that the fracture remains reduced (Fig. 21.25).
- The table must allow for movement of the C-arm from the knee to the hip.
- Allow enough room between the patient and C-arm for the surgeon to work.

Screws are inserted into the femur and through the nail to fix the nail in place. When lining up the screw holes in the nail, the hole should be perfectly round and not oblong. Center the screw hole on the monitor. The magnification feature may be used to give the surgeon a better view. The C-arm may need to be tilted or rotated to obtain perfect circles. The surgeon also manipulates the leg to help align the screw holes. After the screws are inserted, check the length of the screws by placing the C-arm in PA projection. Screws should not protrude excessively from the cortical bone (Fig. 21.26).

Fig. 21.24 (A) C-arm positioned between patient's legs for PA projection during femoral nailing. *Arrow* is pointing to femur. (B) C-arm rotated under femur *(arrow)* for lateral projection.

Fig. 21.25 Image of femur fracture during canal reaming.

Structures shown

All parts of the femur, including the greater and lesser trochanters, femoral neck, shaft, and condyles, are seen in the PA and lateral positions. Different instrumentation is in the IM canal beginning with a guide rod that is used to help reduce the fracture and provide a means for the canal reamers to pass through the fracture site (Fig. 21.27). After reduction, the nail and screws are seen.

EVALUATION CRITERIA

- Appropriate projections are seen unobstructed and in correct plane on the monitor.
- Screw holes are perfectly round and in the center of the monitor.
- Sterile field is maintained.
- Proper radiographic technique is maintained.
- Radiation protection is provided for the surgical team.

Fig. 21.26 PA projection of proximal screw in a femoral nail.

Fig. 21.27 PA projection of femur fracture reduced with guide rod and distal interlocking screws inserted.

TIBIA (NAIL)

Position of patient

The patient is supine with the affected leg exposed. The knee is flexed to allow access to the tibial tuberosity without injuring the patella. The injured leg is on the opposite side of the table so that the C-arm does not interfere with the surgical team.

Position of C-arm

Cover the C-arm with a sterile drape. Move the C-arm into the field perpendicular to the patient. Center the beam over the leg and tilt the tube to match the angle of the leg (Fig. 21.28). No obstructions should be under the table to avoid interfering with the C-arm movement. Rotate the C-arm under the table and into the lateral position, taking care not to disturb any instrumentation protruding from the operative site. Center the leg on the monitor by raising or lowering the C-arm. The surgeon manipulates the leg, and the radiographer tilts or rotates the C-arm to obtain round holes (Figs. 21.29 and 21.30). The magnification feature can be used to enlarge the image if necessary. Advance the C-arm until its tube side is far enough from the injured leg to allow the surgeon to fit the drill and drill bit into the area.

- Along its shaft the tibia is triangular, so when checking the length of the screws the C-arm may have to be rotated forward or back to get a true length.
- Center the beam on the fracture site during canal reaming. When the leg is in the center of the monitor, turn the wheels of the C-arm horizontally to allow the machine to move longitudinally down the shaft of the leg without moving out of the field of view.

Fig. 21.28 C-arm positioned for tibial nailing. The radiographer tilted the fluoroscopic image intensifier to be parallel with the long axis of the leg.

Fig. 21.29 Image of tibial nail screw holes in incorrect alignment and oblong in shape.

Fig. 21.30 Image of tibial nail screw holes perfectly round and magnified to assist proper alignment.

Structures shown

Structures shown include the tibia and fibula, the tibial shaft along with any fracture, the tibial plateau, tibial tuberosity, distal tibia, and ankle joint (Fig. 21.31). After hardware is inserted, the tibial nail fills the IM canal, with proximal and distal screws prominent.

A

B

Fig. 21.31 (A) Improper alignment of distal screw holes. (B) Screw holes properly aligned with screwdriver over distal screw hole.

HUMERUS

Position of patient

The patient is supine or in a reclining or beach chair position (Fig. 21.32). The injured arm may be resting on a Mayo stand with the surgeon's assistant holding the arm to stabilize and align the humerus. The patient should be positioned with the shoulder off the side of the table. This position allows the humerus to be seen in its entirety without being obscured by the table.

Position of C-arm

Cover the C-arm with a sterile drape. Enter the field parallel to, or at a 45-degree angle to, the patient. The assistant rotates the arm medially with the elbow bent 90 degrees. The C-arm is tilted and rotated to obtain a true lateral projection, depending on the angle of patient position. The arm is held at the elbow to provide support, and the arm is rotated until the hand is pointing upward. The C-arm is tilted to obtain PA projection according to the patient's angle. Center the beam on the humerus.

- When installing a nail or rod into the humerus and trying to locate and center the distal screws, place a sterile drape over the tube or pull the sheets draping the patient over the tube. Touch only the underside of the sheets when placing them over the tube. Raise the tube to magnify the screw holes and to allow the surgeon to work.

Fig. 21.32 (A) C-arm positioned for PA projection of the shoulder with patient in beach chair position for preliminary imaging. (B) C-arm positioned for axillary projection.

NOTE: Do not leave any drape over the tube for a long time to prevent unnecessary heat buildup in the tube.

• Be careful not to strike the patient's head with the image intensifier.

Structures shown

This procedure should show all parts of the humerus, including the head, neck, greater and lesser tubercles, shaft, and distal portion of the humerus. Any fractures and the hardware used for repair (Fig. 21.33) are also seen.

■ Angle of humerus and C-arm coincide to obtain true PA and lateral projections.
■ When nailing the distal screws, holes should be perfectly round to allow screws to pass through the nail.
■ Humerus is in the center of the monitor to maintain radiographic technique.
■ Image is rotated in the same plane as the humerus.
■ Sterile field is maintained, especially with the proximity of possibly nonsterile portions of the tube to the sterile field.
■ Radiation protection is provided for the surgical team.

Fig. 21.33 (A) Images of humeral fracture with nails used to reduce fracture of the humeral head. (B) Image of clavicle fracture with plate and screw fixation.

FEMORAL/TIBIAL ARTERIOGRAM

Position of patient

The patient is supine with the affected leg exposed from the groin area to the foot. There should be enough room under the table to allow the C-arm to move from the hip to the foot. The leg may be rotated medially or laterally to keep the femur or tibia from obscuring any vasculature (Fig. 21.34).

Position of C-arm

Cover the C-arm with a sterile drape and enter the field perpendicular to the patient. When the leg is in the center of the monitor, turn the wheels of the C-arm horizontally to allow the machine to move to the left or right without taking the leg out of the field of view. Use the subtraction or road-mapping feature to remove all structures except the contrast medium that is injected into the artery (Fig. 21.35). This feature shows any stenoses or injuries to the artery.

Fig. 21.34 Subtraction image of surgical femoral artery angiogram with stenosis *(arrow)*.

Structures shown

The bones of the leg are seen before subtraction. After contrast medium is introduced, the femoral artery and its branches are seen, and, following the contrast medium down the leg, the popliteal and tibial arteries are seen. The contrast images show any pathologic defects in the arterial structures.

EVALUATION CRITERIA

- All pertinent vasculature must be shown without being obscured by the table or bones of the leg.
- Integrity of the mask image should be maintained by not moving the leg or the C-arm during subtraction or road mapping.
- Proper radiographic technique is maintained.
- Sterile field is maintained.
- Radiation protection is provided for the surgical team.

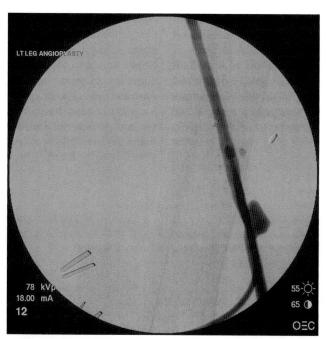

Fig. 21.35 Subtraction image of surgical femoral artery angiogram after balloon angioplasty.

Mobile Radiography Procedures for the Operating Room
CERVICAL SPINE

Image receptor: The IR should be a 10- × 12-inch (24- × 29-cm) grid IR crosswise.

Position of patient

The patient is upright, prone, or supine. In the upright and prone positions, the patient's head is held in a traction device to align the spine. In the supine position, the chin is elevated and held with a strap or tape.

Position of image receptor and portable machine

- Place the grid IR in the IR holder and cover with a sterile drape (Fig. 21.36).
- Position the IR holder on the opposite side of the patient. The surgical technician moves the sterile back table so that the radiographer does not compromise the sterile field.
- Direct the beam perpendicular to the IR and parallel to the floor.
- The beam enters perpendicular to the IR to eliminate grid cutoff.
- Raise or lower the tube and IR to center on the cervical spine.

Structures shown

- Cervical spine in lateral projection (Fig. 21.37).
- Degenerative or pathologic defects, such as osteophytes, fractures, or subluxation.
- Radiograph may be taken at the beginning of the case to verify the correct portion of the spine to be repaired. Instruments are placed to designate the level of the spine (Fig. 21.38).

EVALUATION CRITERIA

- Entire spine is on the radiograph.
- Spine is in the center of the radiograph and is not rotated.
- Proper radiographic technique is used.
- Radiation protection is provided.
- All hardware that may be used should be included.
- Grid cutoff is absent.

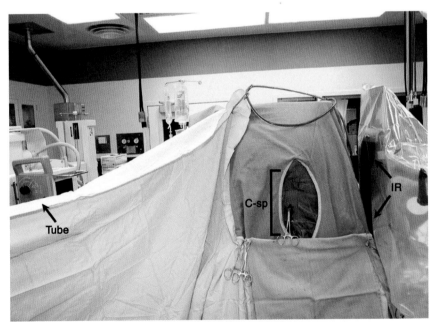

Fig. 21.36 Mobile radiographic machine (*arrow*) in position for upright lateral cervical spine. A surgical clamp, which is attached to the spinous process of interest, extends from the incision site. IR draped and in holder (*double arrow*) is centered to the patient.

Fig. 21.37 Lateral cervical spine radiograph (patient in sitting position for surgery) showing localization marker in place on the spinous process of C6.

Fig. 21.38 Lateral projection of the cervical spine with patient supine. This was done to verify the correct position of instruments before continuing surgery. Often a spinal needle is placed in the disk space to show position. Note that even though a 14 × 17 wireless DR detector is used, the radiographer has properly coned to pertinent anatomy.

THORACIC OR LUMBAR SPINE

Image receptor: The IR should be a 14- × 17-inch (35- × 43-cm) grid IR crosswise.

Position of patient

The patient is prone or supine with the arms placed up by the head. The chest and abdomen are supported by a frame or chest roll to flex the spine into anatomic position. A radiograph may be done to verify that the surgeon is working on the correct vertebra or to show the position of hardware (Fig. 21.39).

Lateral projection

Place grid IR in IR holder and cover with a sterile drape. Position the holder next to the patient and move the IR up or down to center on the lumbar spine. Direct the beam perpendicular to the IR and parallel to the floor (Fig. 21.40). Respiration should be suspended during exposure.

PA projection

For the PA radiograph, slide IR in the slot under the table and center on the spine. Cover field with sterile drape. Center the beam to the IR and perpendicular to the long axis of the spine.

Structures shown

- The lumbar spine in PA and lateral projections.
- Vertebral bodies, spinous processes, facets, and lamina.

- Hardware to repair any defects. Bone grafts or interbody fusion devices may be used.
- Instrumentation is often seen on radiograph.
- PA projection may be obscured by the patient support.

EVALUATION CRITERIA

- Spine is in the center of the radiograph and in true PA or lateral projection.
- Spine bodies are seen without any rotation.
- All hardware used must be seen on radiograph.
- All unnecessary instrumentation is removed to avoid obscuring spine.
- Proper radiographic technique is used.
- Radiation protection is provided for the surgical team.

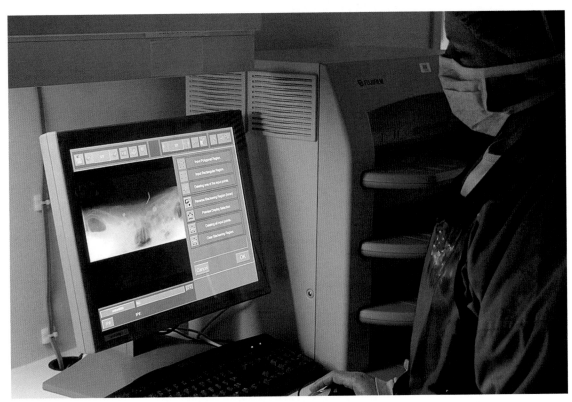

Fig. 21.39 Lateral lumbar spine with intraoperative marker to verify correct level of interest. CR and DR allow postprocessing adjustments.

Fig. 21.40 (A) Mobile x-ray machine correctly positioned for cross-table lateral lumbar spine. (B) Radiographer positioning mobile unit intraoperatively for lateral lumbar spine procedure.

Fig. 21.41 PA projection of a hip joint replacement with plate and screw fixation following a periprosthetic femur fracture.

EXTREMITY EXAMINATIONS

Image receptor: Choose the appropriate-size IR to include all appropriate anatomy and hardware.

Position of patient

The patient is supine, prone, reclining, or in the beach chair position. Portable machines approach perpendicular to the patient. Institutions may cover the tube or sterile field, or both, with a sterile drape. Angle the tube to match the IR or desired projection. The surgeon may choose to hold the patient's limb in position during the exposure. To reduce exposure to the surgeon, positioning aids, such as sterile towels, sponges, or mallets, may be used.

The surgeon may also cover the field with a cloth sterile drape rather than a plastic sterile drape. If so, the surgeon marks the location of the part to ensure proper centering. Lighting may also need to be adjusted for better visualization of the field. For cross-table examinations, the beam is directed perpendicular to the IR and parallel to the floor. Center the beam to the IR and raise or lower the tube to the center of the part.

Fig. 21.42 AP and lateral postreduction images of a comminuted ankle fracture. Some casting materials require an increase in technical factors for correct penetration and image quality.

Structures shown

- All pertinent anatomy in correct alignment.
- Hardware including plates, wires, pins, screws, external fixation, and joint replacement components used to repair fractures or degenerative problems (Figs. 21.41 through 21.47).

Fig. 21.43 AP and lateral image of the ankle with antibiotic beads. Antibiotic beads are placed at the site of infection to promote healing.

Fig. 21.44 AP and lateral projection of proximal tibia with plate and screw fixation used to repair tibial plateau fracture.

Fig. 21.45 AP and lateral projection of elbow with plate and screws used to reduce forearm fracture.

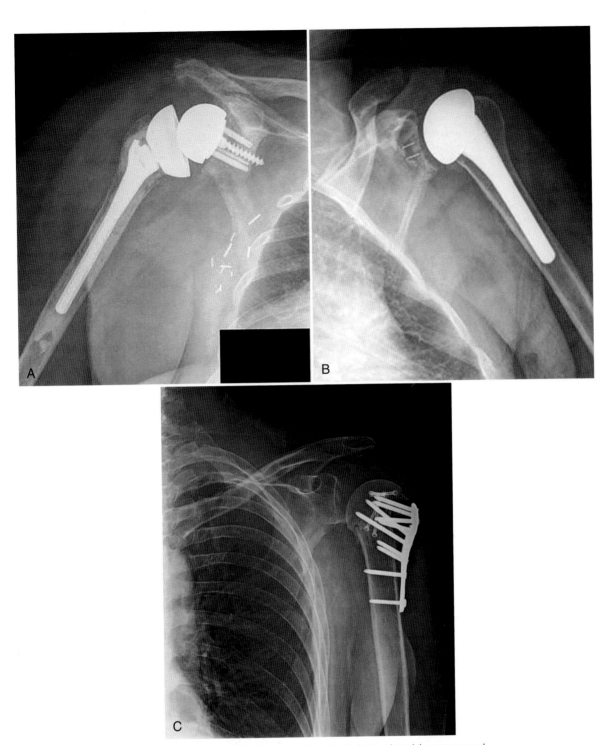

Fig. 21.46 (A) Total shoulder arthroplasty with polyethylene glenoid component. (B) Reverse total shoulder arthroplasty. (C) Shoulder with plate and screws fixation. Creative patient positioning or tube angulation may be necessary to achieve optimal images on complex comminuted fractures.

EVALUATION CRITERIA

- Complete joint including all hardware is seen on the image.
- Proper radiographic technique is used.
- Sterile field is maintained.
- Radiation protection is provided.
- Collimation to include all hardware used.
- No unnecessary instruments are in field.

NOTE: Often to save time or cost, multiple projections are done on one imaging plate. Be careful not to superimpose any of the projections. Many surgeons request different projections depending on the individual case. When performing a wrist examination, the arm is positioned on one side of the imaging plate with the wrist in the AP or PA projection. Center the beam and collimate to the wrist to include all hardware. When the exposure is complete, the surgeon moves the arm to the other side of the imaging plate in the lateral position. Center the beam on the wrist and collimate (Figs. 21.48 and 21.49).

Fig. 21.47 AP (A) and lateral (B) postreduction images of a fifth metatarsal nonhealing fracture.

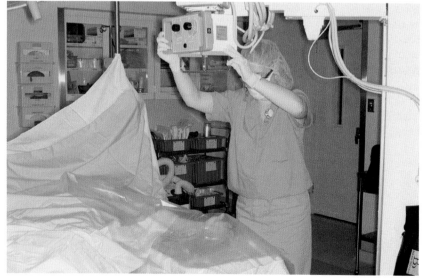

Fig. 21.48 Radiographer positioning a mobile machine for lateral projection of wrist.

Fig. 21.49 PA, lateral, and tilt lateral projections of wrist. Note proper radial tilt of 22 degrees shows joint space clear of reduction screws.

Definition of Terms

antisepsis Chemical disinfection of the skin.

asepsis Absence of infection or germs or elimination of infectious agents.

aseptic technique Principles involved with manipulation of sterile and non-sterile items to prevent or minimize microbiologic contamination.

contamination Presence of pathogenic microorganisms.

microbial fallout Microorganisms normally shed from skin that can contaminate sterile surfaces or areas.

restricted area Operating rooms, clean core or sterile storage areas.

semirestricted area Area of peripheral support, such as hallways or corridors leading to restricted areas.

sterile Substance or object that is completely free of living microorganisms and is incapable of producing any form of organism.

teamwork The Association of Surgical Technologists (AST) Standards of Practice Standard I states: "Teamwork is essential for perioperative patient care and is contingent on interpersonal skills. Communication is critical to the positive attainment of expected outcomes of care. All team members should work together for the common good of the patient, for the benefit of the patient and the delivery of actions with the health care team, the patient and family, superiors, and peers. Personal integrity and surgical conscience are integrated into every aspect of professional behavior."

unrestricted area Areas in which street clothes are permitted, such as outer hallways, family waiting areas, locker rooms, and employee lounges.

Selected bibliography

Anderson AC: *The radiologic technologist's handbook of surgical procedures*, Philadelphia, 2000, CRC Press.

Fortunato N: *Berry & Kohn's operating room technique*, ed 9, St Louis, 2000, Mosby.

Huth-Meeker M, Rothrock JC: *Alexander's care of the patient in surgery*, ed 10, St Louis, 1995, Mosby.

Huth-Meeker M, Rothrock JC: *Alexander's care of the patient in surgery*, ed 11, St Louis, 1999, Mosby.

Permar JA, Wetterlin KJ: Surgical radiography. In Frank ED, et al, editors: *Merrill's atlas of radiographic positions and radiologic procedures* (vol 3). ed 11, St Louis, 2007, Mosby.

Wetterlin KJ: Mobile radiography. In Frank ED, et al, editors: *Merrill's atlas of radiographic positions and radiologic procedures* (vol 3). ed 9, St Louis, 2007, Mosby.

22
PEDIATRIC IMAGING

RAYMOND THIES • DEREK CARVER • ANGELA FRANCESCHI

Introduction to Pediatric Imaging

Imaging children is one of the most fascinating and worthwhile specialties in radiography. To witness their cheerful resilience and the acceptance of immense challenges by the parents is a privilege. At the same time, pediatric imaging can be one of the most confounding experiences. Radiographers gain skills in multitasking, such as quickly engaging and reassuring the child using an age-appropriate approach, then switching gears to gain the confidence of the parents, explaining and instructing them on immobilization techniques for the exam, all the while keeping in mind that other patients are waiting. It is important to be mindful of the various stressors parents may have endured before finding their way to the imaging room. In addition to the stress of a pending diagnosis, parents may have experienced an early and long commute, an unsettled child, a busy parking lot, and difficulty navigating their way through the institution. Do not personalize family moods. Your primary job is to actively listen, communicate, and understand the parents and their child. This is the primary path to achieving cooperation and quality diagnostic radiography. Children take their behavioral cues from facial expressions, intonations, and body postures; an ill-at-ease parent will convey that mood to the child, making the exam more difficult to perform. The sooner you can win the child's trust and turn his or her attention to the task at hand, the more successful the exam results will be and the family will leave praising your efforts. Part radiographer, psychologist, physicist, and caregiver, your job is always full of surprises and can be immensely satisfying. Whether you are an imaging professional looking for guidance on pediatric imaging or a student exploring career possibilities, this overview will give you (1) a broad look at the specialty, (2) details on how to conduct the most common pediatric exams including positioning and projections, and (3) an understanding of the more prevalent pathologies and syndromes.

WAITING ROOM

Waiting and procedure rooms that are well equipped can reduce anxiety and act as a diversion for both the parents and the children. Children are attracted to and amused by toys, thus leaving the parents free to check in, register, and ask pertinent questions. Gender-neutral toys or activities, such as coloring with crayons located at a small age-appropriate table, are most appropriate. (Children should be supervised to prevent them from putting the crayons in their mouths.) Books or magazines for older children are also good investments. The Child Life Department of the hospital can provide advice and make appropriate recommendations (Figs. 22.1 through 22.3).

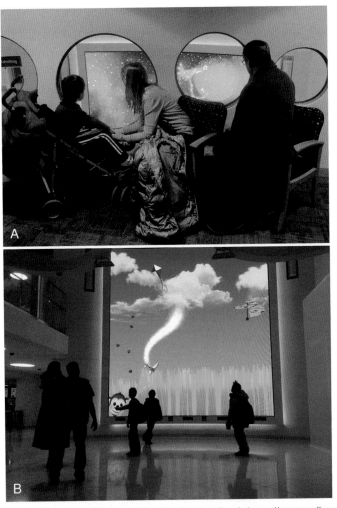

Fig. 22.1 (A) Radiology outpatient and family viewing the interactive media wall. (B) The interactive media wall from the first floor lobby.

Specific Pediatric Considerations

SAFETY

- Never leave your patient unattended.
- Keep items that could be swallowed out of reach.

COMMUNICATION

- Introduce yourself while making eye contact (if culturally appropriate) with patient and parents.
- Explain the radiography team role.
- Always speak to a child using language appropriate for the child's developmental level.
- Explain the exam.
- Take history (as required), and discuss pertinent medical information on a level the family can understand.
- Avoid medical jargon and unfamiliar terms. If a medical term cannot be avoided, explain in lay terms.

- Be mindful not to engage in conversations that are inappropriate in the presence of the patient.
- Before beginning the exam, ask if there are any questions or concerns.
- Use family teaching sheets when applicable. (These are web-based outlines of your hospital's procedures for the patient/family.)

RESPECT FOR PATIENT/PARENT RIGHTS AND DIGNITY

- Listen to patient's/parent's questions and concerns.
- Some patients/parents speak English as a second language, which may impede their complete understanding of the exam and communication of exam results. To better serve the family and for medicolegal reasons, have an interpreter present.
- Be mindful of cultural preferences and taboos. Ask your interpreter, the family, or seek out resources within your institution.
- Always knock before entering, and avoid entering an imaging room while an exam is in progress.

PROVISION OF ADEQUATE CARE AND SERVICE TO THE PATIENT AND FAMILY

- Create a child-friendly environment.
- Use appropriately sized equipment.
- Remember, parents know their children best, so seek and make use of their advice.
- Utilize your child life specialist (CLS); they are invaluable for facilitating cooperation.
- If not contraindicated by the study, use a soft pad with a sheet on the exam table for patient comfort.
- Place the patient on the exam table when ready to proceed.

Fig. 22.2 Nuclear medicine waiting room.

Fig. 22.3 Transition hallway from nuclear medicine to ultrasound.

Age-Based Development

The pediatric patient may not always fit neatly into the following developmental stages for a variety of reasons (e.g., pathology, developmental delays, parenting, chronic illness or prolonged hospital stay, or mood at the time of exam), but there are some universal approaches to interacting with children that will always apply (e.g., setting limits, making eye contact, and addressing their fears). Be observant, take your queues from the patient and family, and tailor your approach to them. Watch their eyes and body postures. Are the parents gripping things tightly? Do you need to set limits for their children? Is the child clinging to the parent's leg? Is the child tense? Listen to the child's choice of words.

With a team approach (gastrointestinal/genitourinary [GI/GU] exams, survey studies), pass on your experience in connecting with the family in a final strategy session before the team enters the exam room. Introductions should always be made in a slow and relaxed fashion so the family and patient understand them. Cultural norms are important, and although the family might make allowances for your ignorance, it is best to educate yourself on the norms and appropriate behavior in the family's country. Learn a few words or phrases in the languages most common to your patient's demographic. Cultural biases can also work in reverse; the family might make assumptions about you and how they treat you based on your sex or their socioeconomic status in their country of origin. Consulting your interpreter for advice is the first place to start.

PREMATURE INFANTS

Generally, bedside radiography and procedures in GI and GU using fluoroscopy encompass the majority of the contact radiographers will have with premature infants in the department. Elevate the room temperature 10 to 15 minutes prior to the patient's arrival. When these babies are in radiology for a procedure, an intensive care unit (ICU) nursing team will accompany them. The nursing team will provide care for the patient, but you will need to explain the procedure and how the nursing team can help. Obtain the current status of the patient and any special requests from the nursing staff. As with any exam, suction and oxygen must always be available and the room well stocked. Leave the patient in the incubator/warmer until just before the procedure. Depending on the exam, you may be able to use a radiolucent cushion on the exam table for patient comfort. Discuss the patient immobilization plan (who will hold, how, what body part) with the nursing staff to ensure that you accommodate the patient's medical condition. Have warming lights available, wash hands, glove, and adhere to all isolation precautions.

NEONATE (0 TO 28 DAYS)

The neonatal period is a time of transition from the uterine environment to the outside world. During this first month the newborn is forming attachments with caregivers. They are sensitive to the way they are held, rocked, and positioned. They love to be swaddled, which gives them a sense of security and keeps them from being disturbed by their own startle reflex. Newborns startle easily when moved quickly or upon hearing a loud noise, and bright lights cause them to blink frequently or close their eyes. Understandably, the hospital environment creates particular stressors that can affect those at this very young age, which should be minimized whenever possible.

Because newborns are most secure and comfortable when swaddled, keep them in this position until just before you are ready for imaging. Decrease noise levels and bright lights whenever possible, maintain a warm room, and always use warming lights unless the nursing team directs otherwise. Speak soothingly and try to avoid sudden, quick movements. Let the caregivers know exactly what is expected during imaging and involve them in soothing and calming their infant. Pacifiers, oral sucrose (check with the nursing team), a personal blanket, and quiet singing can all help to sooth newborns, enabling them to feel safe and secure.

INFANT (28 DAYS TO 18 MONTHS)

During different periods of infancy, babies experience stranger and separation anxiety. When working with infants, involve the parents whenever possible; the comfort of seeing the parent's/caregiver's face, hearing that familiar voice, and feeling the caregiver's touch can be invaluable when calming the infant.

The radiographer and the CLS play important roles in establishing a relationship with the infant by talking and smiling; this will help put the parents at ease and demonstrate care and concern for their baby. The caregiver knows the infant best, so ask what soothes and comforts the baby when he or she is distressed. Personal objects, such as a pacifier or a blanket, can distract and soothe the infant during the exam. To ease the transition from the parent's arms to the exam table, it is advisable to decrease stimuli and eliminate loud noises. Keeping the baby swaddled or in their carrier until just prior to imaging minimizes transitions and reduces the baby's time on the exam table. The first rule of imaging infants is never leave the infant unattended; the radiographer or parent should always have a hand on the infant. The second rule is always cushion the exam table under the infant's skull. Be sure not to flex the head forward, which may cause respiratory difficulties.

TODDLER (18 MONTHS TO 3 YEARS)

Toddlers can be a challenge for both radiographers and staff. Toddlers are not abstract thinkers and are unable to understand the concept of "inside their body." They operate very much in the "here and now." They are seldom able to keep their bodies still, which can make imaging problematic, and they also have a short attention span and become overwhelmed quickly. Toddlers are fearful of medical experiences and often become unruly while they are being positioned for an exam. Unfamiliar exam positions and faces can escalate their movement.

In an effort to provide adequate care and minimize reactions, keep language brief and use concrete words. Because keeping their body still is most often an issue, efficiency is crucial. Be sure the room is organized before the patient and family enter. If the toddler has a toy or blanket, keep it within reach during the examination if possible. Distraction techniques can be extremely helpful in keeping the toddler calm. A screaming toddler can often be distracted and calmed by being allowed to blow bubbles or use a tablet computer with an age-appropriate application.

After the imaging has been completed, let children know they did a great job, that you are proud of them, and that they should be proud of themselves. Praise may be in the form of positive statements or a small reward like a sticker or balloon.

PRESCHOOLER (3 TO 5 YEARS)

New places, faces, and experiences can be overwhelming to preschoolers. Unfamiliar sights, sounds, and faces can be quite intimidating and can leave the preschooler feeling frightened. In addition, preschoolers are establishing routines and greatly benefit from structure and knowing what to expect. For preschoolers, the medical environment is unpredictable, so often these patients need time to explore and familiarize themselves with the imaging room, even if it is brief. They also need to feel comfortable with the clinicians who will be working with them. Taking the time to establish rapport will be instrumental in making preschoolers feel comfortable, thus enhancing their coping ability (Fig. 22.4).

Additional steps include letting them know exactly what to expect and what you expect of them. For example, mention the loud sounds of the "camera," show the movement of the "camera," the coldness of a solution or cotton ball they may feel, and most important, assure them that you will let them know before you do anything. These simple courtesies facilitate trust and cooperation and help the child feel more comfortable. Some preschoolers may have difficulty understanding the exam through dialogue. Therefore, when speaking with them about imaging or "taking pictures," it may be helpful to model this process using a doll or stuffed animal.

Although preschoolers are developing independence and want to establish themselves as separate from their parents, they can become fearful if separated from them; utilizing parents can be instrumental to the success of the exam. If the parents are not able to remain with the child during imaging, be sure they can be first to pick up and comfort the child when the procedure is completed.

When working with patients of this age, use directive statements in an effort to facilitate cooperation; for example, "It's time to" or "You can help me by" are directive statements that will limit their response, leaving them more likely to comply. Open-ended questions that begin with "Do you want to (get on the table, get changed, etc.)" leave preschoolers feeling as if they have a choice when in reality getting on the table or having the exam is not a choice. Open-ended statements confuse preschoolers and can leave them feeling overwhelmed. Preschoolers are constantly seeking approval from others and respond well to positive affirmations. Praise and encouragement are beneficial for this age group, as they will create a positive experience and help to boost the preschooler's confidence for future medical appointments.

Fig. 22.4 The radiographer should make an introduction to the child and show the child how the collimator light is used.

SCHOOL AGE (6 TO 12 YEARS)

School-age children are becoming logical thinkers and have a fear of failure, so positive affirmations and reassurances are extremely beneficial. They are curious and full of questions; take the opportunity to connect using age-appropriate explanations. Break down the exam into steps, let them know exactly what to expect and what you expect of them, and, most important, let them know before you do anything. These simple courtesies will facilitate trust and cooperation and help the child feel more comfortable.

Avoid unfamiliar medical jargon, as this will only confuse school-age children and can decrease their ability to cope. School-agers are very literal, so it is crucial to avoid words that can be misconstrued like shoot, shot, or dye. School-age patients benefit from being given choices; this will give them a sense of control and entitlement, which inevitably enhances their coping abilities. However, be cautious to only give realistic choices; cajoling the child using open-ended questions could mislead the child.

It is important to make imperative or interrogative statements, such as "It's time to get changed; would you like the green gown or the blue one?" or "You need to get on the table; would you like me to help you or would you like your mom to help you?" These choices are direct and allow for a realistic choice. Coping and distraction techniques available to patients and staff like taking deep breaths, blowing bubbles, listening to music, watching a movie, or playing games with a tablet can be instrumental in helping children cope during exams.

ADOLESCENT (12 TO 18 YEARS)

When imaging adolescents, respect their need for privacy; a private area for changing, knocking before entering their exam room, and limiting the number of staff involved will help to alleviate stress. If you have clinicians (GI/GU, MR, CT), and radiographers of both sexes and time permits, ask the patient if he or she would feel more comfortable with a male or female performing the exam. In many pediatric centers, girls who have reached the age of 10 to 12 years must be asked if there is any chance they might be pregnant. You may also ask if the girl has started menstruating. A truthful response is more probable if the parent is not present when these questions are asked. The patient's response will dictate whether further explanation is required. For example, you may need to add, "We ask these same questions of all girls because unborn babies are extremely sensitive to radiation exposure."

If it is necessary for adolescent patients to disclose their medical history, speak directly to them and their parents rather than just the parents. Radiographers have a tendency to ask the parents this information, and it is important to remember that adolescents most often know their body best. As adolescents, they do not always discuss things with their parents for reasons of embarrassment or shame. In addition, before beginning the exam, ask the adolescent patient if they would like to have a parent present during imaging. This gives adolescents a choice and also lets them know it is okay to ask parents to step out.

It is not uncommon for the adolescent patient to respond negatively to having an exam. In addition to being extremely modest, they see themselves as invincible and often do not believe that anything could possibly be wrong with them. Adolescents also fear "being different" and are afraid of something happening to their bodies that would alter their appearance or make them unlike their peers. Validating their feelings and letting them know you want to help will reassure them, for example: "I understand the way you are feeling; lots of teenagers have this test done and they feel the same way" or "I am here to help you as best I can." Assisting adolescents with preparation, explaining the rationale for why the exam is taking place, and giving them tools for coping will facilitate cooperation and decrease fears. Deep breathing, listening to music, or having a conversation with a caregiver can help to put the patient at ease.

Patients With Special Needs

The radiographer should consider age and behavior when approaching children with physical and mental disabilities. School-age children with disabilities strive to achieve as much autonomy and independence as possible. They are sensitive to the fact that they are less independent than their peers. The radiographer should observe the following guidelines:

- Introduce yourself and identify the patients at their level (you may have to kneel down), then briefly explain the procedure to the child and parents. All children appreciate being given the opportunity to listen and respond. As with all patients, children want to be spoken to rather than talked about.
- If this approach proves ineffective, turn to the parents. Generally, the parents of these patients are present and can be very helpful. In strange environments, younger children may trust only one person—the parent. In that case, the medical team can gain cooperation from the child by communicating through the parent. Parents often know the best way to lift and transfer the child from the wheelchair or stretcher to the table. Children with physical disabilities often have a fear of falling and may want only a parent's assistance.
- Place the wheelchair or stretcher parallel to the imaging table, taking care to explain that you have locked the wheelchair or stretcher and will be getting help for the transfer. These children often know the way they should be lifted—*ask them*. They can tell you which areas to support and which actions they prefer to do themselves.

Finally, children with spastic contractions are often frustrated by their inability to control movements that are counterproductive to the exam. Gentle massage or a warm blanket should be used to help relax the muscles.

Communicating with a child who has a mental disability can be difficult, depending on the severity of the disability. Some patients react to verbal stimuli, whereas loud or abrupt noises may startle and agitate them. Ask the parent or caregiver if there is anything you should know about the child that would help achieve a quick and accurate exam. They will alert you to psychological, behavioral, or physical impairments that may not be obvious or referenced on the exam order.

AUTISM SPECTRUM DISORDERS[a]

Medical imaging of individuals with autism spectrum disorders (ASDs) can be difficult. In addition to difficulties with communication, there are also behavioral issues, medical issues, and environmental concerns that need to be considered. There are important steps that should be taken before the patient is brought into the examination room and, in some cases, before they come to the imaging facility.

According to the Centers for Disease Control and Prevention (CDC), ASDs are a group of developmental disabilities that can cause significant social, communication, and behavioral challenges. People with ASDs handle information in their brain differently than other people. A spectrum means that autism can range from very mild to severe. There are some similar symptoms, such as problems with social interaction; however, there are differences in time of onset, severity, and the nature of the symptoms. One popular saying within the autism community is "If you know one person with autism, then, you know one person with autism." This makes creating treatment plans difficult for parents, caregivers, and physicians. What works well for one individual may not be effective for another. This also makes imaging individuals with ASDs challenging.

The prevalence of autism is on the rise; in 1998 the rate of autism was 1 in 110, and by 2000 it had risen to 1 in 88. More recent studies have indicated that it may be as high as 1 in 35 for males and 1 in 50 for all children. It is five times more common in males than females, and on average the diagnosis is earlier for those with more severe symptoms. Parents may notice the difference as early as 6 months, whereas high-functioning individuals, such as those with Asperger syndrome, are diagnosed at around 6 years of age.

Most patients with ASDs will be identified before scheduling imaging procedures. The CDC has several publications on the diagnosis for ASD; however, for facilitating imaging the following are commonly recognized signs of autism:
1. Difficulty with social interaction
2. Problems with verbal and nonverbal communication
3. Repetitive behaviors or narrow, obsessive interests

Special considerations for imaging

Once an ASD patient is identified, there are many things we can do to provide for a successful imaging experience for both radiographer and patient. Whether or not the patient is in the department, we should begin by asking more questions. Box 22.1 is an example of a patient questionnaire. It might be beneficial to schedule the exam at a time when the department is not busy. Loud noises or visual overstimulation can be distracting and in some cases can cause severe behaviors. This can be especially true during the adolescent years. Because these children are larger, aggressive or violent behavior can be dangerous for the patient or staff. It is wise to prepare for all possibilities. A good patient questionnaire can help gather resources and prepare the environment. You can use the questionnaire to eliminate noises when needed and adjust lighting.

---

[a]Written by Jerry Tyree.

> **BOX 22.1**
>
> Autism patient questionnaire
>
> ---
>
> Is your child sensitive to fluorescent lighting?
> Is your child comfortable in a dimly lit room?
> Is your child tactile defensive, or sensitive to touch?
>   If yes, explain.
> Is your child sensitive to loud noises?
>   High frequencies?
>   Low frequencies?
> Is your child uncomfortable in cool or cold situations?
> Is your child uncomfortable in warm or hot situations?
> Do you have any calming objects you would like the child to have in the imaging suite?
> Will your child find a video played during the procedure calming?

Try to give the patient with an ASD the first or last appointment of the day. People with an ASD find waiting around for an appointment extremely stressful. Waiting in busy hospital corridors will increase the stress levels of an already anxious child or adult. If possible, find a small side room the family can wait in. Alternatively, they may prefer to wait outside or in the car and a member of staff should be identified to collect them or call their cell phone when the radiographer is ready. If the appointment is likely to be delayed, the family may wish to leave the building completely and return at a later agreed time.

Temperature is often difficult to adjust, but patient dress can be modified if it is an issue. Many individuals with autism are sensitive to touch. They have difficulty habituating stimuli of any type. Some may wear socks inside out so they cannot feel the seam on their toes. These are serious issues for individuals on the spectrum.

Sometimes we need to modify our positioning techniques for individuals who are tactile defensive, or sensitive to touch. A sensitivity to the "poking" often used to find anatomic landmarks can also be problematic. Some barbers have found that once you touch, you maintain the touch until you are finished with the haircut. One hand must remain on the head until the haircut is complete. We can use this same concept with imaging; once you begin to touch, do not remove your hand until you have all the information you need.

Videos can be a double-edged sword. Although a familiar video can be calming, if it varies in any small way from the one the child is used to, it can actually cause a severe reaction. It might be best if patients bring in videos of their own, especially if the procedure is expected to be long.

Personal space and body awareness

A crowded waiting room may be distressing for people with an ASD who may need their personal space. Similarly, close proximity to the radiographer could be uncomfortable for the patient.

Problems can also occur when trying to explain where pain is experienced. Those who have difficulty with body awareness may not be able to experience where different body parts are.

Touch

Individuals with ASDs may be hyposensitive to touch, or tactile defensive. They may find a light touch very painful. Some of these patients may prefer more deep pressure in touching, or you may not be able to touch them at all.

Patient responses

Do not be surprised if the patient does not make eye contact, especially if he or she is distressed. Lack of eye contact does not necessarily mean the patient is not listening to what you are saying. Allow the patient extra time to process what you have said. Do not assume that a nonverbal patient cannot understand what you are saying.

People with an ASD can have a high pain threshold. Even if the child does not appear to be in pain, he or she may, for example, have broken a bone. ASD patients may show an unusual response to pain that could include laughter, humming, singing, and removal of clothing. Agitation and behavior may be the only clues that the child or adult is in pain.

Communication

Use clear simple language with short sentences. People with an ASD tend to take everything literally. Thus, if you say, "It will only hurt for a minute," they will expect the pain to have gone within a minute.

Make your language concrete and avoid using idioms, irony, metaphors, and words with double meanings (e.g., "It's raining cats and dogs out there"). This could cause the patient to look outside for cats and dogs. Avoid using body language, gestures, or facial expressions without verbal instructions, as the patient may not understand these nonverbal messages.

Consider involving a caregiver to facilitate communication. Many individuals respond slowly, and patience is required.

Noise

Some departments use buzzers to indicate when it is a patient's turn to have an exam. They may also have music playing in a waiting room. Crying babies or children in the waiting room may also be quite noisy. For those with hypersensitive hearing, these types of noises can be magnified and become disturbing or even painful. Also with this heightened volume, surrounding sounds could become distorted. This could make it difficult for the person with an ASD to recognize sounds, such as a name being called. Individuals may respond by putting their fingers in their ears like the child at a racetrack, whereas others may "stim" (flap hands, flick fingers, rock, etc.). This kind of behavior is calming to the individual, so do not try to stop it unless absolutely essential. Individuals with ASDs often retreat when overstimulated.

Injections/needle sticks

If the patient needs an injection or blood test, divert their attention elsewhere. The use of pictures or a doll is a good idea to demonstrate what is going to happen. People with an ASD can be either undersensitive or oversensitive to pain, so that some may feel the pain acutely and be very distressed whereas others may not appear to react at all.

It is advisable to assume that the patient will feel pain. Use a local anesthetic cream, such as a eutectic mixture of local anesthetics, to numb the site of injection. Sand timers and clocks can be used as distracters during procedures, such as injections, so that the person with autism can see a definite end.

Tips for radiographers

Relaxation techniques such as deep breathing, counting, singing favorite songs, talking about a favorite interest, or looking at favorite books/toys could also help during physical examination or treatments. Parents may be instructed to bring a favorite toy or video if a player is available in the procedure room.

Make sure directions are given step by step, verbally, visually, and by providing physical supports or prompts, as needed by the patient. Patients with ASDs often have trouble interpreting facial expressions, body language, and tone of voice. Be as concrete and explicit as possible in your instructions and feedback to the patient. Demonstrating on others or on toys to show what will happen during a physical examination can reassure an individual with an ASD.

Many children with autism fixate on routines. Most medical imaging will fall outside of their routines. Social stories can be used to make something unfamiliar seem more routine. A social story can be a written or visual guide describing various social interactions or situations. These stories can be a book, on flashcards, or the department can have them online so the family can share with the patient what it is like to go to the x-ray department. The caregiver can revisit or practice these social stories prior to the exam. Pictures of the parking garage, waiting room, imaging room, even the individual radiographer can be added. The more accurate these pictures are, the better they will work. It might even be helpful to take pictures from the perspective of the individual with the ASD. If the patient will be lying on an x-ray table, a picture taken up toward the tube or scanner might be appropriate. In this way, a social story can be used to make something the individual has never done before seem routine.

Parents of many children with ASDs create social stories for vacations, plane rides, trips to the amusement park, and so on. Parents and caregivers who use these social stories will vouch for their effectiveness. In addition to social stories, it may be helpful if you can allow the patient with autism and caregiver access to the facility before the exam. This allows a "dry run" of the procedure, which may reduce anxiety during the actual exam.

In summation, a combination of questionnaire, social stories, and the patient application of the aforementioned principles should greatly help when imaging individuals with ASDs. Preparation is key, but it need not be prohibitively time consuming. Creating a social story for every exam an imaging department does is ideal, but simplification is possible. Making social stories accessible online is desirable. Adding pictures and images, especially accurate ones of specific facilities, increases the comfort level of patients. These practices are also good for all patients, not just those with ASDs. Many advocates would say that better serving individuals with ASDs (or others with "different" abilities) has improved schools, social services, and the lives of all they touch. The same could be said of our imaging departments.

Radiation Protection
DOSE AND DIAGNOSTIC INFORMATION

The goal in administering radiation for a specific clinical indication is to ensure that the *diagnostic* information obtained will be of greater value than the potential risks associated with the radiation. To protect our patients, we should identify through scientific testing an acceptable level of quantum mottle for each exam, which will not compromise the diagnostic goal of the image. What we, as medical practitioners, are attempting to do is use the minimum radiation dose required to produce a *clinically diagnostic* image for a specific clinical indication; this is our primary goal as radiographers and radiologists. Radiographers should observe the following steps:

- Direct efforts toward proper centering and selection of exposure factors, and precise collimation, which all contribute to safe practice.
- Use strategic placement of gonadal and breast shielding, and employ effective immobilization techniques to reduce the need for repeat examinations.

Instead of the anteroposterior (AP) projection, use the posteroanterior (PA) projection of the thorax and skull to reduce the amount of radiation reaching the breast tissue and lens of the eye, respectively.

- During radiography of the upper limbs, protect the upper torsos of all children.
- Pulsed fluoroscopy with "last image hold" also reduces patient dose and length of examination.

A cautionary note: The fact that digitally acquired images can be "postprocessed," thereby correcting some exposure errors, does not negate an important truth—images of proper density are achieved by proper positioning. The anatomy to be demonstrated must be in proper alignment with the photocell or ionization chamber.

Child versus adult

The possible long-term stochastic effects of a low linear energy transfer (LET) radiation dose on pediatric patients, if they exist, are much greater than the same dose to an adult because the child has a longer lifetime over which to express any long-term effects, and due to the child's smaller body volume, the potential exists to expose multiple organ systems to radiation for any given exam.

Shielding and dose reduction

A primary radiation shield should always be employed to protect gonadal, breast, and thyroid tissues when the exam protocol allows. Patients should always be shielded, including male breast tissue, unless the shielding will compromise the diagnostic area of interest for the exam (e.g., male or female lateral proximal femurs, female abdominal images, and male or female false profile lateral hips). Initial images for PA scoliosis and female pelvic exams should not be shielded (your clinical setting will have specific guidelines for shielding) (Fig. 22.5). Males can be shielded on the initial AP pelvic image provided the shield is positioned below the pubic symphysis (Fig. 22.6).

Discussing radiation risks and benefits with parents

Just as you have developed exam-based routines, you should have an example-based "script" for discussing the risk/benefit equation of radiation exposure. When parents have questions, listen carefully and hear their questions, fears (which may only be implied), point of reference for understanding radiation dose (usually CT), and educational level. Be aware that people in medical settings, especially when under stress, often hear only 50% of what is being said; additionally, they often give greater weight to negative information. Be knowledgeable and confident with your answers (body language, tone, interest, and clarity of presentation without technical jargon); a rambling or confusing presentation will do more harm than good. "In risk perception theory, perception equals reality. This means there may be no correlation between public perceptions of risk and scientific or technical information. Therefore, you must discuss the risk based on the perception."[1]

Fig. 22.5 Proper positioning of female gonadal shield.

Reframing the way parents and patients understand radiation risks (if they exist) and benefits should be your first goal. Human exposure to x-radiation is usually "understood" through the subjectivity of the lay press, the sensationalism of TV shows, and the half-truths of word of mouth. A wonderfully clear and effective, but often overlooked, approach to help place radiation exposure in perspective is to reference the dose the child will receive for any given exam to the background radiation we all receive daily. Background equivalent radiation time (BERT) equates a particular exam-based radiation dose to the equivalent amount of radiation dose received daily from our natural background (Table 22.1). The BERT method has several advantages: (1) the patient readily understands it; (2) it does not mention radiation risk, which is unknown; and (3) it educates the patient that he or she lives in a sea of natural background radiation.

The lay public's preoccupation with the perceived risks of x-radiation often overshadows the benefits of the diagnostic imaging exam. When a physician orders a radiation-based exam, it is with the confidence that the diagnostic information obtained will outweigh any potential risks (if there are any) of an image. Declining an exam based on perceived risks creates the real risk of a missed diagnosis.

Fig. 22.6 Males can be shielded on the initial AP pelvic image provided the shield is positioned below the pubic symphysis. (A) Shows correct shielding and positioning (femoral heads are centered), but collimation should be tighter and the patient should have been changed prior to imaging. (B) Incorrect shielding; shield covering part of symphysis and inferior rami.

TABLE 22.1

Comparison of pediatric exam dose to background radiation level

Exam	Natural background radiation equivalent[a] (time to receive equivalent background radiation)
Chest CT, high resolution (pulmonary embolism, angiogram)	730 days (6 mSv)
Abdominal CT	365 days (3 mSv)
Abdomen/pelvic radiograph	90 days (0.75 mSv)
Chest radiograph, two view	2.5 days (0.02 mSv)
Natural background radiation	1 day (0.008 mSv)

[a]Using an average background radiation level of 3 mSv/year.
Data from https://www.imagewisely.org/imaging-modalities/computed-tomography/medical-physicists/articles/how-to-understand-and-communicate-radiation-risk. Accessed September 2018; Colang JE, Killion JB, Vano E: Patient dose from CT: a literature review, *Radiol Technol* 79:17, 2007.

Radiographers holding for exams

Effective use of immobilization techniques must always be attempted. Imaging pediatric patients may require the radiographer to hold the patient. Radiographers are encouraged to hold only as a last resort, but there are many challenging exams that would, even with the best of instruction, have a low chance of success using only parents to hold the patient. In deciding whether to hold for an exam, radiographers seek to balance the potential stochastic risks of radiation exposure to themselves (scatter) against the possibility of having to repeat a child's x-ray (primary beam) because of a parent's unsuccessful attempt at immobilization. If our ultimate goal is to reduce the dose to the patient and ourselves, where is the balance?

Evaluating the parents' ability to hold their child firmly enough to prevent movement and achieve correct positioning should begin when you introduce yourself. Is the parent/guardian attentive to what you say? Are they tentative first-time parents? Are they overindulgent and unable to set limits? Are they so concerned with radiation exposure that they have difficulty listening to instructions? Are they overwhelmed with parenting? Do they come with an attitude that will prevent them from listening? Does the patient's physical condition make him or her a challenge to hold? An affirmative answer to any of these questions may suggest that a radiographer does the holding. Allowing a parent who is probably not capable to hold the patient in order to prevent a small, low LET, occupational dose (scatter) to the radiographer is not in the patient's best interest; the patient, now facing a repeat, receives twice the primary beam radiation dose and the radiographer will still end up having to hold. Before making the decision to hold, the radiographer should make every attempt at immobilization or to instruct the parent/caregiver clearly and slowly, using lay terms, while demonstrating the technique. After the parent has attempted to hold the child, the radiographer must decide whether to continue allowing the parent to hold the child or to step in himself or herself, thereby assuring that a diagnostic exam is achieved on the first try. The goal of any radiographic exam is to produce an image with a radiation dose as low as diagnostically achievable while providing good patient and family care. This is a lot to juggle even for the seasoned pediatric radiographer, and it takes a lot of experience to do it well.

Artifacts

The dynamic range of digital radiography has increased the universe (number and type) of artifacts visible on images. With film screen and digital images, the usual suspects are dirt, scratches, the presence of unwanted metallic or radiopaque objects on the patient, processing errors, and motion. The following is a partial list of artifacts unique to digital radiography:

- Soap or starches in patient gowns that appear as long slender irregular densities (Fig. 22.7).
- Silk-screening on t-shirts, and dirt on imaging plates.
- Textured or thick hair, cornrows, dreadlocks, ponytails, bobby pins, hair clips, or any object woven into the hair.
- Clothing seams, sweat pants eyelets, silkscreen designs, appliqué or embroidery, textured t-shirts, onesies, dry or wet diapers, and sanitary pads.
- Glitter, rhinestones, pearls, belly-button rings, or other piercings. You may encounter some resistance from parents concerning the removal of an infant's new ear piercing studs; assure the parent that the holes will not close during the time it takes to generate the exam images.

Fig. 22.7 Soap or starches in patient gowns appear as long slender irregular densities (red arrows).

The ratio of artifact size and body volume is greater in pediatric patients than adults. In other words, given two images, one of an adult and one of an infant and both of the same anatomic area, and given two artifacts of the same size, shape, and density located in the same spot within those same anatomic areas, the likelihood of detecting the artifact in the infant's image would be greater due to the artifact's size relative to the anatomy.

To reduce clothing artifacts, remove any piece of clothing covering the anatomy of interest. Paper shorts are radiolucent and can be used for pelvic and abdominal imaging. Years of experience support this approach; failure to remove clothing will result in repeat images. When there is a need to observe breathing patterns (chests), particularly on children who cannot hold their breath (those younger than 6 or 7 years old), clothes should be removed from the waist up so the radiographer can observe breathing. As noted earlier, it is well documented that patients in a hospital setting hear about 50% of what is said to them, so when the patients/parents enter the exam room after changing, ask them again if they have removed the requested pieces of clothing. Clear communication is paramount, followed closely by checking for compliance. Trust, but verify. Do not assume (Fig. 22.8).

Fig. 22.8 (A) Eyelets on sweatpants *(orange arrow)*. (B) Belly-button ring *(orange arrow)*.

Common Pediatric Positions and Projections
ABDOMEN, GASTROINTESTINAL, AND GENITOURINARY STUDIES
Abdomen

Abdominal radiography in children is requested for different reasons than it is for adults. Consequently, the initial procedure or protocol differs significantly. In addition to supine and upright images, the assessment for acute abdomen conditions or the abdominal series in adult radiography usually includes images obtained in the left lateral decubitus position. Often the series is not considered complete without a PA projection of the chest. To keep radiation exposure to a minimum, the pediatric abdominal series need only include two images: the supine abdomen and an image to show air-fluid levels. The upright image is preferred over the lateral decubitus in patients younger than 2 or 3 years old because, from an immobilization and patient-comfort perspective, it is much easier to perform. The upright image can be obtained with a slight modification of the Pigg-O-Stat (Modern Way Immobilizers, Gainesboro, TN) (Fig. 22.9), whereas the lateral decubitus position requires significant modification of the Pigg-O-Stat. As mentioned for hip radiography, the diaper should be completely removed for all abdominal and pelvic imaging to avoid artifacts.

Fig. 22.9 The Pigg-O-Stat, modified with the seat raised to suit upright abdominal radiography. The sleeves and seat are cleaned, and the seat is covered with a cloth diaper or thick tissue before the patient is positioned. (Note the gonad shield placed anterior.)

Fig. 22.10 Immobilization of the active child: sandbags over the arms, Velcro strips around the knees, and a Velcro band beside the patient's feet to be secured over the legs.

Positioning and immobilization

Young children can be immobilized for supine abdominal imaging with the same methods as those used for radiography of the hips and pelvis (Fig. 22.10), which provide basic immobilization of a patient for supine table radiography. All boys should be shielded using methods described for radiography of the hips and pelvis. The central ray should be located midway at the level of L2. The radiographer should observe the following guidelines for upright abdominal imaging:

- Effectively immobilize newborns and children up to 3 years old for the upright image using the Pigg-O-Stat.
- Raise the seat of the Pigg-O-Stat to avoid projecting artifacts from the bases of the sleeves over the lower abdomen (see Fig. 22.9).
- For the best results in an older child, have the child sit on a large box, trolley, or stool, then spread the legs apart to prevent superimposition of the upper femora over the pelvis.

Lateral images of the abdomen are occasionally required in children, generally to localize something in the AP plane. Immobilization for lateral images is challenging; this difficulty, along with the fact that patient immobilization is the same as for lateral spine images, makes it worthy of mention here. Properly instructed, the parent can be helpful with obtaining this image. The radiographer should observe the following steps:

- Remember that the parent can do only one job.
- Ask the parent to stand on the opposite side of the table and hold the child's head and arms.
- Immobilize the rest of the child's body using available immobilization tools. These tools include large 45-degree sponges, sandbags (large and small), a "bookend," and a Velcro band.

- Accomplish immobilization by rolling the child on the side and placing a small sponge or sandbag between the knees.
- Snugly wrap the Velcro band over the hips; to prevent backward arching, place the "bookend" against the child's back with the 45-degree sponge and sandbag positioned anteriorly (Fig. 22.11).

Note that it is common for pediatric clinicians to request two projections of the abdomen. This should be supported by the clinical indications. A neonatal patient with necrotizing enterocolitis requires supine and left *lateral decubitus* images to rule out air-fluid levels indicative of bowel obstruction. However, the patient with an umbilical catheter needs supine and *lateral* images to verify the location and position of the catheter. *When in doubt, consult the radiologist.*

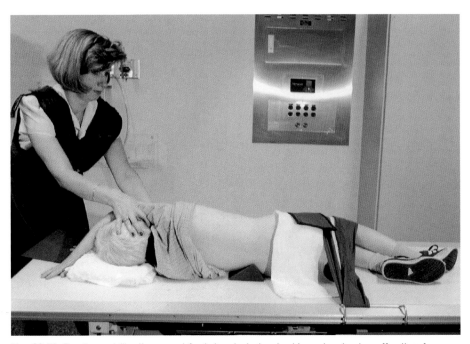

Fig. 22.11 The immobilization used for lateral abdominal imaging is also effective for lateral thoracic and lumbosacral spine images. A 45-degree sponge and sandbag are used anteriorly.

Pathology

Intussusception. Intussusception is the invagination or telescoping of the bowel into itself; the majority of cases (90%) are ileocolic (Fig. 22.12). Idiopathic intussusception is most common and is the most common cause of small intestinal obstruction in the infant-toddler age group, reaching a peak incidence between 2 months and 3 years of age. The majority of cases (60%) occur in males. Intussusception can present with an abrupt onset of abdominal pain that becomes more frequent. There can be bouts of diarrhea, vomiting, and lethargy. Blood and blood clots in stool with the consistency and color of currant jelly are highly suggestive of intussus-

ception. No matter how high the clinical index of suspicion is for intussusception, an abdominal image is always indicated; in some patients this supine image may be negative. Bowel perforation and degree of obstruction are ruled out with a horizontal-beam image, whereas a prone or left-side-down decubitus is more likely to demonstrate a soft tissue mass than the supine position. The combination of diminished colonic stool and bowel gas, especially when accompanied by a visible soft tissue mass, indicates a high likelihood of intussusception. An abdominal physical exam by an experienced surgeon is a useful precaution before proceeding to reduction.

Although there are significant procedural variations among radiologists for the reduction of intussusceptions, many pediatric radiology departments use the pneumatic enema under fluoroscopic guidance as the treatment of choice because of its ease of use, a reduced risk for peritonitis in the event of a perforation (as compared with hydrostatic), reduced time of procedure, and reduced radiation dose. The pneumatic filling of a large portion of the small bowel is usually necessary to confirm reduction. Contraindications to radiologic reduction are intestinal perforation, frank peritonitis, and hypervolemic shock.

Fig. 22.12 (A) Intussusception. (B) Ultrasound image illustrates doughnut-shaped lesion marked for measurement.

(A, From Van Meter K: *Gould's pathophysiology for the health professions*, ed 5, St. Louis, 2014, Elsevier. B, From Eisenberg RL, Johnson NM: *Comprehensive radiographic pathology*, ed 5, St. Louis, 2010, Mosby/Elsevier.)

Pneumoperitoneum. Intraperitoneal air/gas is most commonly the result of perforation of the hollow viscera (stomach or intestines) or can be caused by surgical complications, such as abdominal drainage tubes, percutaneous gastronomy tubes, or insufflation of CO_2 or air during liver and renal biopsies or during laparoscopy (Fig. 22.13A). These causes may have the same radiologic appearances but different clinical significance. Patients normally have pneumoperitoneum following abdominal surgery, which clears more rapidly in children than in adults. Studies have demonstrated clearing of free air in most postoperative children within 24 hours.

Diagnosis of pneumoperitoneum is most easily made with a cross-table horizontal beam projection, which is also indicated to rule out free air or intestinal obstruction, or when small amounts of free air are suspected, the decubitus position is recommended (see Fig. 22.13B). A properly positioned abdominal image, upright, cross-table, or decubitus will include both pubic symphysis and the bases of both diaphragms. In the upright image, free air is easily demonstrated under the diaphragms, displacing the liver on the right, and stomach, liver, and spleen on the left. A child who is younger than 1 year or unable to stand can be examined in the left decubitus position, which allows the liver to fall away from the wall of the peritoneal cavity revealing lucency between the abdominal wall and the liver.

The gridded, tabletop, decubitus view is most successfully achieved when the patient's back is parallel and in contact with the imaging IR. Arms are on either side of the head and above the shoulders with elbows bent one on either side of the head. The patient's pelvis is perpendicular to the table with knees bent and legs stacked one atop the other. The person holding will immobilize the patient's arms and head as one unit (left hand) and hold the lower torso just below the buttocks (right hand). A gonadal shield should be used on males, but make sure to keep it below the pubic symphysis.

The horizontal beam image may be useful in distinguishing a pneumoperitoneum caused by bowel perforation (air fluid levels present) and a dissecting pneumomediastinum presenting with air in the peritoneal space and no fluid levels (this difference is not always present). Pneumomediastinum is usually suspected when there is a history of assisted ventilation or chest trauma and is best visualized in PA and lateral views of the chest.

Fig. 22.13 (A) Pneumoperitoneum resulting from a fundoplication procedure *(orange arrows)*. Rigler's sign (air on both sides of bowel wall) is present at *blue arrow*.
(B) Pneumoperitoneum seen *(orange arrow)* as a complication from percutaneous gastronomy tube procedure.

Gastrointestinal and genitourinary studies

As with any radiology procedure-based modality, a team approach to the care of the patient and family is essential. There are many procedures unique to pediatrics that fall under the headings GI/GU. Although it is beyond the scope of this chapter to delve into the specifics of each of these exams, many of which are complex, we will briefly discuss some of the most common procedures and indications. Common to each of these procedures is the use of a contrast medium, which enhances the visualization of soft tissue. These media can be either water-soluble iodine based or non-water-soluble barium sulfate based. The water-soluble contrast media are used for intravenous (IV) injection and non-IV excretory urography studies, for post-surgical assessments where leakage might occur, and for suspected perforations. They are characterized as being either nonionic (fewer side effects) with low osmolality (low-osmolality contrast agents [LOCAs]) or ionic (increased side effects) with high osmolality (high-osmolality contrast agents [HOCAs]). The choice of which LOCA to use is based on the concentration of iodine desired within the blood plasma and urine, the cost, and safety. Dosage is based on patient weight for IV injections; after injection of a bolus at a moderate rate, contrast excretion begins almost immediately and peaks at 10 to 20 minutes. Studies have shown that the adoption of a LOCA offers a definite improvement in patient experience and safety compared to that of a HOCA. The American College of Radiology (ACR) has specific criteria for the use of LOCAs, which include questions about previous history of contrast reactions, asthma, allergies (especially to shellfish), and cardiac issues. Adverse reactions can be life threatening. When administering a contrast agent, the trained radiographer should have a nurse present and a doctor available.

Barium sulfate-based contrast agents are not water soluble and are for oral or rectal administration to rule out malrotation, investigation of esophageal problems, swallow studies, or to rule out Hirschsprung disease. The patient should be advised to drink plenty of liquids after the study, as the body does not break down barium. Barium is contraindicated for suspected perforations, instances of lower bowel obstructions, or attempted reduction of meconium ileus or meconium plug (Table 22.2).

Radiation protection

When performing exams using conventional fluoroscopic units, it is good practice to cover most of the tabletop with large mats of lead rubber (the equivalent of 0.5 mm of lead is recommended) (Figs. 22.14 and 22.15). Operators and patients can be effectively protected by positioning the mats so that only the areas being examined are exposed.

Fig. 22.14 Another modification of the "bunny" technique. The arms are left free and are raised above the head to prevent superimposition over the esophagus. In this example, tape is used to secure the blanket; however, Velcro strips are easier to use if a parent is not available to assist. (Note lead under patient when tube is under the table.)

Fig. 22.15 The octagonal immobilizer (or, for this child, a "rocket ship") permits the child to be immobilized in a variety of positions. (Note lead under patient when tube is under the table.)

Vesicoureteral reflux

For infants and small children experiencing first-time febrile urinary tract infections (UTIs), the goal after antibiotic treatment is to rule out the possibility of reflux, existing renal scarring, and structural or functional abnormalities of the urinary tract that may predispose the patient to reflux and infection, particularly to anomalies that may require prompt surgical treatment. This is accomplished with an ultrasound (US) and, if indicated, a voiding cystourethrogram (VCUG). Patient assessment may begin with a noninvasive US to assess the upper urinary tracts and kidneys. If the US is negative, the decision to proceed with the VCUG is made after a thorough discussion between the parents, the attending urologist, and the pediatrician. Some radiologists feel that a VCUG for a first-time nonfebrile UTI with a negative US is not indicated. The VCUG is an invasive procedure in which a Foley catheter (5 to 8 French) is inserted into the urethra, advanced into the bladder, and then taped to the inside of the leg in a female or to the shaft of the penis in a male. An iodinated contrast agent (see Table 22.2) designed for the lower urinary tract is instilled into the bladder by gravity. The volume used is based on the patient's age. Bilateral, oblique, pulsed fluoroscopy captures are made to check for reflux (Fig. 22.16A) and assess urinary anatomy. Fluoroscopy captures are made of voiding as the Foley is removed (see Fig. 22.16B). VCUG teams often include an attending fellow or resident, a radiographer, and a CLS with access to a registered radiologist assistant (RRA) as required. The parents are encouraged to participate, as this can help soothe and calm the infant or child. Age-appropriate distraction devices are employed as required.

Fig. 22.16 (A) VCUG, 33-month-old female with bilateral grade 3 reflux as seen in the AP projection under fluoroscopy. Bladder *(B)*, ureter *(U)*, renal pelvis *(RP)*, and renal calyce *(RC)*. (B) VCUG, 8-year-old male with bladder diverticula *(D)* as seen in the LPO projection. Voiding shows moderate dilatation of the posterior urethra *(U)*. Foley catheter *(FC)*, bladder *(B)*, and uncircumcised penis *(P)*.

CHEST

The most frequently ordered and one of the most challenging imaging exams in pediatric imaging is the chest x-ray. Patients between 1 and 4 years can be difficult to immobilize and position because they are strong and in an unfamiliar setting they are scared. The anxiety level created in this situation can be high for parents, students, and the experienced radiographer. Take the time to adequately explain to the parents the goals of the exam and how to correctly hold the child for the exam. Even though you are assured the parent can hold properly, it is essential that you remain vigilant in your transition from the patient to the exposure control station, ensuring that the parents continue to immobilize correctly and effectively. If the parent is struggling and frustrated, consider using the Pigg-O-Stat (Fig. 22.17) or, as a last resort, a radiographer may have to hold the child. Radiation delivered to the patient must always be as low as diagnostically achievable, and every attempt must be made to acquire the image on the first attempt. Quite simply, if you think the positioning is compromised or the immobilization ineffective, do not make the exposure.

TABLE 22.2

Gastrointestinal/genitourinary studies

Indications	Procedure	Contrast agent
Gastrointestinal studies		
R/O esophageal atresia	Swallow	LOMC
Dysphasia	Swallow	Barium
Stridor, R/O retropharyngeal abscess	Airway fluoroscopy	Air
R/O malrotation	UGI	Barium
R/O irritable bowel syndrome	UGISB	Barium
R/O Hirschsprung, low bowel obstruction	Contrast enema	Cysto Conray 17.2%
CF cleanout	Contrast enema	Cysto Conray 17.2% w/ Gastrografin
Meconium ileus	Contrast enema	Gastrografin w/Water 1:1
Intussusception reduction	Air enema	Air
R/O swallowing dysfunction	MBSW	Barium
Genitourinary		
Febrile UTI, R/O reflux, hydronephrosis	VCUG	Cysto Conray 17.2%
Megaureter	VCUG, IVP	Cysto Conray 17.2%
Ectopic ureter	VCUG	Cysto Conray 17.2%
Ureterocele, ureteral duplication	IVP	LOMC, Optiray 320
Neurogenic bladder Bladder diverticula	VCUG	Cysto Conray 17.2%

Fig. 22.17 Position for PA chest image. The Pigg-O-Stat (Modern Way Immobilizers, Clifton, TN) is a pediatric positioner and immobilization tool. The IR is held in the metal extension stand.

The central ray for PA and lateral projections is directed to the level of T6-7 (nipple line), but the collimated field should extend from and include the mastoid tips to 13 cm (2 inches) above the iliac crests. Inclusion of the mastoid tips shows the upper airway; narrowed or stenotic airways are a common source of respiratory problems in pediatric patients. By collimating just above the iliac crests, the radiographer will be sure to include the inferior costal margins. Numerous children arrive in the imaging department with long lung fields resulting from hyperinflation (e.g., patients with cardiac disorders and asthma).

Most radiologists will agree that upright chest images yield a great deal more diagnostic information than supine images. However, it is important that you be able to achieve diagnostic quality in both positions. Infants needing supine and cross-table lateral images can be immobilized using Velcro straps around the knees and a Velcro band across the legs. The patient is supine on a radiolucent pad with the arms held above the head for both the AP and the cross-table lateral. This technique is particularly useful for patients with chest tubes, delicately positioned gastrostomy tubes, or soft tissue swellings or protrusions that may be compromised by the sleeves of the Pigg-O-Stat.

Chest (<1 year)

At Boston Children's Hospital (BCH), all non-bedside, two-view chest x-rays and most decubitus views of infants, 0 to 365 days, are performed using a "baby box" invented by our technical director, Linda Poznauskis (Fig. 22.18). This device has proven invaluable for immobilizing and positioning the infant with minimal discomfort and helping to ensure a diagnostic and reproducible exam in a timely manner. The patient must be nude from the waist up with all heart monitor leads removed (when safe), and lines and tubes (especially nasogastric tubes) positioned away from the chest anatomy. The baby is placed supine on the box, shielded,

Fig. 22.18 The baby box aids in the immobilization of an infant (0 to 12 months) for AP and cross-table lateral chest x-rays, soft tissue neck and C-spine imaging. There is a sliding tray *(orange arrow)* that holds the imaging plate for supine positions, a slot on the side *(blue arrow)* holds the IR for cross-table work, and Velcro straps *(yellow arrow)* are used to immobilize.

and the lower torso immobilized with the attached Velcro (Velcro USA, Inc., Manchester, NH) strap and sandbag as necessary. The parent is directed to slowly raise the baby's arms up and alongside its head. While holding the arms at the level of the elbows, the parent places his or her thumbs at the sides of the head or on the forehead to ensure that the baby's head is in a true supine position with no rotation or obliquity (Fig. 22.19). A small rotation of the head will cause distortion of the infant's lung fields, and if the baby arches its back the image will be rendered lordotic. Special attention should be paid to the tendency of parents to pull the arms

and baby toward them rather than simply holding the arms and head together. This results in the patient being slowly pulled from under the Velcro and off the IR, causing the lung apices to be clipped. Collimate, ensure that the parent continues to immobilize effectively, and expose when the baby's belly is fully distended indicating a full inspiration. Do not be in a hurry here—activate the rotor, pick up the rhythm of the infants breathing, and time your exposure. If the infant is hyperventilating, an inspiratory image will be obtained, although it may not be at full inspiration.

The left, cross-table, lateral projection (Fig. 22.20) is obtained by placing the IR in the baby box's shallow groove on the left side of the baby box. Using the same holding technique, the Velcro is released and the patient is moved closer to the IR, thus minimizing OID (magnification); the Velcro is then refastened. Collimation should allow the x-ray beam to overlap onto the side of the box closest to the x-ray tube to prevent clipping the posterior lung fields. It is imperative, especially for medicolegal reasons, that all first-time AP images and all subsequent images contain the correct marker placement.

Fig. 22.19 (A) Supine AP chest x-ray for an infant younger than 12 months. Parent immobilizes at the elbows with thumbs at or on sides of forehead. (B) AP chest image of infant younger than 12 months.

Fig. 22.20 (A) Left, cross-table, lateral chest projection: same immobilization as for AP, but infant must be moved closer to the IR to reduce OID and avoid clipping the spine. (B) Lateral projection chest image of an infant younger than 12 months.

Chest (>1 year)

This population of little patients will resist any positioning the radiographer attempts by wiggling, twisting, crying, contorting, or all of the above in what appears to be an effort to force a repeat image. The biggest reason for repeats in this age group is that the patient pulls away from the image receptor, resulting in a lordotic image. Properly positioning this age group requires good communication between the radiographer and parents. Parents can be tentative about holding their child firmly. If the child is allowed to twist or lean away from the IR, the image will be non-diagnostic. If the parents are unsuccessful in immobilization, use the Pigg-O-Stat (if age appropriate) or use a radiographer as a last resort.

Chest x-rays (for children 1 to 6 years old) can be obtained by seating the child at the end of the exam table using a custom-made frame that supports the IR and aids in the positioning of the child. The PA chest x-ray is accomplished with the child's arms raised next to the head with instructions to the parent that the child's head and arms be held as a unit (Fig. 22.21). A slight upward pull on the child's body will keep a straight torso. Do not let the patient lean away from the IR, as this will produce a lordotic image; this can be prevented either by moving the patient's bottom away from the IR or by placing a 15-degree positioning sponge between the patient and the IR at the level of the patient's abdomen, with the thicker portion at the level of the pelvic ilia. Patients should be nude from the waist up in order to visualize and time the inspiration. (The Medical Physicist at Boston Children's has approved this position. Primary beam radiation is confined to the imaging cassette and there is no primary beam exposure to the technologist or the parent. This has been the routine standard of care at this hospital for the past 15 years.)

For the sitting left lateral, patients are held from behind or the front, with arms in the same position as used for the PA (Fig. 22.22). A large firm positioning sponge can be placed between the parent's chest and the patient's back, or the positioning can be done without the sponge on older children. While holding the child's head and arms as a unit, the parent is instructed to exert a slight upward pull while keeping the patient's back against the sponge and perpendicular to the IR. If the patient is unruly, a second person will be required to hold down on the child's knees. Make sure you have a clear view of the patient's belly to check for inspiration. Older patients are done standing using an upright bucky.

Image evaluation

The criteria used to evaluate the image are inclusion of the full lung fields, airway, visibility of peripheral lung markings, rotation, inspiration, cardiac silhouette, mediastinum, and bony structures. In the PA chest image, the ideal technical factor is a selection that permits visualization of the intervertebral disk spaces through the heart (the most dense area), while showing the peripheral lung markings (the least dense area). Rotation should be assessed by evaluating midline structures (sternum, trachea, spinous processes, etc.). These anterior and posterior midline structures should be superimposed. Similar to chest radiography in adults, the visualization of eight to nine posterior ribs is a reliable indicator of an image taken with good inspiration (Table 22.3).

Fig. 22.21 (A) Parent holding for a PA chest on a child older than 1 year. (B) Resultant chest image. Care should be taken to tie up textured hair, as it can show as an artifact on digital images.

Fig. 22.22 (A) Parent holding for a lateral chest on a child older than 1 year. (B) Resultant chest image.

TABLE 22.3

Quick reference guide for image assessment

| | Density | | | Contrast | | | |
	Most dense	Least dense	Recorded detail	Long scale >3 shades	Short scale >3 shades	Anatomy	Rotation check
PA chest	Midline; intervertebral disk spaces, heart	Peripheral lung markings	Peripheral lung markings	Airway, heart, apices, bases, mediastinum, lung markings behind diaphragm and heart		Airway to bases	Airway position, SC joints, lung field measurement, cardiac silhouette
PA chest	Heart	Retrocardiac space	Peripheral lung markings	Airway, heart, apices, bases		Airway to bases, spinous process to sternum	Superimposition of ribs, spinous processes on profile
Abdomen	Lumbar spine	Peripheral edges, soft tissue above the iliac crests	Organ silhouettes	Diaphragm, liver, kidney, spine, gas shadows		Right and left hemidiaphragm, pubic symphysis, right and left skin edges	
Limbs	Bone	Soft tissue	Bony trabecular patterns		Bone, muscle, soft tissue	Joints above and below injury, all soft tissue	AP and lateral images must not resemble obliques
Hips	Hip joints	Iliac crests	Bony trabecular patterns		Bone, soft tissue	Iliac crests, lesser trochanter	Symmetric iliac crests
Lateral lumbar spine	L5-S1	Spinous processes	Bony trabecular patterns		Bone	T12 to coccyx, spinous processes to vertebral bodies	Alignment of posterior surfaces of vertebral bodies

Evaluating the image to determine its diagnostic quality is a practiced skill. This chart, designed as a quick reference guide, outlines the five important technical criteria and the related anatomic indicators used in critiquing images.

Chest (3 to 18 years)
Upright

Upright images on children 3 to 18 years old are easily obtained by observing the following steps:

- Help the child sit on a large wooden box, a wide-based trolley with brakes, or a stool, with the IR supported using a metal extension stand. Young children are curious and have short attention spans. By having them sit, the radiographer can prevent them from wiggling from the waist down.
- For the PA position, have the child hold onto the side supports of the extension stand, with the chin on top of or next to the IR. This prevents upper body movement.
- When positioning for the lateral image, have the parent (if his or her presence is permitted) assist by raising the child's arms above the head and holding the head between the arms (Fig. 22.23).

Supine

Infants needing supine and cross-table lateral images can be immobilized using Velcro straps around the knees and a Velcro band across the legs (Fig. 22.24). The patient is elevated on a sponge with the arms held up, and a cross-table lateral is performed. This technique is particularly useful for patients with chest tubes, delicately positioned gastrostomy tubes, or soft tissue swellings or protrusions that may be compromised by the sleeves of the Pigg-O-Stat.

Image evaluation

As in adult chest radiography, the use of kVp is desirable in pediatric chest imaging; however, this is relative. In adult imaging, high kVp generally ranges from 110 to 130, but for pediatric PA projections, kVp ranges from 80 to 90. The use of a higher kVp is not always possible because the corresponding mAs are too low to produce a diagnostic image.

The criteria used to evaluate recorded detail include the resolution of peripheral lung markings. Evaluating any image for adequate density involves assessing the most and least dense areas of the anatomy that is shown. In the PA chest image, the ideal technical factor is a selection that permits visualization of the intervertebral disk spaces through the heart (the densest area) while showing the peripheral lung markings (the least dense area). Rotation should be assessed by evaluating the position of midline structures. Posterior and anterior midline structures (i.e., sternum, airway, and vertebral bodies) should be superimposed. The anatomic structures to be shown include the airway (trachea) to the costophrenic angles. Similar to chest radiography in adults, the visualization of eight to nine posterior ribs is a reliable indicator of an image taken with good inspiration (see Table 22.3).

Fig. 22.23 (A) PA chest images should be performed on the 3- to 18-year-old with the child sitting. (B) The parent, if present, can assist with immobilization for the lateral image by holding the child's head between the child's arms. Metal extension stands (*arrows* on A and B) are commercially available from companies that market diagnostic imaging accessories.

Fig. 22.24 The patient is raised on a sponge with arms held up by the head, and the legs are immobilized using Velcro straps. The IR is in place for the horizontal lateral beam (cross-table lateral).

PELVIS AND HIPS

General principles

The initial radiography examination of the pelvis and hips is routinely done for children older than 1 year. Ultrasonography is used for infants younger than 1 year. With a basic comprehension of the most common pediatric pelvic positions, pathologies, and disease processes, the radiographer can provide the radiologist with the superior diagnostic images required to make an accurate diagnosis.

Despite the importance of radiation protection, little written literature is available to guide radiographers on the placement of gonadal shields and when to use shielding. The radiographer should observe the following guidelines:

- *Always* use gonadal shielding on boys. However, take care to prevent potential lesions of the pubic symphysis from being obscured.
- In girls, use gonadal protection on all images *except* the first AP projection of the *initial* examination of the hips and pelvis.
- After sacral abnormality or sacral involvement has been ruled out, use shielding on subsequent images in girls.
- Before proceeding, check the girl's records or seek clarification from the parents regarding whether this is the child's first examination.
- Because the female reproductive organs are located in the mid-pelvis with their exact position varying, ensure that the shield covers the sacrum and part or all of the sacroiliac (SI) joints, making sure it does not cover the hip joints or pubic symphysis.

NOTE: Many children have been taught that no one should touch their "private parts." Radiographers need to be sensitive and use discretion when explaining and carrying out the procedure.

- *Never touch the pubic symphysis in a child,* regardless of whether you are positioning the patient or placing the gonadal shield.
- The superior border of the pubic symphysis is always at the level of the greater trochanters. Use the trochanters as a guide for positioning and shield placement. The CR should be located midline at a point midway between the anterior superior iliac spine (ASIS) and the symphysis.
- In boys, keep the gonadal shield from touching the scrotum by laying a 15-degree sponge or a cloth over the top of the femora. The top of the shield can be placed 3 cm below the level of the trochanters, and the bottom half of the shield can rest on top of the sponge or cloth (Fig. 22.25).
- In girls, place the top, widest part of the shield in the midline, level with the ASIS.

Initial images

Hip examinations on children are most often ordered to assess for Legg-Calvé-Perthes disease (aseptic avascular necrosis of the femoral head), developmental dysplasia of the hip (DDH), slipped capital femoral epiphyses (SCFE), and to diagnose nonspecific hip pain. These conditions require the evaluation of the symmetry of the acetabula, joint spaces, and soft tissue, therefore symmetric positioning is crucial. The initial examination of the hips and pelvis in children older than 1 year includes a well-collimated AP projection and a lateral projection commonly referred to as a frog lateral. This position is more correctly described as a coronal image of the pelvis with the thighs in abduction and external rotation, or the Lauenstein position (see Chapter 8). This bilateral imaging serves as a baseline for future imaging and allows comparison of right to left hips.

Fig. 22.25 (A) The male gonadal shield should cover the scrotum without obscuring the pubic symphysis. The greater trochanters indicate the upper border of the pubic symphysis; the top of the shield should be placed approximately a ½ inch below this level. The gonadal shield rests on a 15-degree sponge, which prevents the radiographer's hands from coming close to or touching the scrotal area. (B) A 3½-year-old normal pelvis; note the shielding.

Preparation and communication

All images of the abdomen and pelvic girdle should be performed with the child's underwear or diaper removed. Buttons, silk screening, and metal on underwear as well as wet diapers produce significant artifacts on images, often rendering them nondiagnostic. The radiographer should have all required positioning devices on the table prior to the patient's arrival.

Positioning and immobilization

As described previously, *symmetric positioning* is crucial. As in many examinations, the hip positions that are the most uncomfortable for the patient are often the most crucial. When a child has hip pain or dislocation, symmetric positioning is difficult to achieve because the patient often tries to compensate for the discomfort by rotating the pelvis. The radiographer should observe the following steps when positioning the patient:

- As with hip examinations in any patient, check that the ASISs are equidistant from the table.
- After carefully observing and communicating with the patient to discover the location of pain, use sponges to compensate for rotation. Sponges should routinely be used to support the thighs in the frog-leg position. This can help prevent motion artifacts.

- Do not accept poorly positioned images. Repeat instructions as necessary to achieve optimal positioning.

Because *immobilization techniques* should vary according to the aggressiveness of the patient, the radiographer can follow these additional guidelines:

- Make every effort to use explanation and reassurance as part of the immobilization method. A child may require only a Velcro band placed across the legs as a safety precaution.
- For an active child, wrap a Velcro strip around the knees and place large sandbags over the arms (see Fig. 22.10). The Velcro strip over the knees keeps the child from wiggling one leg or both legs out from under the Velcro band and possibly rolling off the table.
- If the child has enough strength to free his or her arms from the sandbags, ask a parent to stand on the opposite side of the table from the radiographer and hold the child's arms. The parent's thumbs should be placed directly over the child's shoulders (Fig. 22.26). This method of immobilization is used extensively. It also works well for supine abdominal images, intravenous urograms (IVUs), overhead GI procedures, and spinal radiography.

Leg-length discrepancies, which can cause hip problems, are diagnosed using a *Scanogram,* a technique in which three exposures of the lower limbs (single exposures centered over the hips, knees, and ankles) are made on a single 35 × 43 cm IR (see Chapter 7). Two radiolucent rulers with radiopaque numbers are included bilaterally and within the collimated field, making it possible for the orthopedic surgeon to then calculate the difference in leg lengths.

Evaluating images

Rotation or symmetry can be evaluated by ensuring that midline structures are in the midline and that the ilia appear symmetric. Depending on the degree of skeletal maturation, visualization of the trochanters can indicate the position of the legs when the image was taken. Symmetry in the skin folds is also an important evaluation criterion for the diagnostician. The anatomy to be shown includes the crests of the ilia to the upper quarter of the femora. The image should demonstrate the bony trabecular pattern in the hip joints, which is the thickest and most dense area within the region. The visualization of the bony trabecular pattern is used as an indicator that sufficient recorded detail has been shown; this should not be at the expense of showing the soft tissues—the muscles and skin folds (see Table 22.3).

Fig. 22.26 If the child is strong enough or aggressive enough to remove the sandbags (see Fig. 22.10), the parent can hold the child's humeri by placing the thumbs directly over the child's shoulders.

LIMB RADIOGRAPHY

Limb radiography accounts for a high percentage of pediatric general radiographic procedures in most clinics and hospitals. Producing a series of diagnostic images will require you to assess the child's age-appropriate development, behavior, and age in order to determine which forms of immobilization you will employ. This is best accomplished in consultation with the parents; an active 3-year-old may require that you use immobilization techniques that are one or two age groups below the patient's chronologic age group.

Immobilization
Newborn to 2 years old

Depending on the exam, swaddling the child in a blanket, towel, or pillowcase will make the child manageable when performing upper limb radiography. This wrapping technique, a modification of the "bunny" method (Fig. 22.27), keeps the infant warm and allows one parent to concentrate on immobilizing the injured limb. When imaging small hands, a piece of Plexiglas can be used to firmly hold the hand while making the exposure. Lower extremities are best imaged with the help of swaddling, a Velcro band, or parent holding over the abdomen with a large sandbag placed over the unaffected leg (Fig. 22.28).

Fig. 22.27 (A) With a simple modification of the "bunny" technique using a towel (or pillowcase), the child can be immobilized for upper limb radiography. Plexiglas *(dashed lines)* and "bookends" *(B)* can be used to immobilize the hands of children 2 years old and younger. Note that after the child is wrapped, a Velcro band is used for safety, and a small apron is placed diagonally over the body to protect the sternum and gonads. The IR is placed on a lead mat, which prevents the image receptor from sliding on the table. (B) Nine-month-old normal right hand.

Fig. 22.28 (A) The challenges of immobilizing lower limbs are greater than those of immobilizing upper limbs. After wrapping both of the patient's arms in a towel and placing a Velcro band over the abdomen, the radiographer can place a large sandbag over the unaffected leg. With careful collimation and proper instruction, the parent can hold the limb as demonstrated. Normal 21-month-old AP (B) and lateral (C) tibia and fibula.

Preschool age

The upper limbs of preschoolers are best imaged with the child sitting on the parent's lap as shown in Fig. 22.29. If the parent is unable to participate, these children can be immobilized as described previously.

With parental participation, radiography of the lower limbs can be accomplished with the child sitting or lying on the table. Preventing the patient from falling from the table is always a primary concern with preschoolers. Instruct the parent to remain by the child's side if the child is seated on the table or stool. If the examination is performed with the child lying on the table, a Velcro band over the abdomen or parent holding should be employed.

NOTE: The child's ankle should be in flexion, not extension.

School age

School-age children generally can be managed in the same way as adult patients for upper and lower limb examinations.

Radiation protection

The upper body should be protected from scatter radiation in all examinations of the upper limbs because of the close proximity of the thymus, sternum, and breast tissue. Child-sized lead aprons with cartoon characters are both popular and practical (Fig. 22.30).

Fractures

Fractures in children's bones occur under two circumstances: abnormal stresses in normal bone and normal stresses in abnormal bone. A fracture is defined as the breaking or rupture of a bone caused by mechanical forces either applied to the bone or transmitted directly along the line of the bone. Children's bone fractures differ from those of adults because growth is active and favors rapid repair and remodeling. In general, children's bones are less dense than those of adults, and the ability to visualize soft tissue and bony detail are of utmost importance; in particular, small linear fractures are difficult to discern without good soft tissue detail. Fat pad displacement and tissue swelling may be the only radiographic signs of injury. Such subtle findings can disguise an epiphyseal growth plate fracture, which if left untreated could result in irregular or cessation of growth in the affected bone. Overriding and distraction deformities may correct without residual deformity, but rotational deformities will not. Consequently, images of the fractured bone showing the relative position of the two ends of the bone (AP, lateral, oblique) are necessary for evaluation of rotation; preliminary assessment may require the *contralateral* side to be examined for comparison.

The earlier in a child's life this epiphyseal fracture occurs, the better the chances of spontaneous correction of angulation fractures.

Here is an abbreviated list of some of the more common pediatric extremity fractures.

Fig. 22.29 Preschoolers are best managed sitting on a parent's lap. A lead mat is used to keep the IR from sliding. Note the use of Plexiglas to immobilize fingers. (The parent's hands are shown without lead gloves and not draped in lead for illustration purposes only.)

Fig. 22.30 The teddy bear on this full-length apron *(left)* makes it appropriate for young children.

Salter-harris

About one-third of all skeletal injuries to children are at the epiphyseal growth plates, especially in the ankle and wrist. Salter and Harris described these fractures in 1963 as Salter-Harris types I through V (Fig. 22.31).

Plastic or bow

The bones of children, as compared to those of adults, can absorb and deflect more energy without breaking due to a lower bending resistance. Plastic or bowing fractures occur in children when this bending resistance is exceeded and the bone or bones bow without breaking. The bowing fracture is a bending deformity, which usually occurs in the forearm. There is no grossly visible fracture in the tubular structure of the bone; however, microfractures are visible using microscopy. The bowing is appreciable on plain images and often requires a comparison view to confirm the deformation. A bowing fracture is usually reduced under general anesthesia, as the force required to reduce the bowing is substantial.

Greenstick

A green stick fracture occurs when one cortex of the bone's diaphysis breaks and the side remains intact.

Torus

The torus fracture is a type of greenstick fracture in which the load on the bone is in the same direction as the diaphysis, causing the cortex to fold back on itself.

Toddler's fracture

A toddler's fracture is described as a subtle, nondisplaced, oblique fracture of the distal tibia in children 9 months to 3 years of age; the fracture may only be seen on one view of the lower shaft of the tibia. If AP, lateral, and oblique projections are radiographically negative, but there is strong suspicion of a toddler's fracture, a radionuclide scan may be indicated. The child's age and the presentation are significant to this diagnosis. It is important to realize that this is a common accidental injury, which the parents may not have witnessed. If the onset of symptoms (pain, non-weight-bearing) is rapid and the patient's age is within the noted range, a toddler's fracture has a high index of suspicion. Remember, however, that a similar fracture in a very young infant who is not yet a "toddler" cannot be ascribed to accidental falls and, therefore, would be suspicious of abuse.

Fig. 22.31 Salter-Harris fractures. The black lines represent the fracture lines. (A) A type I fracture occurs directly through the growth plate. (B) A type II fracture extends through the growth plate and into the metaphyses. (C) A type III fracture line extends through the growth plate and into the epiphyses. (D) A type IV fracture line extends through the metaphyses, across or sometimes along the growth plate, and through the epiphyses. (E) A type V fracture involves a crushing of all or part of the growth plate. Fractures that occur through the epiphyses are significant injuries because they can affect growth if not recognized and treated properly. A proper radiographic technique is required for the demonstration of both soft tissue and bone. This is especially important with type I fractures in which the growth plate is separated as a result of a lateral blow, and type V fractures in which the growth plate has sustained a compression injury. Types I and V fractures do not occur through the bone.

Supracondylar fracture

More severe than the toddler's fracture, the supracondylar fracture is the most common elbow fracture in children, accounting for 60% of all pediatric elbow fractures (Fig. 22.32). Occurring frequently in children between the ages of 3 and 10, it is caused by the child falling on an outstretched hand with hyperextension of the elbow. The most extensively displaced of these fractures can cause serious vascular and nerve damage. Great care should be taken when positioning for this fracture.

Image evaluation

Among the many striking differences in radiographic appearance between adult and pediatric patients are the bone trabeculae and the presence of epiphyseal lines or growth plates in pediatric patients. As they gain experience in evaluating pediatric images, radiographers develop a visual appreciation for these differences. To the uneducated eye, a normally developing epiphysis, for example, may mimic a fracture. For this reason, and because fractures can occur through the epiphyseal plate, physicians, and to a certain degree radiographers, must learn to recognize epiphyseal lines and their appearance at various stages of ossification. Fractures that occur through the epiphysis are called *growth plate fractures* (Salter-Harris). Because the growth plates are composed of cartilaginous tissue, the *density* of the image must be such that soft tissue is shown in addition to bone (see Table 22.3). Visualization of the bony trabecular pattern is used as an indicator that sufficient *recorded detail* has been achieved. Because of the small size of pediatric extremities, an imaging system with superior resolution is required. Generally, the speed of the imaging system should be half that used for spines and abdomens.

Fig. 22.32 (A and B) AP and lateral projections of a supracondylar fracture *(arrows)*.

SKULL AND PARANASAL SINUSES

Skull

The two most common indications for a pediatric, radiographic skull series are to rule out craniosynostosis and fracture. Synostosis is the fusion of two bones, and it can be normal or abnormal. The term *craniosynostosis,* or *premature cranial suture synostosis,* describes the premature closure of one or more of the cranial sutures and may be isolated or part of a craniofacial syndrome; both result in the deformity of the calvaria's shape. Etiologically, abnormal synostosis is described as either primary or secondary. Primary craniosynostosis is characterized by some type of defect in one or more of the cranial sutures and can be intrinsic or familial. The familial form manifests as a component of a craniofacial syndrome (Pfeiffer, Apert, Crouzon, Beare-Stevenson) and may be the result of one of several genetic mutations. Secondary craniosynostosis is the result of some underlying medical condition, which can be systemic or metabolic (hyperthyroidism, hypercalcemia, vitamin D deficiency, sickle cell, or thalassemia). Microcephaly, encephalocele, and shunted hydrocephalus can diminish the growth stretch at sutures, which can lead to craniosynostosis secondarily.

Calvarial growth takes place perpendicular to the suture lines. The suture lines involved, time of onset, and the sequence in which individual sutures fuse will determine the nature of the deformity. When sutures fuse prematurely, calvarial growth occurs along the axis of the fused suture. The altered skull shape is diagnostic. Restoring growth is dependent on the early release of all fused sutures.

The birth prevalence of craniosynostosis ranges from approximately 3 to 5 cases per 10,000 live births. The isolated variety (only one suture affected) constitutes 80% to 90% of cases, and the sutures most commonly involved, in descending order of frequency, are the sagittal, coronal, metopic, and lambdoid. The syndromic variety accounts for up to 10% to 20% of cases. Coronal synostosis is more frequently seen in females, whereas sagittal synostosis is more common in males. Most cases are diagnosed early in life. Skull images of infants are obtained in the supine position. Radiographic views include (1) a supine AP projection obtained to demonstrate the calvaria, (2) one or both lateral projections obtained to demonstrate the calvaria and skull base (both lateral projections are indicated in trauma and focal lesion evaluation), and (3) an AP axial Towne projection, but only with a 30-degree caudad angle (due to differing skull morphology in pediatric patients younger than age 10 years) is obtained to demonstrate the occipital bone and foramen magnum.

Skull fractures occurring in children are usually the result of blunt force trauma and include both accidental and nonaccidental trauma, as well as those sustained from forceps extraction at birth. Fractures can occur with minimal force in the abnormally fragile bone associated with osteogenesis imperfecta (OI). Diastatic fracture lines (breaks along the sutures) present as more lucent, more linear, and exhibit no interdigitations, which distinguish them from sutures. Depressed skull fractures appear dense due to the overlapping bone fragments. Skull radiography will demonstrate horizontal linear fracture lines that may not be visible on CT when the fracture is parallel to the CT axis. All skull imaging is done with a grid, large focal spot, using a set technique (can use AEC for AP), and with no clothing from the waist up. Immobilizing an infant for a skull series is accomplished most efficiently by using the "bunny immobilization" technique (Fig. 22.33), as all three projections can be accomplished with minimal help, or the parents can be drafted to immobilize the shoulders, torso, and legs (sand bags will work if the patient is younger than 2 years); however, this technique requires a lot more instruction and is less reliable.

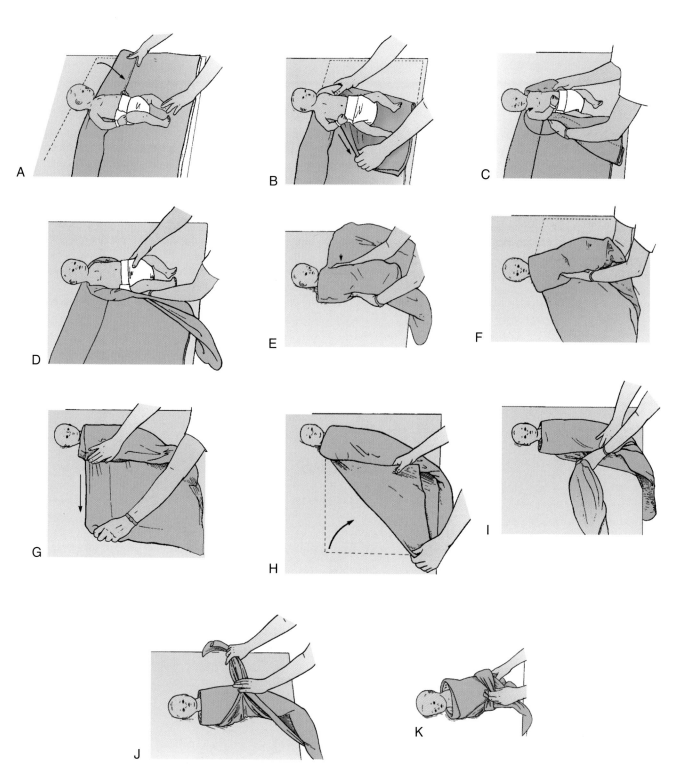

Fig. 22.33 The "bunny" method used to immobilize the patient for cranial radiography. (A) to (D) focus on immobilization of the shoulders, (E) to (G) concentrate on the humeri, and (H) to (K) illustrate the way the sheet is folded and wrapped to immobilize the legs. (A) Begin with a standard hospital sheet folded in half lengthwise. Make a 6-inch fold at the top, and lay the child down about 2 feet from the end of the sheet. (B) Wrap the end of the sheet over the left shoulder, and pass the sheet under the child. (C) This step makes use of the 6-inch fold. Reach under, undo the fold, and wrap it over the right shoulder. (Steps B and C are crucial to the success of this immobilization technique because they prevent the child from wiggling their shoulders free.) (D) After wrapping the right shoulder, pass the end of the sheet under the child. Pull it through to keep the right arm snug against the body. (E) Begin wrapping, keeping the sheet snug over the upper body to immobilize the humeri. (F) Lift the lower body and pass the sheet underneath, keeping the child's head on the table. Repeat steps (E) and (F) if material permits. (G) Make sure the material is evenly wrapped around the upper body. (Extra rolls around the shoulder and neck area produce artifacts on 30-degree fronto-occipital and submentovertical images.) (H) Make a diagonal fold with the remaining material (approximately 2 feet). (I) Roll the material together. (J) Snugly wrap this over the child's femora. (The tendency to misjudge the location of the femora and thus wrap too snugly around the lower legs should be avoided.) (K) Tuck the end of the rolled material in front. (If not enough material remains to tuck in, use a Velcro strip or tape to secure it.).

(From the Michener Institute for Applied Health Sciences, Toronto, Ontario, Canada.)

The AP skull (Fig. 22.34A) is positioned with the orbitomeatal line (OML) perpendicular to the IR using two round, 10-cm, radiolucent sponges, one on either side of the head. It is important when using these sponges to use your palms rather than pressing your fingers into the sponge (which will appear on the image). The axial Townes method (see Fig. 22.34B) is also done supine using the "mouse ears" sponges to bring the chin toward the chest so that the OML is perpendicular to the exam table and IR. The central ray is directed 30 degrees caudad and enters 2.5 to 5 cm above the glabella. The lateral skull can be imaged using one of two methods. The first projection is a left, cross-table lateral (see Fig. 22.34C) with the infant supine and elevated on a radiolucent pad and positioned supine. The grid holder with IR is parallel to the skull and extends to the tabletop (below the pad) to avoid clipping of the posterior skull. The infant's shoulder is in contact with IR (Fig. 22.35). The central ray is perpendicular and enters 1 cm superior to the external auditory meatus (EAM). Use the flat surface of the hand to position one round "mouse ear" sponge just superior to the vertex of the skull and the other hand to hold the mental protuberance of the mandible. Leave the infant supine and rotate the skull to a lateral position with the side of interest down. The central ray enters 1 cm superior to EAM. Position one "mouse ear" sponge just posterior to

Fig. 22.34 (A) AP skull. (B) Townes 30 degrees. (C) Lateral (method 1 as mentioned previously).

the vertex of the skull (use a flat hand) and the other hand will hold the mental protuberance of the mandible. This is an awkward position for infants so expect them to struggle (Table 22.4).

Paranasal sinuses

The main indication for performing a paranasal sinus series on the pediatric patient is to rule out sinusitis. However, radiographic opacification is not a clear indication of sinus disease; incidental findings of mucosal thickening with magnetic resonance imaging (MRI) are common in children younger than 5 years when examined for other indicated reasons according to Caffey. Because errors in positioning may simulate pathologic change in this age group, demonstrating air-fluid level in an upright exam with compelling clinical and laboratory support would probably warrant the diagnosis of sinusitis without resorting to CT. The maxillary, ethmoid, and sphenoid sinuses are present and aerated at birth, whereas the frontal sinuses do not usually appear until the second year.

Fig. 22.35 Effective immobilization for lateral skull images with a horizontal beam can be achieved using the infant head and neck immobilizer.

TABLE 22.4
Summary of skull projections

AP skull	No angle on central ray, which enters at the nasion with the orbitomeatal line perpendicular to the imaging plate
AP axial Townes	Central ray 30-degree caudad, enters at the nasion
Lateral 1	Dorsal decubitus projection (cross-table lateral); central ray enters superior to external auditory meatus
Lateral 2	Supine with side of interest down; central ray enters superior to external auditory meatus

The paranasal sinus protocol may include three views: Caldwell (Fig. 22.36), Waters (Fig. 22.37), and a left lateral projection (Fig. 22.38), which should include frontal sinus anatomy, C-spine, and airway to the thoracic inlet. Proper collimation to the area of interest is the single most common shortcoming. To preserve image quality, consider precollimating before moving the patient into position; collimate to the area of interest only. Adjusting your light field on the back of the head does not allow for divergence of the central ray, thus too much of the skull is included. Experience has shown that in children younger than 8 years, the Caldwell method requires no central ray angulation and can be positioned with forehead and nose against the bucky. This is possibly due to the immature and varying morphology of the pediatric skull (Fig. 22.39).

The central ray is horizontal and exits at the nasion for the Caldwell method. For the Waters method, the child's nose and chin touch the bucky and the central ray remains horizontal exiting at the acanthion, projecting the petrous ridges below the maxillary sinuses. The major pitfall is too much central ray angulation, which causes the sinuses to either not be visualized or falsely appear to be obliterated. The left lateral is really a soft tissue neck (STN), which includes the vertical plate of the frontal bone (where frontal sinuses will be seen, but not usually prior to 2 years), the nasal shadow, the C-spine, and the thoracic inlet. With both the Waters and the Caldwell methods, ask the patient to move away from the bucky or upright grid once you have determined the appropriate receptor height, precollimate to the area of interest, and then place the patient back in the light field. The image quality will be improved and radiation to the patient will be reduced. This technique takes some getting used to because the projected light field on the back of the head will appear too small; trust science, the beam will diverge. Place your marker so it will not appear over an area of interest.

Fig. 22.36 (A) Caldwell without 15-degree angle. Note that both nose and forehead touch the grid at this age. (B) Caldwell image.

Fig. 22.37 (A) Waters method with chin and nose touching grid. (B) Waters image.

Fig. 22.38 Lateral projection for sinus series. The indication for the exam is normally noisy breathing with suspected adenoid hypertrophy. Often collimation includes from the frontal sinus to the thoracic inlet on inspiration through the nose in cases of other possible causes such as foreign bodies and retropharyngeal space anomalies (e.g., abscess). This collimation is also used for soft tissue neck for similar reasons.

SOFT TISSUE NECK

Indications for the STN include foreign bodies (FBs), stridor, laryngo- and tracheal malacia, laryngotracheal bronchitis, epiglottitis, and adenoid hypertrophy. The diagnostic quality of this exam requires careful instructions, neck extension, an inspiratory exposure, and complete immobilization. These requirements are more easily achieved with the infant or child in the supine position, although the exam can be done successfully with the patient in the upright position depending on how much the child will cooperate. The only contraindication to the supine position is the presence of the epiglottitis (Fig. 22.40); these patients must always be imaged in the sitting or upright position. *Never place these patients in the supine position as a swollen epiglottis can block the airway.* A "baby box" can be used for STN exams with infants and small children (6 months to 3 years). A 15-degree radiolucent sponge is placed under the infant/child's shoulders to achieve a slight extension of the neck and airway (shielding and immobilization are identical to the chest x-ray). A parent will hold the patient at the shoulders, pulling down slightly. The second holder, using two round, Mickey Mouse ear sponges (using flat hands), one on either side of the head and above the sella turcica, will hold the head in a true lateral position in extension and without rotation (Fig. 22.41). Collimation should be from the nasion (including complete nasal passage) to the thoracic inlet, including the entire C-spine. The head in flexion or an expiratory image may cause a false positive for enlargement of the retropharyngeal soft tissues. The lateral projection should be done with a set technique, no grid, at 182 cm SID.

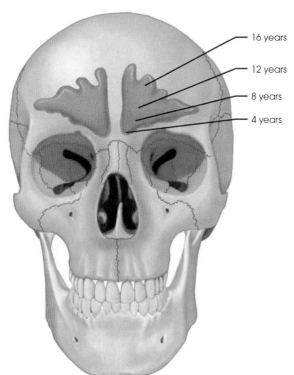

Fig. 22.39 Frontal sinus development correlated with age—green, 4 years; blue, 8 years; purple, 12 years; pink, 16 years.

16 years
12 years
8 years
4 years

(From Fonseca RJ, Barber DH, Powers M, Frost DE: *Oral and maxillofacial trauma,* ed 4, St. Louis, 2013, Elsevier.)

Fig. 22.40 There is diffuse swelling of the epiglottis, aryepiglottic folds, and the retropharyngeal soft tissues. These findings are consistent with epiglottitis.

The AP STN projection must be performed with a 102-cm SID grid. Patients from infants to adolescents should be positioned with the patient's occlusal plane perpendicular to the image receptor (exact positioning will vary with age) to prevent the occipital bone from superimposing the airway (overextension). Flexion will also cause superimposition of the airway.

The thick part of a 15-degree radiolucent sponge placed under the patient's shoulders will help position the skull for the AP supine extension (Fig. 22.42; using a 15-degree extension of the skull). A small cephalad angle can also be used with the AP projection to better visualize C-1 and C-2.

Fig. 22.41 (A) Soft tissue neck (STN) with a Fuji Synapse soft tissue preset. (B) STN without preset.

Fig. 22.42 A well-positioned and collimated AP projection with a 15-degree wedge radiolucent sponge placed under the patient's shoulders and a small cephalad angle.

Foreign Bodies

AIRWAY FOREIGN BODY

Airway FBs occur with frequency in children ages 6 months to 3 years, although it is not uncommon in teenagers. Radiolucent objects include firm vegetables, peanuts, hard candy, peas, carrots, and raisins. Round-shaped foods are the most frequently aspirated. Radiopaque FBs (Fig. 22.43) include coins (most common), hair clips, safety pins, and small toys. Splintered wood and glass have also been discovered, usually as the result of traumatic injury. Balloons are most likely to result in death. A young child with a persistent cough but without a fever carries a high index of suspicion for FB aspiration. Clinical presentations may also include stridor, a wheezing cough, recurrent pneumonia, or hemoptysis. If a radiolucent FB is in the trachea, the chest image may be normal and require a CT, or it may demonstrate bilateral over- or under-inflation (air trapping). More commonly, the FB is found in the bronchial tree, and most frequently the right main stem bronchus, which is larger and more in line with the trachea. On images the FB presents most commonly as a unilateral hyperlucent lung (see Fig. 22.43A).

The STN is accomplished with the help of an infant head and neck immobilizer (see Fig. 22.35). If an FB is suspected clinically, inspiratory and expiratory images may be obtained to rule out air trapping, as younger children will be unable to cooperate with inhalation and expiration commands; right and left decubitus views would then be indicated. The hyperinflated lung will not deflate when the patient is lying on the affected side. A routine protocol for imaging FB includes an AP chest to include the full airway, an abdomen to include lung bases and pubic symphysis, and a lateral STN (nasion to thoracic inlet including C-spine). All images must overlap. This survey ensures that multiple objects are not missed and provides a complete imaging of the airway and alimentary tract. If the FB is suspected of being in the airway, then bilateral decubitus views would be indicated.

INGESTED FOREIGN BODY

Whereas older children and parents might provide a history of FB ingestion, young children may simply present with unexplained drooling or the inability to swallow solids. The image readily demonstrates a radiopaque object, of which coins are the most common. A coin in the esophagus will usually lie in the coronal plane (Fig. 22.44), whereas a coin in the trachea will be visualized in the sagittal plane; a nonradiopaque FB may require an esophagogram for visualization. If a contrast study is indicated, a small amount of low-osmolar, nonionic, water-soluble contrast should be used like Iohexol (Omnipaque 350). Pica, or the compulsive ingestion of nonfood articles, may be common in those with serious mental impairment or developmental delay (Fig. 22.45). Pica is the Medieval Latin name for the bird called the magpie that, it is claimed, has a penchant for eating almost anything.

Fig. 22.43 (A) A foreign body in the right main stem bronchus. There is atelectasis (collapse) predominantly affecting the right lower lobe *(yellow arrow)*. Note the distinct right heart border on the AP *(red arrow)* and unilateral hyperlucent lung *(green outline)*. (B) Note the patchy opacities below the foreign body in the lateral view *(yellow arrows)*.

(Used with permission from Lifeinthefastlane.com at http://lifeinthefastlane.com/ lower-airway-foreign-body/.)

Fig. 22.44 (A) Ingested earring. Reference earring placed lateral to the patient *(yellow arrow)* to assist in confirmation. (B) Coin in the coronal plane.

Fig. 22.45 Gastrointestinal pica with paper clip *(green arrow)* and coin *(yellow arrow)*.

Selected Pediatric Conditions and Syndromes

CYSTIC FIBROSIS

Cystic fibrosis (CF) is an autosomal recessive disorder of the exocrine system caused by mutations located on chromosome 7. Generally speaking, these mutations affect the sodium and chloride ion transport system, which operates at the surface level of epithelial cells, resulting in thick mucus that cannot be cleared. These cells line the airways, sweat glands, GI tract, and the GU system. The organ systems most impacted are the lungs, sinuses, pancreas, intestines, hepatobiliary tree, the spermatic ducts in the male (vas deferens), and reduced fertility rates in the female. There are approximately 30,000 CF patients in the United States and 70,000 worldwide. The median survival age as at 2010 was 37.4 years with 40% of patients older than 18. One of the earliest manifestations of CF is meconium ileus in the neonate. Most patients are diagnosed in the first year with 50% presenting with a chronic cough by 10 months.

Pulmonary complications are the leading cause of morbidity and mortality with CF. In a healthy person, the surfaces of the respiratory tract are bathed in a salty surfactant that traps and, with the help of cilia, removes pathogens and foreign substances from the lungs. This system is compromised in the CF patient, allowing microbes such as *Pseudomonas aeruginosa, Staphylococcus aureus,* and *Haemophilus influenza* to flourish in stagnant mucus leading to inflammation and bronchoconstriction, ultimately causing irreversible lung damage. Due to its low radiation dose, chest radiography is the modality of choice for evaluating respiratory complications resulting from CF. The earliest sign of irreversible lung disease in these patients is bronchiectasis. Radiographic findings include bronchial thickening and dilation, peribronchial cuffing, mucoid impaction, and cystic radiolucencies (Fig. 22.46).

Nonrespiratory manifestations include a whole range of GI complications from meconium ileus in neonates to adult gastroesophageal reflux and rectal mucosal prolapse. As the patient ages, GU complications include renal compromise, nephrolithiasis (3% to 6% of patients), and diabetic nephropathy. Musculoskeletal disorders include abnormal bone mineralization of unknown etiology and metabolic bone disease due to malnutrition and decreased lung function. Reproductive manifestations include late onset puberty (1 to 4 years), a 95% to 99% infertility rate in male patients due to blockage or absence of the spermatic ducts (vas deferens), and incomplete epididymides.

Depending on the course and severity of the disease, CF can develop into one of the most debilitating illnesses of adolescence. It is important that radiographers understand the challenges facing these teenagers.

Standard precautions for CF patients include the following:
1. Departments sending a CF for imaging must call ahead to place a room on hold.
2. Check-in sends the arriving patient immediately to the room on hold.
3. The patient is assigned a "fast pass," which pushes him or her to the front of the imaging cue.
4. The patient is changed appropriately (chest or KUB).
5. The radiographer is gowned and gloved and should attempt to maintain a 3-foot separation from the patient.
6. The radiographer, in the presence of the patient, should clean all surfaces that the patient will contact during the exam.
7. Gown and gloves must be replaced if the radiographer must leave the room.
8. Upon completion of the exam, the patient is sent back to the ordering department and all horizontal surfaces that were within 6 feet of the patient as well as surfaces the patient contacted must be disinfected.

Fig. 22.46 AP chest of patient with CF.

DEVELOPMENTAL DYSPLASIA OF THE HIP

DDH is the malformation of the acetabulum in utero and is usually the result of fetal positioning or a breech birth. The acetabulum fails to form completely and the femoral head(s) are displaced superiorly and anteriorly. The ligaments and tendons responsible for proper alignment are often affected. Females are affected at a rate five times more than males, the left hip is involved more than the right, and 5% to 20% of cases occur bilaterally. The clinical diagnosis is made when there is partial or complete displacement of the femoral head from the acetabulum relative to the pelvis. With infants younger than 6 months of age, the modality of choice is US due to its lack of radiation and because the cartilaginous nature of the hip is better visualized at this stage of development. US is used for infant follow-up until 6 months, at which time images can be used to confirm placement of the femoral head(s).

Radiographic exams used to diagnose DDH include the frog lateral and the von Rosen positions. There is some discussion among radiologists that because the frog lateral position is used to reduce the dysplasia, the von Rosen should be the preferred position. Treatment of DDH varies with the diagnosis. Subluxation of the hip in the neonate may be stabilized in weeks if the femora are abducted in flexion, aided by double and triple diapering. A dislocated or dislocatable hip may be reduced and immobilized by the use of a Pavlik harness worn for 1 to 2 months; more complex cases may require surgery and a spica cast. During follow-up imaging, care should be taken when the spica cast is removed to keep the legs abducted to ensure hip stability. Later interventions include periacetabular osteotomy surgery to correct the developmental dysplasia (Fig. 22.47).

Fig. 22.47 Follow-up image post left periacetabular osteotomy surgery to correct DDH. The right femur also suffers from a lack of acetabular coverage due to a malformed acetabulum.

Nonaccidental Trauma (Child Abuse)

Although no *universal* agreement exists on the definition of child abuse, the radiographer should have an appreciation of the all-encompassing nature of this problem. *Child abuse* has been described as "the involvement of physical injury, sexual abuse or deprivation of nutrition, care or affection in circumstances, which indicate that injury or deprivation may not be accidental or may have occurred through neglect."[2] Although diagnostic imaging staff members are usually involved only in cases in which physical abuse is a possibility, they should realize that sexual abuse and nutritional neglect are also prevalent.

It is mandatory in all states and provinces in North America for health care professionals to *report suspected cases of abuse or neglect*. The radiographer, while preparing or positioning the patient, may be the first person to suspect abuse or neglect (Fig. 22.48). The first course of action for the radiographer should be to consult a radiologist (when available) or the attending physician. After this consultation, the radiographer may no longer have cause for suspicion because some naturally occurring skin markings mimic bruising. *If the radiographer's doubts persist, the suspicions must be reported to the proper authority, regardless of the physician's opinion.* Recognizing the complexity of child abuse issues, many health care facilities have developed a multidisciplinary team of health care workers to respond to these issues. Radiographers working in hospitals have access to this team of physicians, social workers, and psychologists for the purposes of reporting their concerns.

The ACR defines a skeletal survey as "a systematically performed series of radiographic images that encompasses the entire skeleton or those anatomic regions appropriate for the clinical indications." There are three indications for a skeletal survey according to the ACR: suspected nonaccidental trauma (abuse), skeletal dysplasias, syndromes and metabolic disorders, and neoplasms. Fractures in the first year of life are relatively rare, so their occurrence might warrant a skeletal survey to rule out child abuse. Although 64% of all reported cases of maltreatment with major physical injury occur in patients 0 to 5 years of age, those with radiologic evidence of abusive injury will be younger than 2 years of age. Pediatric imaging departments have specific protocols that protect the patient when there is a suspicion or evidence of child abuse. The diagnosis of abuse becomes more

Fig. 22.48 A 7-year-old with loop marks representative of forceful blows by a looped belt.

likely when there is a discrepant history of minor trauma in a child with complex, multiple fractures. Although policies vary from institution to institution, the goal is always protection of the child. The nonaccidental traumas often present in the emergency room (ER) for other indications and when imaged are found to have fractures of a suspicious nature. A scenario may go something like this:

1. Parent and 9-month-old infant are seen in the ER, where the infant presents with shortness of breath, wheezing, and low-grade fever for 2 days.
2. The patient is assigned to an exam room for nurse/doctor interview, assessment, and physical examination.
3. Routine standard-of-care chest x-rays are ordered to rule out pneumonia.
4. Radiographer alerts radiologist to the presence of what appears to be two healing posterior rib fractures (Fig. 22.49) and corner fractures (Fig. 22.50).
5. Radiologist consults with a child protection team and ER attending.
6. Hospital social services are called to conduct an interview with the parent.
7. The hospital's child protection team, ER attending, and social worker explain the findings to the parent. The family is then escorted, by security, to radiology for an immediate skeletal survey.

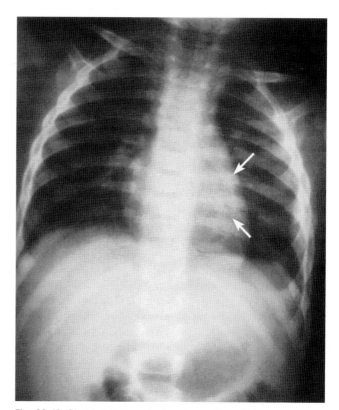

Fig. 22.49 Chest radiograph showing different stages of healing posterior rib fractures (arrows).

Depending on the findings, the infant may be admitted for care or removed from the home by Child Protective Services. Children presenting with emergent head trauma would be admitted and transferred to a surgical ICU. The abuse of a child is so repugnant that the urge to judge the parents will almost be reflexive; try to resist this temptation and stay focused on the very difficult and emotional task of providing medical care to the patient. Give a thorough explanation of what the skeletal survey entails: the time involved, the special accommodations that are provided for their infant, and inform them that the infant will cry. Allowing the parents to participate in the exam is a judgment call; overly emotional parents may be more of a hindrance, whereas calm parents may

help to sooth their infant. The parents who will not be helping should be escorted to a nearby waiting room. The survey can be accomplished quickly and efficiently with experienced radiographers.

Due to the medicolegal sensitivity of the skeletal survey and to expedite the exam, it is always best to have three radiographers working the exam: one immobilizes and positions; the second sets technique, positions, shields, collimates, and makes the exposure; the third supplies the two-person team with image plates if CR, immobilization devices, processes, and assesses the quality of each image. A skeletal survey for nonaccidental trauma on infants younger than 1 year should be done on high-resolution mammography imaging plates using a dedicated

processor. The table should have a pad with sheet, chucks, positioning sponges, pacifier, Sweeties (if not contraindicated), and gonadal shield. Have all supplies at the table or readily accessible within the room. The room should be warmed as appropriate and warming lights used as required. The radiology nurse should be aware that a survey is ongoing. All images are made with the infant lying on the IR (nothing is placed between the IR and patient). The patient can stay in a diaper, which will be removed when the abdomen/pelvis/femurs are imaged. Imaging should be timely, efficient, and repeats avoided. The radiologist accesses the images when the imaging is complete and will request additional images as needed.

Fig. 22.50 Images demonstrating physical abuse. Left and right corner fractures (*arrows,* A and B) and bucket-handle fractures (*arrow,* C) are considered classic indicators of physical abuse in children. The bucket-handle appearance is subtle and demonstrated only if the "ring" is seen on profile *(arrow).*

Imaging protocol at Boston Children's Hospital

- For efficiency and for medicolegal reasons, two radiographers should be in the room when imaging.
- Only AP projections are required for long bones unless there is a positive finding (Boxes 22.2 and 22.3).
- Equivocal findings in a long bone may necessitate a lateral projection.
- Hand images should be slightly obliqued rather than PA.
- Use mammography-imaging plates (increased resolution) and expose one body part per plate.
- Reduce motion by using the large focal spot, exposing only on expiration, with complete immobilization.
- All skeletal survey images should be done with 60 kVp (increased bony detail for CR-based systems).
- The 2-week follow-up exam does not require skull images.
- There should be nothing between the IR and the body part.
- Chest and abdominal images should overlap.

Box 22.2 is a skeletal survey protocol for nonincidental traumas of infants younger than 12 months and is tabletop at 102 cm SID, using a large focal spot with bone technique and mammography imaging plates. Box 22.3 lists radiologic findings.

BOX 22.2
Survey skeletal projections

AP and lateral skull (a positive finding may require right and left laterals and Townes)
AP and lateral chest
Bilateral shallow obliques of chest to show ribs
Abdomen (to overlap with chest)
AP bilateral femurs
AP bilateral tibias
AP bilateral feet
AP bilateral humeri
AP bilateral forearms
Bilateral hands, oblique 20 degrees
Lateral C spine
Lateral L spine

A positive finding may require laterals of extremities.

BOX 22.3
Specificity of radiologic findings

High specificity
Metaphyseal lesions
Rib fractures, especially posterior
Scapular fractures
Spinous process fractures
Sternal fracture

Moderate specificity[a]
Multiple fractures, especially bilateral
Fractures of different ages
Epiphyseal separations
Vertebral body fractures and subluxations
Fractures of the digits
Complex skull fractures

Low specificity (but common)[a]
Clavicle fractures
Long bone shaft fractures
Linear skull fractures
Subperiosteal new bone formation

---

[a]Moderate and low-specificity lesions become high when history of trauma is absent or inconsistent with injuries.
Used with permission of Dr. Paul Kleinman, Boston Children's Hospital, Boston, MA, United States.

Childhood Pathologies

OSTEOGENESIS IMPERFECTA

OI means "imperfectly formed bone." It is a serious but rare heritable or congenital disease of the skeletal system (20,000 to 50,000 cases in the United States). It results from a genetic defect on two genes that encode for type 1 collagen, the main collagen of osseous tissue, tendons, teeth, skin, inner ear, and sclera of the eyeballs. Although people with OI may have different combinations of symptoms, they all have weaker bones. Some common symptoms of OI include the following:

1. Short stature
2. Triangular-shaped face
3. Breathing problems
4. Hearing loss
5. Brittle teeth
6. Bone deformities, such as bowed legs or scoliosis

There are several types of OI, which vary in severity and symptoms and are classified as types I to IV.

Type I

Type I is the most common and mildest form. In this type the collagen is normal but is produced in reduced quantities. There is little or no bone deformity, although the bones remain fragile and easily broken. Teeth are prone to carries and are easily broken. The sclera of the eyes may have a purple, blue, or gray tint.

Type II

Type II is the most severe form of the disease, and many infants do not survive. The collagen suffers from the genetic defect, and bones may break in utero (Fig. 22.51).

Type III

Type III patients have improperly formed collagen, often with severe bone deformities, as well as other complications. The infant is often born with numerous fractures and tinting of the sclera. Children are generally shorter and have spinal deformities, respiratory complications, and brittle teeth.

Type IV

Type IV is moderately severe, and the collagen defect and bones, although easily fractured, are only mildly to moderately deformed. Some people may be shorter than average with brittle teeth.

Use verbal communication when imaging the patient with OI, being careful not to physically move or position the body. Let the patient position him- or herself or with the help of a parent to avoid causing new fractures. The caregiver or parent should do the transfer, changing, and aid in positioning. The exam table will require a radiolucent pad with sheet, a pillow, or towel under the patient's head, and radiolucent positioning devices to help support the patient. The radiographer should communicate the exact positioning required and then review the position before exposure. Positioning devices may be employed, but the family should place them. The radiographer will use his or her positional skills with the radiographic tube (move tube not patient) to obtain two projections differing by 90 degrees, thereby avoiding manipulating the part of interest. One of the reasons it is so important to ask the patient, "Is there anything I should know about your medical condition that would help me to help you?" is because the patient might have OI and it may not be indicated on the exam requisition. Although the omission of such critical information is hard to believe, it does happen; this is why we have "time-outs" before invasive procedures.

Fig. 22.51 AP (A) and lateral (B) projections of the left tibia and fibula. Patients with OI are not only fragile, but their anatomy can be misshaped, making it difficult to determine the correct position for AP and lateral projections.

PATHOLOGIC FRACTURES AND BENIGN AND MALIGNANT NEOPLASMS

Long bones, ribs, and facial bones are susceptible to fibrous displacement of their osseous tissue creating a benign condition called fibrous dysplasia. As these neoplasms grow, they erode the bone, causing the cortices to thin and weaken, which may lead to pathologic fracture. These dysplasias can become filled with fluid and are then known as bone cysts, often occurring in the upper ends of the humeri, femurs, and tibias of children, which are usually located beneath the epiphysis traveling down the metaphysis as they grow. The cysts often appear as incidental findings from another exam or following a pathologic fracture. Radiographically they present as thin-walled lucencies with sharp boundaries.

Osteochondroma

One of three types of chondromas, also known as osteochondromas, does not appear in the fetal skeleton and is virtually nonexistent until the second year of life. Growing from the bone's shaft, the tumor widens the bone, weakening the cortex (Fig. 22.52). Covered in periosteum that is continuous with the bone shaft and with its tip covered by a proliferative cartilage cap, the exostosis usually grows away from the joint using a similar mechanism to that of the epiphysis; there is no involvement of the bone's epiphyseal ossification center. When the person reaches maturity, bone growth ceases as it does in the tumor. There can be secondary vascular and neural manifestations, the patient can present with pain and swelling, or, alternately, the patient may be asymptomatic.

Fig. 22.52 (A) A 14-year-old with a right, distal, tibial, pedunculated osteochondroma, and deformation of distal fibula. (B) Bilateral osteochondromas.

(Courtesy Dr. George Taylor, Radiology, Boston Children's Hospital.)

Aneurysmal bone cyst

Aneurysmal bone cyst (ABC) occurs in children and young adults and has an unknown etiology. Secondary ABCs make up about 50% of all cases, and there is preponderance in females. The most commonly affected sites are both long and short tubular bones (Fig. 22.53A), neural arches of the vertebral bodies, pelvic, and facial bones. The cyst is composed of blood and connective tissue with connective tissue predominating as the ABC ages (see Fig. 22.53B). The most characteristic radiologic finding is a thin shell of bone containing the dilated cyst. ABCs are classified into five types, I through V, and should be removed immediately due to their potential for rapid and extensive damage.

Osteoid osteoma

A small, benign, ovoid tumor rarely exceeding 1 cm in diameter, osteoid osteomas occur most commonly in the tibia, femur, and the tubular bones of the hands (basal phalanges) and feet including their respective epiphyses (Fig. 22.54A). About 90% of these lesions occur in the first two decades of life. Radiographically they appear as a well-circumscribed radiolucency with a density at the center (nidus) in the midst of extensive bony thickening and sclerosis. These tumors are hard to penetrate radiographically and may require an increased technique. Although the lesion rarely exceeds 1 cm in diameter, the sclerosis that accompanies it can reach to 2 cm. A lesion larger than 2 cm is most likely an osteoblastoma. Treatment of osteoid osteomas includes, but is not limited to, tetracycline localization in the nidus. Radiofrequency (RF) ablation is another treatment option, in which an electrode tip at 90-degree centigrade is placed into the nidus for 6 minutes (see Fig. 22.54B).

Fig. 22.53 (A) ABC of the left proximal humerus *(orange arrow)*. (B) ABCs in the tarsus *(orange parentheses)*.

Fig. 22.54 (A) AP and lateral views of distal radial osteoid osteoma. (B) Radio frequency ablation of an osteoid osteoma of the right tibia.

Malignant neoplasms
Osteosarcoma

Alternatively known as osteogenic sarcoma, it is the most common of the primary malignant tumors. Usually appearing in the second decade of life, it often begins in the center of the metaphysis, enlarges, and destroys the bone. Males seem to have a slight preponderance. The most common sites are the metaphysis of the proximal humeri and proximal tibias, and the femurs. The earliest presentations of this rapidly growing tumor are pain and swelling at the site. Pathologic fractures are not uncommon, and systemic signs attesting to its rapid growth are weight loss, anemia, and dilated surface veins at the site. The chief radiologic finding is an increase in ossification of the tumor tissue, which may present as an irregularly radiolucent, multiloculated mass. Metastases occur early, usually in the lungs, and chemotherapy increases the risk for secondary tumors, both sarcomas and osteosarcomas, after the treatment of the primary tumor. Bone sarcomas show a chromosome band that supports a recessively transmitted predisposition for this tumor and for retinoblastomas.

Ewing sarcoma

Occurring usually at the end of the first decade or beginning of the second, Ewing sarcoma is the second most common malignant tumor in children, and almost any bone in the body may be affected. These tumors grow most frequently in the ilium, femurs, humeri (Fig. 22.55), and tibias. Unlike most of the primary malignancies, Ewing sarcoma does present with fever, weakness, pallor, and lassitude in contrast to most of the primary malignancies. It is not an osteogenic tumor, and the distinctive radiographic findings are the normally opaque spongiosa and cortical bone replaced by more radiolucent tumor tissue with bone destruction, layered periosteal new bone (onion-skin), and overlying large and swollen soft-tissue mass.

PNEUMONIA

Pneumonia is the most frequent type of lung infection, resulting in inflammation with compromised pulmonary function. It ranks sixth among the leading causes of mortality in the United States and is the most lethal nosocomial infection. Viruses are the most common cause of both upper and lower respiratory tract infections, whereas bacteria account for about 5% of all childhood pneumonias. In children younger than 2 years old, 90% of cases are viral, with the respiratory syncytial virus responsible for about a third of these cases. Viral or interstitial pneumonias are more common, are usually less severe than bacterial pneumonia, and are frequently caused by influenza. Radiographic findings are minimal, and the infection is usually confirmed clinically or through serologic tests.

Although chest images are important in determining the location of the inflammation, they are not definitive as to whether the causative agent is viral or bacterial; some knowledge of the suspected pathogens and their radiographic appearances can offer clues (Fig. 22.56). Pneumonias appear as soft, patchy, ill-defined alveolar infiltrates or pulmonary densities. The inflammation may affect the entire lobe of a lung (lobar pneumonia), a segment of a lung (segmental pneumonia), the bronchi and associated alveoli (bronchopneumonia), or the interstitial lung tissue (interstitial pneumonia).

Fig. 22.55 Neutral view of right humerus postosteotomy and plating for Ewing osteosarcoma. (*Orange arrow* points to osteotomy site.)

The single most common pneumonia-producing bacterial agent in school-age children is *Mycoplasma pneumonia* (present in 40% to 60% of cases). Pneumococcal (lobar) pneumonia is the most common bacterial pneumonia, probably because the bacteria are present in our healthy throats. It presents on the image as a collection of fluid in one or more lobes; the degree of segmental involvement can usually be identified with a lateral view. Staphylococcal and streptococcal bacterial pneumonias are far less common. Staphylococcal pneumonia occurs infrequently except during an epidemic of influenza, when it can be common and life threatening, especially in infants. Streptococcal pneumonias are even rarer, accounting for less than 1% of all hospital admissions for acute bacterial pneumonia. Radiographic findings are localized around the bronchi, usually of the lower lobes.

Mycoplasma pneumonia is caused by mycoplasmas and is most common in older children and young adults. This disease appears as a fine reticular pattern in a segmental distribution, followed by patchy areas of air space consolidation. In severe cases, the radiographic appearance may mimic tuberculosis. The morbidity rate associated with mycoplasma pneumonia is very low, even when the disease is not treated. Aspiration (chemical) pneumonia or chemical pneumonitis is caused by aspirated vomitus and appears on the image as densities radiating from either hila.

One of the most common challenges facing the radiologist is to rule out pneumonia. In most cases, the PA and lateral positions of the chest will suffice. In equivocal cases, the decubitus views are helpful in clarifying a suspected pulmonary abnormality. Images should be made with short exposure times (large focal spot) and must be inspiratory. Artifacts, possibly leading to a false positive, can be avoided with careful patient positioning, a peak inspiratory image, and ensuring the neonate's head is midline without any rotation. Pathologic conditions, such as CF and asthma with atelectasis, will distort the lung fields and could lead to an erroneous finding of pneumonia. Comparison to earlier images is essential to rule out residual or recurrent problems that might suggest an underlying abnormality. A pneumatocele (a thin-walled, radiolucent, air-containing cyst) is the characteristic radiographic lesion and is more typically seen in children. In later stages of the disease, these can enlarge, forming empyemas.

Fig. 22.56 PA (A) and lateral (B) chest images of an adolescent with pneumonia (*orange arrows*).

PROGERIA

Progeria is a rare combination of dwarfism and premature aging also known as Hutchison-Gilford syndrome. It is one of the many genetically based premature aging disorders that occur sporadically, with an incidence of 1 in 8 million births and a male-to-female ratio of 1.5 : 1. There is a strong racial susceptibility for Caucasians who represent 97% of patients. Derived from the Greek, meaning "prematurely old," the progeria patient ages up to 7 years for every year of life. These children fall within the expected growth percentile at birth, but after the first decade they have only achieved the stature of a 3-year-old. The child's average life span is 13 years (range 7 to 27 years).

There is no cure for progeria, and death is mainly due to cardiovascular complications like myocardial infarction or congestive heart failure. Symptoms include scleroderma, loss of hair and subcutaneous fat, short stature (average 100 cm), low weight (12 to 15 kg), abnormal dentition, an increased prominence of scalp veins, coxa valga, and osteopenia (Fig. 22.57). Progeria is probably an autosomal recessive syndrome affecting the *LMNA* gene that produces a defective lamina A protein resulting in a weakened cell nucleus. This unstable nucleus apparently results in premature aging.

SCOLIOSIS

Scoliosis is an abnormal lateral curvature of the spine in excess of 10 degrees, which has a component of rotation, bringing the ribs anteriorly in the direction of the rotation, and affecting lung function in more serious cases (Fig. 22.58). The scoliotic curve may be simple or may involve a compensating curve resulting in an "S" shape; the spinal curvature may occur on the right, the left, or both sides. In the greater population, between 3 and 5 children out of every 1000 develop a scoliosis that requires treatment. It affects girls about seven times more than boys, and idiopathic scoliosis tends to run in families, although no genetic link has been found. Scoliosis occurs, and is treated, as three main types.

Idiopathic

The most common type occurs mostly in preadolescent and adolescent girls; however, most cases either remain asymptomatic or the curves are too small to require treatment. Idiopathic scoliosis is comprised of three subtypes:

Adolescent. Represents the majority of cases, mostly in girls between 10 and 13 years old, and often requires no treatment.

Juvenile. Represents about 10% of cases in the age range of 3 to 9 years.

Infantile (early onset). Accounts for about 5% of cases, occurring in boys from birth to 3 years old and is mostly self-resolving.

Fig. 22.57 A progeria patient with osteopenia.

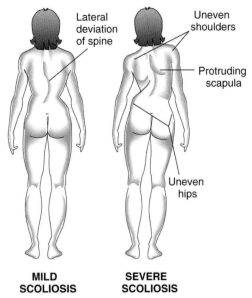

Fig. 22.58 Symptoms that suggest scoliosis.

(From VanMeter: *Gould's pathophysiology for the health professions,* ed 5, St. Louis, 2014, Elsevier.)

Neuromuscular

This refers to scoliosis that is associated with disorders of the nerve or muscular systems (e.g., cerebral palsy [CP], spina bifida, muscular dystrophy, or spinal cord injury).

Congenital

This is the least common form and occurs in utero between 3 and 6 weeks causing partial, missing, or fused vertebrae.

Scoliosis imaging

Usually indicated are standing *erect* AP and lateral images of the entire spine from the EAM to the SI joints at 182 cm (see Volume I, Chapter 9, scoliosis projections, for references). The first PA image is without breast shields to allow for visualization of the ribs and spine in their entirety. The lateral view should always be protected, whether the patient is male or female, by the use of a shadow shield to cover the face and breast tissue, while being careful to avoid clipping the anterior C-spine and the anterior L-spine in lordotic patients, and must include the EAM. In subsequent PAs, breast tissue should be protected for both male and female patients by using a shadow shield; the inexperienced radiographer should consult the patient's previous PA images to determine the location and severity of the curve before shielding (Fig. 22.59).

Filtration should always be used to compensate for thickness and density differences of the C-spine and thoracic cavity, respectively. The C-spine filter is placed at the x-ray tube window, and its projection should begin at the top of the shoulders and extend superiorly. The thoracic filter, again mounted at the x-ray tube window, begins at the mid-horizontal line and extends superiorly. A hypersthenic patient will dictate the need for additional C-spine compensating filters. The patient should remove all piercings, be undressed, wearing only underwear or boxers (check to make sure females have removed their bras), a hospital gown, and socks. Posture should be as the patient normally carries himself or herself and erect. Sitting images are more involved and require care in patient transfer to the special scoliosis-imaging chair. Holding help will most likely be required, and the lateral position should have a positioning sponge between the patient's back and the holder for support. The patient's pelvis should be as close to the grid or sponge as possible. This can be difficult with CP patients, as they tend to slide away from a support and may require that their knees be held so they cannot slide forward. If the patient's wheelchair has removable sides, some patients can be imaged in their chairs, but great care should be made to maintain *erect* posture. Make every attempt to shield these patients, although breast protection may not be possible due to the severity of the curve(s) and pelvic structure. A more advanced modality is the slot-scan EOS system (Biospace Med, Paris, France), which is covered later under "Advances in Technology."

Fig. 22.59 (A) Often the initial PA scoliosis image is made without shielding to reveal the relationships of spine, ribs, and pelvis. (B) Follow-ups require breast shields. (C) Shadow shields for breast tissue and eyes and a secondary stand-shield are used with all lateral views unless ordered otherwise.

Cobb angle, patterns of scoliosis, and estimation of rotation

The degree of curvature is measured from the PA view using the Cobb method. The image is examined to see what type of curve is present—acute (possible fracture?), smooth and arcuate, lumbar or thoracic, single or double—and whether there are any rib or vertebral anomalies. To measure the Cobb angle, one identifies the curve's superior and inferior end vertebrae, which are the two vertebrae that tilt most severely toward the concavity of the curve. Straight lines are then drawn across the superior and inferior end plates of the curve's upper and lower end vertebrae; the lines extend toward the concavity. These lines will intersect off the image, making the Cobb angle impossible to measure, so to the right of the spine from each end plate line extend a perpendicular line until they both intersect. The angle superior to the intersection represents the Cobb angle. Once the Cobb angle is determined, an estimation of the degree of rotation can be determined with reference to the vertebrae at the apex of the curve.

Lateral bends

Pediatric patients scheduled for surgery will have bending images to assess the rigidity and flexibility of the curve(s). A left thoracolumbar curve would be considered the major curve (structural) if it failed to correct with either right or left bends. The lumbar curve on the same patient would be considered a compensatory curvature (nonstructural) if it corrects on the right bend. Once the patient has reached skeletal maturity, curves of less than 30 degrees will not progress.

Skeletal maturity

In pediatric radiology, evaluation of skeletal maturity is made on the basis of bone growth in an image of the left hand and wrist. In children with endocrine abnormalities and growth disorders, the determination of skeletal maturation (bone age) is important in their diagnosis and treatment. In clinical practice, bone age is most often obtained by comparing the image with a set of reference hand images from the atlas by Greulich and Pyle. This reference work is the result of a 1950s survey of a healthy, white, middle to upper class population. A study by Zhang[3] questioned the validity of using the Greulich and Pyle atlas for an ethnically diverse population and found that ethnic and racial differences in growth patterns exist at certain ages with both Asians and Hispanics; this was seen in both male and female subjects, especially in girls aged 10 to 13 years and boys aged 11 to 15 years. A recent paper by Tsai et al.[4] in *Pediatric Radiology* provides strong support for using fibular shaft length as a more accurate alternative to current methods for bone age estimation with infants aged less than 1 year.

Treatment options

Options for treatment of scoliosis range from observation and monitoring to physical therapy, bracing, casting, and surgery. Invasive treatments may include spinal fusion/instrumentation, dual posterior growing rods to control spinal deformity, rod lengthening for infantile scoliosis, thoracoscopic anterior spinal surgery and instrumentation, osteotomy, or a combination of surgical procedures.

Advances in Technology

RADIOGRAPHY

Although this technology has been available in Europe for some time, it has been approved in North America more recently. The EOS system (Biospace Med) (Figs. 22.60 and 22.61) for orthopedic imaging has three advantages over conventional x-ray-based systems according to the company:

1. Greatly reduced dose to patient
2. Allows three-dimensional modeling for the evaluation of rotation, torsion, and orientation
3. Imaging is always on-axis and distortion free

EOS allows the slot-scan-based image to be made weight bearing, sitting (without assistance), and without the need for stitching. Various clinical parameters useful in evaluating and developing a patient's path to recovery are calculated automatically, including a patient report with images. Lower limb modeling is not adapted for patients younger than 15 years. Spine modeling is not adapted for patients aged 7 and younger or for the following pathologies: supernumerary vertebrae, congenital deformities, and spondylolisthesis.

MAGNETIC RESONANCE IMAGING

Many imaging centers routinely sedate young children before an MRI, incurring anesthesia costs, overnight admissions for infants, costs associated with sedation, anesthesia preparation, and recovery, and reduced patient and family satisfaction.

To this end, BCH conducted two pilot studies during 2009 and 2010 to assess the feasibility of pediatric scans without sedation ("Try Without," unpublished); in the initial pilot, children between the ages of 5 and 7 were assessed, and in the second pilot children from 4 to 6 years and infants 0 to 6 months were assessed. With adequate preparation and age-appropriate distractions, some children under the age of 7 remained still without sedation for 20 to 60 minutes. Results showed that 88% of children between the ages of 5 and 7 and 82% of children 4 to 6 years old including infants 0 to 6 months completed their scans without sedation. Since 2010, 3300 children have completed their MRI scans without sedation. You will see more of this cost/benefit/patient satisfaction analysis in the future of health care.

Fig. 22.60 EOS slot-scan standing scoliosis images of a 13-year-old female CP patient, with 3D remodeling showing axial rotation of individual vertebrae (e) and large lateral ejection of the apical vertebrae (f).

(Courtesy EOS Imaging, Cambridge, MA.)

Fig. 22.61 Patient positioned for simultaneous acquisition of PA and lateral full spine views for scoliosis.

A "noiseless" MRI system (Silent Scan, GE Healthcare, Waukesha, Wisconsin), which scans at a noise level of about 4 dB, compared to 86 to 110 dB with current technology, is available commercially; the reduced noise is the result of 3D MR acquisition, in combination with proprietary high-fidelity gradient and RF system electronics according to the company (Fig. 22.62). If this technology meets expectations, it could offer the potential for further reductions in sedation for younger patients.

ULTRASOUND

A wireless transducer (Siemens) is available that will transmit over a distance of 3 meters, which may assist with imaging infants and children. Called a point-of-care system, the transducer will expand the use of US in both interventional radiology and therapeutic applications. US has made huge advances through the years, but it is still largely constrained by bandwidth (0 to 50 MHz) and sensitivity. In a collaborative effort to overcome these limitations, Texas A&M University,

King's College London, the Queen's University of Belfast, and the University of Massachusetts, Lowell, have developed a new meta-material that converts US waves into optical signals, making images with greater detail (0 to 150 MHz) possible, maintaining sensitivity, and allowing one to see deeper into tissues.

COMPUTED TOMOGRAPHY

In pediatric patients, CT has been useful in diagnosing congenital anomalies, assessing metastases, and diagnosing bone sarcomas and sinus disease. Young children have difficulty following the instructions needed for a diagnostic scan. Suggestions regarding approach and atmosphere are presented at the beginning of this chapter. As in the care of any pediatric patient, the role of the CT radiographer is essential to the success of the examination; the radiographer must gain the respect and confidence of the young patient and the caregiver, if present. The CT scanner itself is an imposing piece of equipment that needs careful explanation to help allay the patient's fears. One of the most signifi-

cant fears is claustrophobia, which can be reduced by the use of distraction devices like virtual goggles and music and creative room décor (Fig. 22.63).

Toshiba has unveiled its Aquilion One Vision 640-slice CT scanner. This new system is equipped with a gantry rotation of 0.275 seconds, a 100-kw generator, and 320 detector rows (640 unique slices) covering 16 cm in a single rotation, with the industry's thinnest slices at 500 microns (0.5 mm). The One Vision uses an alternating focal spot that allows 16-cm z-axis coverage to be sampled twice, generating 640 slices in one rotation. The system can accommodate larger patients with its 78-cm bore and fast rotation, including bariatric patients and patients with high heart rates. More slices and shorter scan times reduce the possibility of patient motion (cardiac CT) and allow for scanning bariatric patients or those with larger anatomy. The faster scan times should reduce the number of patients requiring sedation. The Image Gently campaign has suggested CT protocols for reducing CT dose to patients.

Fig. 22.62 MRI suite with Siemens Skyra scanner. This machine can be used for adults and children.

Fig. 22.63 A Siemens Sensation CT scanner decorated for children.

INTERVENTIONAL RADIOLOGY

Image-guided, minimally invasive IR has dramatically changed the role of the radiology department in teaching and nonteaching hospitals and clinics. In the past, the justifications and rationales for radiology departments were diagnostic ones. Radiology departments with interventional staff now offer hospitals therapeutic services in addition to diagnostic procedures. This heightened awareness has largely resulted from the nature and efficacy of interventional procedures. Therapeutic procedures performed in IR provide an attractive alternative to surgery for the patient, parent, hospital, and society. A procedure performed in IR is much less invasive and expensive than one performed in the operating room. Shortened inpatient stays for IR procedures translate into economic savings for the parents and the hospital.

For simplicity, interventional radiology can be divided into vascular and nonvascular procedures. Vascular procedures are generally performed in angiographic suites. During these therapeutic interventions, angiography and ultrasonography are also performed for diagnostic and guidance purposes. Angiography can be arterial or venous; pediatric vasculature is well suited to both. IV injection of contrast media is favored in infants because their relatively small blood volume and rapid circulation allow for good vascular imaging. In infants, hand injections are often preferred over power injections to help avoid extravasation. Intra-arterial digital subtraction angiography (DSA) (see Chapter 27) has become a valuable tool. DSA is performed using a diluted contrast medium, which can reduce pain. Road mapping is a software tool, available on newer angiographic equipment, that uses the *intra-arterial* contrast injection and fluoroscopy to display arterial anatomy—a useful tool for imaging tortuous vessels.

Vascular procedures can be neurologic, cardiac, or systemic in nature. Nonvascular procedures often involve the digestive and urinary systems; examples include the insertion of gastrostomy tubes to supplement the nutrition of pediatric patients, and the insertion of cecostomy tubes in chronically constipated patients with spina bifida. Vascular access devices are of three types: nontunneled, tunneled, and implanted. The selection of device is often determined by a combination of factors, including the purpose of the access and estimated indwelling time. The physician or patient may choose a particular device after assessing issues of compliance or underlying clinical factors.

Nontunneled catheters are commonly referred to as *peripherally inserted central catheters (PICCs)*. They are available with single or multiple lumens. The insertion point is usually the basilic or cephalic vein, at or above the antecubital space of the nondominant arm. Multiple lumens are desirable when a variety of medications (including total parenteral nutrition) are to be administered (Fig. 22.64). These devices must be strongly anchored to the skin because children often pull on and displace the catheters, resulting in damage to the line and potential risk to themselves.

Fig. 22.64 (A) Postinsertion image of a double-lumen PICC in a 7-year-old boy (shown in the interventional suite). Conscious sedation was used for this procedure. (B) Left-sided PICC. *Orange arrows* track the double lumen PICC to its terminus *(yellow arrow)* in the superior vena cava.

Tunneled catheters, as with PICCs, can have multiple lumens. In contrast to PICCs they are not inserted into the peripheral circulation; rather, they are inserted via a subcutaneous tunnel into the subclavian or internal jugular veins. The tunneling acts as an anchoring mechanism for the catheter to facilitate long-term placement (Fig. 22.65). Tunneled catheters are used to administer chemotherapy, antibiotics, fluids, and hemodialysis, and are referred to as Hickman lines when placed in subclavian or internal jugular veins.

Implanted devices are often referred to as ports. These are titanium or polysulfone devices with silicone centers attached to catheters. The whole device is implanted subcutaneously with the distal end of the catheter tip advanced to the superior vena cava or right atrium. A port is the device of choice for noncompliant patients, and children and adults who are undergoing chemotherapy, and for aesthetic purposes or long-term use, would rather not have the limb of a catheter protruding from their chest (Fig. 22.66).

Vascular access devices have dramatically changed the course of treatment for many patients in a positive way. Patients who would have previously been hospitalized for antibiotic therapy can now go home with the device in place and resume normal activity. The increased prevalence of these devices means that patients with vascular access devices are in the community and visiting radiology departments everywhere. PICCs have a smaller likelihood of introducing catheter-related infections; tunneled lines present a greater risk.

Radiographers must recognize vascular access devices and treat them with utmost care. They should report dislodged bandages and sites showing signs of infection (i.e., redness, exudate immediately). Catheter-related infections constitute the largest nosocomial source of infection; they can be life threatening and cost hospitals hundreds of thousands of dollars each year.

Postprocedural care vascular access devices currently represent a significant and ongoing challenge for all personnel who treat, manage, and come in contact with these patients.

Fig. 22.65 External appearance of tunneled, double-lumen central venous access device. These catheters are used for long-term therapy. Their short track to the heart can increase the risk of infection, necessitating proper care for maintenance.

Fig. 22.66 Digital image of port *(arrow)*. Ports are vascular devices that must be accessed subcutaneously. They are preferred for active children and for aesthetic reasons.

ACKNOWLEDGMENTS

To all who came before us and shared their knowledge and the many people who gave willingly of their time, experience, and expertise: George Taylor, MD, Department of Radiology, Boston Children's Hospital (BCH); Jeanne Chow, MD, Department of Radiology, BCH; Carol Barnewolt, MD, Department of Radiology, BCH; Alison Ames, RT(R), outpatient supervisor, Department of Radiology, BCH; Judith Santora, RT(R), inpatient supervisor, Department of Radiology, BCH; Richard Cappick, RT(R), CT, CT modality operations manager, Department of Radiology, BCH; Diane Biagiotti, BS, RT(R), MRI modality operations manager, Department of Radiology, BCH.

References

1. American College of Radiology: Image Wisely (website). Available at: https://www.imagewisely.org/imaging-modalities/computed-tomography/medical-physicists/articles/how-to-understand-and-communicate-radiation-risk. Accessed September 2018.
2. Robinson MJ: *Practical pediatrics*, ed 6, New York, 2007, Churchill Livingstone.
3. Zhang A, Sayre JW, Vachon L, et al: Racial differences in growth patterns of children assessed on the basis of bone age, *Radiology* 250(1):228–235, 2009.
4. Tsai A, Stamoulis C, Bixby SD, et al: Infant bone age estimation based on fibular shaft length: model development and clinical validation, *Pediatr Radiol* 46(3):342–356, 2016.

Selected bibliography

Centers for Disease Control: Autism Spectrum Disorders. Available at: http://www.cdc.gov/ncbddd/autism/facts.html. Accessed January 2014.

Coley BD: *Caffey's pediatric diagnostic imaging*, ed 12, St. Louis, MO, 2013, Elsevier.

Erikson EH: *Childhood and society*, New York, 1993, WW Norton.

Godderidge C: *Pediatric imaging*, Philadelphia, 1985, WB Saunders.

Gray C, White AL: *My social stories book*, 2002, Jessica Kingsley.

Hudson J: *Prescription for success: supporting children with ASD in the medical environment*, Shawnee, KS, 2006, Autism Asperger Publishing Company.

Kleinman PK: *Diagnostic imaging of child abuse*, Baltimore, 1987, Williams & Wilkins, p 2.

Kreiborg S: Postnatal growth and development of the craniofacial complex in premature craniosynostosis. In Cohen MM, Jr, MacLean RE, editors: *Craniosynostosis: diagnosis, evaluation and management*, New York, 2000, Oxford University Press, pp 158–170.

Kwan-Hoong NG, Cameron JR: Using the BERT concept top promote public understanding of radiation. International conference on the radiological protection of patients. In *C&S paper*, Series 7, Malaga, Spain, 2001, Organized by the International Atomic Energy Agency, pp 784–787.

Mace JD, Kowalczyk N: *Radiographic pathology for technologists*, ed 4, St. Louis, MO, 2004, Mosby, pp 23–24.

Morton-Cooper A: *Health care and the autism spectrum: a guide for health professionals, parents and careers*, 2004, Jessica Kingsley. Available from the NAS Publications Department.

Silverman F, et al: The limbs. In *Caffey's pediatric x-ray diagnosis: an integrated approach*, (vol 2). ed 9, St. Louis, MO, 1993, Mosby, pp 1881–1884.

Volkmar FR, Wiesner LA: *Healthcare for children on the autism spectrum: a guide to medical, nutritional and behavioural issues*, Bethesda, MD, 2004, Woodbine House.

Advances in Technology

23

GERIATRIC RADIOGRAPHY

CHERYL MORGAN-DUNCAN

Geriatrics is the branch of medicine dealing with the aged and the problems of aging individuals. The field of *gerontology* includes illness prevention and management, health maintenance, and promotion of quality of life for aging individuals. The ongoing increase in the number of people older than age 65 in the US population is well known. An even more dramatic aging trend exists among people older than 85 years. The number of people 100 years old is approximately 100,000 and increasing. Every aspect of the health care delivery system is affected by this shift in the general population. The 1993 Pew Health Commission Report noted that the "aging of the nation's society and the accompanying shift to chronic care that is occurring foretell major shifts in care needs in which allied health professionals are major providers of services." As members of the allied health professions, radiographers are an important component of the health care system. As the geriatric population increases, so does the number of medical imaging procedures performed on older adult patients. Students and practitioners must be prepared to meet the challenges that this dramatic shift in patient population represents. An understanding of geriatrics can foster a positive interaction between the radiographer and the older adult patient.

Demographics and Social Effects of Aging

The acceleration of the "gray" American population began when individuals born from 1946 to 1964 (known as the "baby boomers") began to turn age 50 in 1996. The number in the age 65 and older cohort is expected to reach 70.2 million by 2030 (Fig. 23.1). The US experience regarding the increase in the older adult population is not unique; it is a global one. As of 1990, 28 countries had more than 2 million persons older than 65, and 12 additional countries had more than 5 million people older than 65. The entire older adult population of the world has begun a predicted dramatic increase for the period 1995–2030.

Research on a wide variety of topics ranging from family aspects of aging, economic resources, and the delivery of long-term care states that gender, race, ethnicity, and social class have consistently influenced the quality of the experience of aging. The experience of aging results from the interaction of physical, mental, social, and cultural factors. Aging varies across cultures. Culturally, aging and the treatment of health problems in older adults are often determined by the values of an ethnic group. Culture also may determine the way the older person views the process of aging and the manner in which he or she adapts to growing older. A more heterogeneous older adult population than any generation that preceded it can be expected as a result of increasing immigration from nonwhite countries and a lower fertility and reproductive rate among the white population. This group will contain a mix of cultural and ethnic backgrounds. The United States is a multicultural society in which a generalized view of aging would be difficult. *Health care professionals need to know not only diseases and disorders common to a specific age group but also the disorders common to a particular ethnic group.* An appreciation of diverse backgrounds can help the health care professional provide a personal approach when dealing with and meeting the needs of older adult patients. Many universities are incorporating cultural diversity into their curricula.

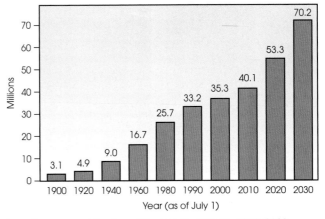

Fig. 23.1 Number of persons older than 65 years in millions, 1900–2030.

(Reprinted from U.S. Department of Commerce, Economics and Statistics Administration: 65+ in the United States. Washington, DC, 1996, U.S. Bureau of the Census.)

The *economic status* of older adults varies and has an important influence on their health and well-being (Fig. 23.2). Most older adults have an adequate income, but many minority patients do not. Single older adults are more likely to be below the poverty line. Economic hardships increase for single older adults, especially women. Of the population older than age 85, 60% is composed of women, making women twice as likely as men to be poor. By age 75, nearly two thirds of women are widows. Financial security is extremely important to an older adult. Many older adults are reluctant to spend money on what others may consider necessary for their well-being. A problem facing aging Americans is health care finances. Older adults often base decisions regarding their health care not on their needs but exclusively on the cost of health care services.

An increase in health care and the aging population go hand in hand. Heart disease, cancer, and stroke account for 7 of every 10 deaths among people older than 65. By 2025, an estimated two thirds of the US health care budget will be devoted to services for older adult patients.

Fig. 23.2 The economic status of older adults varies and is an important influence on their health and well-being.

Aging is a broad concept that includes physical changes in people's bodies over adult life; psychological changes in their minds and mental capacities; social psychological changes in what they think and believe; and social changes in how they are viewed, what they expect, and what is expected of them. Aging is a constantly evolving concept. Notions that biologic age is more critical than chronologic age when determining health status of the older adult are valid. Aging is an individual and extremely variable process. The functional capacity of major body organs varies with advancing age. Environmental and lifestyle factors affect the age-related functional changes in the body organs. Advancements in medical technology have extended the average life expectancy in the United States by nearly 20 years since the 1960s, which has allowed senior citizens to be actively involved in every aspect of American society. People are healthier longer today because of advanced technology; the results of health promotion and secondary disease prevention; and lifestyle factors, such as diet, exercise, and smoking cessation, which have been effective in reducing the risk of disease (Fig. 23.3). Most older adult patients seen in the health care setting have been diagnosed with at least one chronic condition. Individuals who in the 1970s would not have survived a debilitating illness such as cancer or a catastrophic health event such as a heart attack can now live for more extended periods, sometimes with various concurrent debilitating conditions. Although age is the most consistent and strongest predictor of risk for cancer and for death from cancer, management of an older adult cancer patient becomes complex because other chronic conditions, such as osteoarthritis, diabetes, chronic obstructive pulmonary disease, and heart disease, must also be considered in their care. Box 23.1 lists the top 10 chronic conditions for people older than 65 years.

Fig. 23.3 (A) Lifestyle factors—such as diet, exercise, and smoking cessation—reduce the risk of disease and increase life span. (B) Yoga emphasizes breathing and slow, low-impact motion, which are good for those with arthritis.

BOX 23.1
Top 10 chronic conditions of people older than 65 years

Arthritis
Hypertension
Hearing impairment
Heart disease
Cataracts
Deformity or orthopedic impairment
Chronic sinusitis
Diabetes
Visual impairment
Varicose veins

Elder Abuse

Another emerging worldwide issue of older adults is elder abuse. It has been estimated that 2.1 million cases of elder abuse are reported each year. These numbers may be suspect, however, because studies estimate that only one in five cases is reported to the authorities. It is thought that elder abuse is approximately as common as child abuse. Elder abuse is defined as the knowing, intentional, or negligent act by a caregiver or any other person that causes harm or a serious risk of harm to a vulnerable adult. Box 23.2 lists the various types of abuse. The typical victim of abuse is older than 75 years. Most studies of elder abuse show the incidence to be gender neutral. Physical abuse is usually received from the victim's spouse (50%), less often from the victim's children (23%), and only in 17% of cases is the abuse from nonfamily caregivers.

The radiologic technologist should be aware that the presence of injury is not proof of abuse. It is important to be watchful for the warning signs of abuse or neglect listed in Box 23.3. The older adult is often embarrassed by the situation and may be hesitant to communicate his or her concerns for fear of retaliation. The technologist needs to employ excellent communication skills, accurate documentation, and quality radiographs, and the technologist should report any suspicions of neglect or abuse. Injuries sustained by older adult victims are typically to the head, face, and neck as well as defensive injuries.

Attitudes Toward the Older Adult

The attitudes of health care providers toward older adults affect their health care. Research indicates that health care professionals have significantly more negative attitudes toward older patients than younger ones. This attitude must change if health care providers are to have positive interactions with older adult patients. These attitudes seem to be related to the pervasive stereotyping of the older adult, which serves to justify avoiding care and contact with them, as well as the older adults being reminders of one's own mortality. *Ageism* is a term used to describe the stereotyping of and discrimination against older adults and is considered to be similar to that of racism and sexism. Ageism emphasizes that frequently older adults are perceived to be repulsive and that distaste for the aging process itself exists. Ageism suggests that most older adults are senile, miserable most of the time, and dependent rather than independent individuals. The media have also influenced ongoing stereotypic notions about older adults. Commercials target older adults as consumers of laxatives and wrinkle creams and other products that promise to prolong their condition of being younger, more attractive, and desirable. Television sitcoms portray the older adult as stubborn and eccentric. Health care providers must learn to appreciate the positive aspects of aging so that they can assist older adult patients in having positive experiences with imaging procedures.

BOX 23.2

Forms of elder abuse

Physical: inflicting physical pain or injury
Sexual: nonconsensual sexual contact of any kind
Neglect: failure by those responsible to provide food, shelter, health care, or protection
Exploitation: illegal taking, misuse, or concealment of funds, property, or assets of a senior
Emotional: inflicting mental pain, anguish, or distress through verbal or nonverbal acts
Abandonment: desertion of a vulnerable older adult by anyone who has assumed the responsibility for care or custody of that person
Self-neglect: failure of a person to perform essential, self-care tasks, which threatens his or her own health or safety

---

BOX 23.3

Warning signs of elder abuse

- Bruises, pressure marks, broken bones, abrasions, and burns may be an indication of physical abuse, neglect, or mistreatment
- Unexplained withdrawal from normal activities, sudden change in alertness, and unusual depression may be indicators of emotional abuse
- Bruises around the breasts or genital area may occur from sexual abuse
- Sudden changes in financial situations may be the result of exploitation
- Bedsores, unattended medical needs, poor hygiene, and unusual weight loss may be indicators of possible neglect
- Behavior such as belittling, threats, and other uses of power and control by a caregiver may be an indicator of verbal or emotional abuse
- Strained or tense relationships, frequent arguments between caregiver and older adult

A 1995 study by Rarey concluded that most of 835 radiographers surveyed in California were not well informed about gerontologic issues and were not prepared to meet the needs of their patients older than age 65.[1] Further studies prove that medical students generally have poor knowledge and understanding of older adults, and this translates to inferior quality of care for older patients. Researchers contend that knowledge is a critical determinant of healthcare trainees' and professionals' attitudes toward aging; accurate knowledge begets positive attitudes, whereas inaccurate knowledge begets negative attitudes.[2] More education in gerontology is necessary for radiographers and physicians. Education would enable health care providers to adapt imaging and therapeutic procedures to accommodate mental, emotional, and physiologic alterations associated with aging and to be sensitive to cultural, economic, and social influences in the provision of care for older adult patients.

Physical, Cognitive, and Psychosocial Effects of Aging

The human body undergoes a multiplicity of physiologic changes second by second. Little consideration is given regarding these changes unless they are brought on by sudden physical, psychological, or cognitive events. Each older adult is a unique individual with distinct characteristics. These individuals have experienced a life filled with memories and accomplishments.

Young or old, the definition of quality of life is an individual and personal one. Research has shown that health status is an excellent predictor of happiness. Greater social contact, health satisfaction, low vulnerable personality traits, and fewer stressful life events have been linked to successful aging. *Self-efficacy* can be defined as the level of control one has over one's future. Many older adults feel they have no control over medical emergencies and fixed incomes. Many have fewer choices about their personal living arrangements. These environmental factors can lead to depression and decreased self-efficacy. An increase in illness usually parallels a decrease in self-efficacy.

Older adults may experience changing roles from a life of independence to dependence. The family dynamic of a parent caring for children and grandchildren may evolve into the children caring for the aging parent. Older adulthood is also a time of loss. Losses may include the death of a spouse and friends and loss of income owing to retirement. Loss of health may be the reason for the health care visit. The overall loss of control may lead to isolation and depression in the older adult. Death and dying are also imminent facts of life.

A positive attitude is an important aspect of aging. Many older people have the same negative stereotypes about aging that young people do.[3] For them, feeling "down" and depressed becomes a common consequence of aging. One of five people older than age 65 in a community shows signs of clinical depression. Yet health care professionals know that depression can affect young and old. Research has shown most older adults rate their health status as good to excellent. How older adults perceive their health status depends largely on their successful adaptation to disabilities.

Radiographers need to be sensitive to the fact that an older adult may have had to deal with many social and physical losses in a short period. More important, they must recognize symptoms resulting from these losses to communicate and interact effectively with these patients.

Although as a health care provider the radiographer's contribution to a patient's quality of life may be minimal, it is not insignificant. The radiographer must remember that each older adult is unique and deserves respect for his or her own opinions.

The aging process alone does not likely alter the essential core of the human being. Physical illness is not aging, and age-related changes in the body are often modest in magnitude. As one ages, the tendencies to prefer slower-paced activities, take longer to learn new tasks, become more forgetful, and lose portions of sensory processing skills increase slowly but perceptibly. Health care professionals need to be reminded that *aging and disease are not synonymous.* The more closely a function is tied to physical capabilities, the more likely it is to decline with age, whereas the more a function depends on experience, the more likely it will increase with age. Box 23.4 lists the most common health complaints of older adults.

Joint stiffness, weight gain, fatigue, and loss of bone mass can be slowed through proper nutritional interventions and low-impact exercise. The importance of exercise cannot be overstated. Exercise has been shown to increase aerobic capacity and mental speed. Exercise programs designed for older adults should emphasize increased strength, flexibility, and endurance. One of the best predictors of good health in later years is the number and extent of healthy lifestyles that were established in earlier life.

An older adult may show decreases in attention skills during complex tasks. Balance, coordination, strength, and reaction time all decrease with age. Falls associated with balance problems are common in the older adult population, resulting in a need to concentrate on walking. *Not overwhelming older adults with instructions is helpful.* Their hesitation to follow instructions may be a fear instilled from a previous fall. Sight, hearing, taste, and smell all are sensory modalities that decline with age. Older people have more difficulty with bright lights and tuning out background noise. Many older adults become adept at lip reading to compensate for loss of hearing. For radiographers to assume that all older adult patients are hard of hearing is not unusual, but they are not all hard of hearing. Talking in a normal tone, while making volume adjustments only if necessary, is a good rule of thumb. Speaking slowly, directly, and distinctly when giving instructions allows older adults an opportunity to sort through directions and improves their ability to follow them with better accuracy (Fig. 23.4).

Cognitive impairment in older adults can be caused by disease, aging, and disuse. *Dementia* is defined as progressive cognitive impairment that eventually interferes with daily functioning. It includes cognitive, psychological, and functional deficits including memory impairment. With normal aging comes a slowing down and a gradual wearing out of bodily systems, but normal aging does not include dementia. Yet the prevalence of dementia increases with age. Persistent disturbances in cognitive functioning, including memory and intellectual ability, accompany dementia. *Fears of cognitive loss, especially Alzheimer disease, are widespread among older people.*

Alzheimer disease is the most common form of dementia. Health care professionals are more likely to encounter people with this type. Most older adults work at maintaining and keeping their mental functions by staying active through mental games and exercises and keeping engaged in regular conversation. When caring for patients with any degree of dementia, verbal conversation should be inclusive and respectful. One should never discuss these patients as though they are not in the room or are not active participants in the procedure.

BOX 23.4

Most common health complaints of older adults

Weight gain
Fatigue
Loss of bone mass
Joint stiffness
Loneliness

Fig. 23.4 Speaking slowly, directly, and distinctly when giving instructions allows older adults an opportunity to sort through directions and improves their ability to follow them with better accuracy.

One of the first questions asked of any patient entering a health care facility for emergency service is, "Do you know where you are and what day it is?" Health care providers need to know just how alert the patient is. Although memory does decline with age, this is experienced mostly with short-term memory tasks. Long-term memory or subconscious memory tasks show little change over time and with increasing age. There can be various reasons for confusion or disorientation. Medication, psychiatric disturbance, or retirement can confuse the individual. For some older people, retirement means creating a new set of routines and adjusting to them. Most older adults like structure in their lives and have familiar routines for approaching each day.

Physiology of Aging

Health and well-being depend largely on the degree to which organ systems can successfully work together to maintain internal stability. With age, there is apparently a gradual impairment of these homeostatic mechanisms. Older adults experience nonuniform, gradual, ongoing organ function failure in all systems. Many of the body organs gradually lose strength with advancing age. These changes place older adults at risk for disease or dysfunction, especially in the presence of stress. At some point, the likelihood of illness, disease, and death increases. Various physical diseases and disorders affect the mental and physical health of people of all ages. They are more profound among older adults because diseases and disorders among older people are more likely to be chronic in nature. *Although aging is inevitable, the aging experience is highly individual and is affected by heredity, lifestyle choices, physical health, and attitude.* A great portion of usual aging risks can be modified with positive shifts in lifestyle.

AGING OF THE ORGAN SYSTEMS
Integumentary system disorders
Disorders of the integumentary system are among the first apparent signs of aging.

The most common skin diseases among older adults are herpes zoster (shingles), malignant tumors, and decubitus ulcers. With age comes flattening of the skin membranes, making it vulnerable to abrasions and blisters. The number of melanocytes decreases, making ultraviolet light more dangerous, and the susceptibility to skin cancer increases. Wrinkling and thinning skin are noticeable among older adults; this is attributable to decreases in collagen and elastin in the dermis. A gradual loss of functioning sweat glands and skin receptors occurs, which increases the threshold for pain stimuli, making an older adult vulnerable to heat strokes. With age comes atrophy or thinning of the subcutaneous layer of skin in the face, back of the hands, and soles of the feet. Loss of this "fat pad" can cause many foot conditions in older adults.

The most striking age-related changes to the integumentary system are the graying, thinning, and loss of hair. With age, the number of hair follicles decreases, and the follicles that remain grow at a slower rate with less concentration of melanin, causing the hair to become thin and white. A major problem with aging skin is chronic exposure to sunlight. The benefits of protecting one's skin with sunscreen and protective clothing cannot be overemphasized and become more evident as one grows older. The three most common skin tumors in older adults are basal cell carcinoma, malignant melanoma, and squamous cell carcinoma.

Nervous system disorders
The nervous system is the principal regulatory system of all other systems in the body. It is probably the least understood of all body systems. Central nervous system disorders are among the most common causes of disability in older adults, accounting for almost 50% of disability in individuals older than age 65. Loss of myelin in axons of the nervous system contributes to the decrease in nerve impulse velocity that is noted in aging. One such condition of the nervous system decline is Alzheimer disease, which is known to be

the most common form of dementia. More than 5 million Americans currently suffer from the disease, and it is estimated that this number will rise to about 13 million by 2050. Although there exist drug remedies and therapies, and lifestyle modification to stifle its progress, there is no cure for the disease.

In the healthy brain, an intricate network of billions of nerve cells communicate using electrical signals that regulate thoughts, memories, sensory perception, and movement. In Alzheimer's patients, brain cells die when genes and other factors cause the formation of an amyloid protein, which eventually breaks up and forms plaques—the hallmark of Alzheimer's disease (Fig. 23.5). These plaques ultimately lead to the destruction of brain cells. Once the brain cells are destroyed, neural connections are shut down, causing decreased cognitive functions. Other known risk factors of this disease are, of course, age and family history. The greatest risk factor for this disease is increasing age. After age 65, the risk doubles every 5 years. After age 85, the risk is nearly 50%.

Although family history increases the risk for getting the disease, there are a large number of Alzheimer's patients with no family history, suggesting that there are other factors influencing the development of the disease. In addition to the Alzheimer's gene, there is some evidence that some forms of the disease may be due to a "slow virus"; it is also possible that the disorder is caused by an accumulation of toxic metals in the brain or by the absence of certain kinds of endogenous brain chemicals.

Health experts inarguably propose that as the baby boomers become closer to the age where they may contract the disease, Medicare will become burdened with an estimated $626 billion dollars more in Alzheimer's-related health care cost. There is also the considerable psychological burden that is attached to this debilitating disease: adults are becoming more concerned that the disease will affect them or someone they know.

Current attempts to detect Alzheimer disease include imaging procedures such as structural imaging with magnetic resonance imaging (MRI) or computed tomography (CT). These tests are currently used to rule out other conditions that may cause symptoms similar to Alzheimer's but require different treatment options. As for functional imaging of Alzheimer disease, position emission tomography (PET) scans show diminished brain cell activity in the regions affected. Molecular imaging research studies are aggressively being pursued, because they promise to detect biologic cues indicating early stage Alzheimer's before it alters the brain's structure or function and causes irreversible loss of memory or the ability to reason and think.

Similar to any other organ system, the nervous system is vulnerable to the effects of atherosclerosis with advancing age. When blood flow to the brain is blocked, brain tissue is damaged. Repeated episodes of cerebral infarction can eventually lead to multi-infarct dementia. The changes in the blood flow and oxygenation to the brain slow down the time to carry out motor and sensory tasks requiring speed, coordination, balance, and fine motor hand movements. This decrease in the function of motor control puts the older adult at a higher risk for falls. Healthy changes in lifestyle can reduce the risk of disease. High blood pressure is a noted risk and can be decreased with medication, weight loss, proper nutritional diet, and exercise.

Sensory system disorders

All of the sensory systems undergo changes with age. Beginning around age 40, the ability to focus on near objects becomes increasingly difficult. The lens of the eye becomes less pliable, starts to yellow, and becomes cloudy, resulting in farsightedness *(presbyopia)*. Distorted color perception and cataracts also occur. Changes in the retina affect the ability to adapt to changes in lighting, and the ability to tolerate glare decreases, making night vision more difficult for older adults.

Hearing impairment is common in older adults. The gradual progressive hearing loss of tone discrimination is called *presbycusis*. Men are affected more often than women, and the degree of loss is more severe for high-frequency sounds. Speech discrimination is problematic when in noisy surroundings, such as a room full of talking people.

There is a decline in sensitivity to taste and smell with age. The decline in taste is consistent with a decreased number of taste buds on the tongue, decreased saliva, and dry mouth that accompany the aging process.

Hyposmia is the impairment of the ability to smell. It accounts for much of the decreased appetite and irregular eating habits that are noted consistently in older adults. Similar to taste, the degree of impairment varies with a particular odor, and the ability to identify odors in a mixture is gradually lost with age.

Fig. 23.5 Pathologic changes in Alzheimer disease (AD). (A) A mature plaque with central amyloid core next to a neurofibrillary tangle (NFT). (B) Comparison of normal and AD brains. *Top,* normal brain. *Bottom,* brain of a patient with Alzheimer disease. The AD brain shows gyral atrophy and sulcal widening greater than that seen in a person with no cognitive impairment.

(From Naidich TP, Castillo M, Cha S, Smirniotopoulos J: *Imaging of the brain,* ed 7, Philadelphia, 2013, Elsevier.)

Musculoskeletal system disorders

Musculoskeletal dysfunction is the major cause of disability in older adults. Osteoporosis, the reduction in bone mass and density, is one of the most significant age-related changes. Women are four times as likely as men to develop this disease. Risk factors for osteoporosis include estrogen depletion, calcium deficiency, physical inactivity, testosterone depletion, alcoholism, and cigarette smoking. The rate of new bone resorption surpasses the rate of new bone formation at approximately age 40. This accounts for a subsequent loss of 40% of bone mass in women and 30% of bone mass in men over the course of the life span. Osteoporosis is associated with an increased risk of fractures. Common fracture sites are the vertebral bodies, distal radius, femoral neck, ribs, and pubis. Changes in the shape of the vertebral bodies can indicate the degree and severity of osteoporosis. Advanced cases may show complete compression fractures of the vertebral bodies. Compression fractures can result in severe kyphosis of the thoracic spine (Fig. 23.6).

The incidence of degenerative joint disease, osteoarthritis, increases with age. Osteoarthritis is the chronic deterioration of the joint cartilage, and the weight-bearing joints are the most commonly affected. Obesity is probably the most important risk factor. Osteoarthritis of the joint cartilage causes pain, swelling, and a decrease in range of motion in the affected joint. Osteoarthritis is the second most common cause of disability in the United States, affecting more than 50 million Americans. At age 40, most adults have osteoarthritic changes visible on radiographic images of the cervical spine. The most progressive changes occur in weight-bearing joints and hands as age increases (Fig. 23.7).

Total joint replacement or arthroplasty procedures are common among older adult patients. Joint replacement may offer pain relief and improve joint mobility. Joint replacements can be performed on any joint including the hip, knee, ankle, foot, shoulder, elbow, wrist, and fingers. Hip and knee replacements are the most common and the most effective (Fig. 23.8).

With age, women are more likely to store fat in their hips and thighs, whereas men store fat in their abdominal area. Without exercise, muscle mass declines, resulting in decreased strength and endurance, prolonged reaction time, and disturbed coordination. It cannot be overemphasized that regular physical training can improve muscle strength and endurance, along with cardiovascular fitness, even in the oldest individuals.

Cardiovascular system disorders

The cardiovascular system circulates the blood, which delivers oxygen and nutrients to all parts of the body and removes waste products. Damage to this system can have negative implications for the entire body. Decreased blood flow to the digestive tract, liver, and kidneys affects the absorption, distribution, and elimination of substances, such as medications and alcohol.

Cardiovascular disease is the most common cause of death worldwide. The maximum heart rate during exercise decreases with age; older adults become

Fig. 23.6 Lateral chest radiograph of a geriatric patient with kyphosis and compression fractures.

Fig. 23.7 Lateral knee radiograph showing severe arthritis.

short of breath and tire quickly. Loss of arterial elasticity results in elevated systolic blood pressure, increasing the risk for heart disease and stroke. Another prevalent problem is postural hypertension, in which there is a decrease in systemic blood pressure when rising from a supine to a standing position. The predominant change that occurs in the blood vessels with age is atherosclerosis, a development of fatty plaques in the walls of the arteries. These fatty plaques within the artery wall can lead to ulcerations of the artery wall, subsequently making the artery prone to the formation of blood clots. The plaques also cause destruction of the artery wall, causing it to balloon, increasing the risk of an aneurysm. Complications can lead to an embolism, heart attack, or stroke.

Congestive heart failure is due to an inability of the heart to propel blood at a sufficient rate and volume. This pathology is more common in older adults, particularly individuals 75 to 85 years old. People who are most at risk for developing congestive heart failure include individuals who have been diagnosed with coronary artery disease, heart attack, cardiomyopathy, untreated hypertension, and chronic kidney disease. Radiographically, the heart is enlarged, and the hilar region of the lungs is congested with increased vascular markings. Exposure factors must be adjusted to visualize the heart borders despite the pulmonary edema.

Preventive health measures, such as control of high blood pressure, diet, exercise, and smoking cessation, decrease the risk of cardiovascular disease. These interventions are more effective if initiated earlier in life.

Gastrointestinal system disorders

Gastrointestinal disorders in older adults include malignancies, peptic ulcer disease, gastrointestinal bleeding, pancreatitis, difficulty swallowing, diverticulitis, gastric outlet obstruction, esophageal foreign bodies, constipation, and fecal incontinence. Mouth and teeth pain, side effects of medication, decreased saliva, and dry mouth can lead to nutritional deficiencies, malnutrition, and dehydration problems. Most gastrointestinal disorders are related to an age-related decrease in the rate of gastric acid production and secretions and decreased motility of the smooth muscle in the large intestine. A decrease in acid production and secretion can lead to iron-deficiency anemia, peptic ulcers, and gastritis. Diverticulosis, a common problem in older adults, develops when the large intestine herniates through the muscle wall. Gallstone disease, hepatitis, and dehydration tend to be more common in older adults. Healthy lifestyle habits, such as smoking cessation, low alcohol intake, a high fiber–low sugar diet, and regular exercise, can decrease the risk of gastrointestinal problems. Gastrointestinal malignancies are second only to lung cancer as a cause of cancer mortality. Survival after colon and rectal cancer is increased with inexpensive early detection. Stool samples and rectal examinations are effective in detecting early cancer (Fig. 23.9).

Fig. 23.8 AP proximal femur radiograph showing a total hip arthroplasty procedure.

Fig. 23.9 Postoperative image of an older adult patient showing an AP abdomen with surgical staples and nasogastric tube.

Immune system decline

Age takes its toll on the immune system. To be immune to an infection implies protection from that infection. The ability of one's body to remain free of infections requires the immune system to distinguish healthy cells from invading microorganisms or altered cancer cells. The age-related decline of immune system function makes older adults more vulnerable to diabetes mellitus, pneumonia, and nosocomial infections. The incidence of infectious disease increases. Influenza, pneumonia, tuberculosis, meningitis, and urinary tract infections are prevalent among older adults. The three general categories of illness that preferentially affect older adults are infections, cancer, and autoimmune disease.[4]

Respiratory system disorders

Throughout the aging process, the lungs lose some of their elastic recoil, trapping air in the alveoli. This reduced elasticity decreases the rate of oxygen entering the bloodstream and the elimination of carbon dioxide. The muscles involved in breathing become a little more rigid, which can account for shortness of breath with physical stress. In the wall of the thorax, the rib cage stiffens, causing kyphotic curvature of the thoracic spine. Respiratory diseases that increase in frequency with aging include emphysema, chronic bronchitis, pneumonia, and lung cancer.

Chronic obstructive pulmonary disease refers to a variety of breathing disorders that cause a decreased ability of the lungs to perform ventilation. Emphysema is the permanent destruction and distention of the alveoli. Cigarette smoking is the most significant risk factor in the development of emphysema and is the leading cause of chronic bronchitis. Chronic bronchitis is an inflammation of the mucous membrane of the bronchial tubes. These two conditions are considered irreversible. Chest radiographs may show hyperinflation of the lungs (Fig. 23.10).

Pneumonia is the most frequent type of lung infection and among the leading causes of death in older adults. This population is also at an increased risk for aspiration pneumonia secondary to slower swallowing reflexes and other health conditions. Radiographically, pneumonia may appear as soft, patchy alveolar infiltrates or pulmonary densities (Fig. 23.11).

Lung cancer is the second most common cancer and the most common cause of cancer-related death in men and women. More Americans die each year from lung cancer than from breast, prostate, and colorectal cancers combined.

There is a strong association between low lung function and the future development of coronary heart disease. Research has shown that the total amount of air inhaled in one's deepest breath and the fastest rate at which one can exhale are powerful predictors of how many more years one will live. Sedentary lifestyle is the greatest risk factor in lung function, and lifestyle habits are the crucial factors over which one has control.

Fig. 23.10 PA chest radiograph showing emphysema.

Fig. 23.11 PA chest radiograph with right middle lobe pneumonia and accompanying abscess.

Hematologic system disorders

A major hematologic concern in older adults is the high prevalence of anemia. Individuals with anemia often have pale skin and shortness of breath, and they fatigue easily. As bone ages, the marrow of the bone has a harder time maintaining blood cell production than young bone marrow when the body is stressed. The high incidence of anemia in older adults is believed to be a result not of aging per se, but rather of the high frequency of other age-related illnesses that can cause anemia. Anemia is not a single disease but a syndrome that has several causes. Insufficient dietary intake and inflammation or destruction of the gastrointestinal lining leading to inability to absorb vitamin B_{12} causes a type of anemia that affects older adults. Because of other physiologic stresses affecting marrow production, older adults have an increased incidence of various blood disorders.

Genitourinary system disorders

Familiar age-related genitourinary changes are those associated with incontinence. Changes in bladder capacity and muscle structure predispose older adults to this problem. Urinary and bowel incontinence can also lead to social and hygiene concerns. Along with structural changes in the genitourinary system, the number of nephrons in the kidneys decreases dramatically after the onset of adulthood. This decreased reserve capacity of the kidneys could cause what would otherwise be a regularly prescribed dose of medication to be an overdose in an older adult. The role of the kidneys to maintain the body's water balance and regulate the concentration according to the body's need diminishes with age. Acute and chronic renal failure affects many older adults.

Benign prostatic hyperplasia can affect 70% of men older than age 70. Benign prostatic hyperplasia is enlargement of the prostate gland, which can cause obstruction of the flow of urine. Surgical resection of the prostate may be necessary. Prostate cancer is primarily a disease of later life, and more than 80% of tumors are found in men older than 65 years. Prostate cancer is the most common cancer in men and the third most common cause of cancer deaths in men. Radiographic imaging of the male reproductive system comprises ureterograms, intravenous urography, and CT. Ultrasound is commonly used to evaluate testicular masses and prostate nodules.

Endocrine system disorders

The endocrine system is another principal regulatory system of the body. Age-related changes in thyroid function result from inadequate responses of target cells to thyroid hormone. The most common age-related disease associated with the endocrine system is diabetes mellitus. Non–insulin-dependent diabetes mellitus increases in frequency with age and accounts for about 90% of all cases. Regular exercise and weight loss can significantly reduce the risk and delay the onset of non–insulin-dependent diabetes.

SUMMARY

Aging is the one certainty in life. It starts at conception and continues throughout the life cycle. No two people age in the same way. As stated earlier, aging is individualized and is affected by heredity, lifestyle choices, physical health, and attitude. Despite the changes that occur in the body systems observed with aging, most older adults view themselves as healthy. They learn to adapt, adjust, and compensate for the disabilities secondary to aging. *Older people are stereotyped into two groups: diseased and normal.* The normal group is at high risk of disease but is just not there yet. By categorizing these older adults as normal, health professionals tend to underestimate their vulnerability. Modest increases in blood pressure, blood sugar, body weight, and low bone density are common among normal older adults. These risk factors promote disease, and yet they can be modified. They may be age-related in industrial societies, but they are not age-determined or harmless. Positive lifestyle changes, such as diet, exercise, and smoking cessation, reduce the risk of disease and improve the quality of life. Good health cannot be left to chance, and staying healthy depends to a large degree on lifestyle choices and attitude.

SUMMARY OF PATHOLOGY: GERIATRIC RADIOGRAPHY

Condition	Definition
Alzheimer disease	Progressive, irreversible mental disorder with loss of memory, deterioration of intellectual functions, speech and gait disturbances, and disorientation
Atherosclerosis	Condition in which fibrous and fatty deposits on the luminal wall of an artery may cause obstruction of the vessel
Benign prostatic hyperplasia	Enlargement of prostate gland
Chronic obstructive	Chronic condition of persistent obstruction of bronchial airflow pulmonary disease
Compression fracture	Fracture that causes compaction of bone and decrease in length or width
Congestive heart failure	Heart is unable to propel blood at sufficient rate and volume
Contractures	Permanent contraction of a muscle because of spasm or paralysis
Dementia	Broad impairment of intellectual function that usually is progressive and interferes with normal social and occupational activities
Emphysema	Destructive and obstructive airway changes leading to increased volume of air in the lungs
Kyphosis	Abnormally increased convexity in the thoracic curvature
Osteoarthritis	Form of arthritis marked by progressive cartilage deterioration in synovial joints and vertebrae
Osteoporosis	Loss of bone density
Renal failure	Failure of the kidney to perform essential functions
Urinary incontinence	Absence of voluntary control of urination

Geriatric Radiography

Patient Care

Box 23.5 lists quick tips for working with older adult patients. These tips are discussed in the following pages.

PATIENT AND FAMILY EDUCATION

Educating all patients, especially older adult patients, about imaging procedures is crucial to obtain their confidence and compliance. More time with older adult patients may be necessary to accommodate their decreased ability to process information rapidly. Most older adults have been diagnosed with at least one chronic illness. They typically arrive at the clinical imaging environment with a natural anxiety because they are likely to have little knowledge of the procedure or the highly technical modalities employed for their procedures. A fear concerning consequences resulting from the examination exacerbates their increased levels of anxiety. Taking time to educate patients and their families or significant caregivers in their support system about the procedures makes for a less stressful experience and improved patient compliance and satisfaction.

BOX 23.5

Tips for working with older adult patients

Take time to educate the patient and the family.

Speak lower and closer.

Treat the patient with dignity and respect.

Give the patient time to rest between projections and procedures.

Avoid adhesive tape: older adult skin is thin and fragile.

Provide warm blankets in cold examination rooms.

Use table pads and handrails.

Always access the patient's medical history before contrast medium is administered.

COMMUNICATION

Good communication and listening skills create a connection between the radiographer and the patient. Older people are unique and should be treated with dignity and respect. Examples of appropriate communication may include addressing the patient by his or her title and last name. It is inappropriate to call someone "honey" or "dear." Each older adult is a wealth of cultural and historical knowledge that becomes a learning experience for the radiographer. If it is evident that the patient cannot hear or understand verbal directions, it is appropriate to speak lower and closer. Background noise can be disrupting to an older person and should be eliminated if possible when giving precise instructions. Giving instruction individually provides the older adult time to process a request. An empathetic, warm attitude and approach to a geriatric patient result in a trusting and compliant patient.

TRANSPORTATION AND LIFTING

Balance and coordination of an older adult patient can be affected by normal aging changes. The patient's anxiety about falling can be diminished by assistance in and out of a wheelchair and to and from the examination table. Many older adult patients have decreased height perception resulting from some degree of vision impairment. Hesitation of the older adult patient may be due to previous falls. Assisting an older patient when there is a need to step up or down throughout the procedure is more than a reassuring gesture. Preventing opportunities for falls is a responsibility of the radiographer. The older adult patient often experiences vertigo and dizziness when moving from a recumbent position to a sitting position. Giving the patient time to rest between positions mitigates these disturbing, frightening, and uncomfortable sensations. The use of table handgrips and proper assistance from the radiographer create a sense of security for an older adult patient. A sense of security results in a compliant and trusting patient throughout the imaging procedure.

SKIN CARE

Acute age-related changes in the skin cause it to become thin and fragile. The skin becomes more susceptible to bruising, tears, abrasions, and blisters. All health care professionals should use caution in turning and holding an older adult patient. Excessive pressure on the skin causes it to break and tear. *Adhesive tape should be avoided because it can be irritating and can easily tear the skin of an older person.* The loss of fat pads makes it painful for an older adult patient to lie on a hard surface and can increase the possibility of developing ulcerations. Decubitus ulcers, or pressure sores, are commonly seen in bedridden people and people with decreased mobility. Bony areas such as the heels, ankles, elbow, and lateral hips are frequent sites for pressure sores. A decubitus ulcer can develop in 1 to 2 hours. Almost without exception, tables used for imaging procedures are hard surfaced and cannot be avoided. The use of a table pad can reduce the friction between the hard surface of the table and the patient's fragile skin. Sponges, blankets, and positioning aids make the procedure much more bearable and comfortable for the older adult patient.

Because skin plays a crucial role in maintaining body temperature, the increasing thinning process associated with aging skin renders the patient less able to retain normal body heat. The regulation of body temperature of an older adult varies from that of a younger person. To prevent hypothermia in rooms where the ambient air temperature is comfortable for the radiographer, it may be essential to provide blankets for the older adult patient.

CONTRAST AGENT ADMINISTRATION

Because of age-related changes in kidney and liver functions, the amount, but not the type, of contrast media is varied when performing radiographic procedures on an older adult patient. The number of functioning nephrons in the kidneys steadily decreases from middle age throughout the life span. Compromised kidney function contributes to the older adult patient being more prone to electrolyte and fluid imbalance, which can create life-threatening consequences. They are also more susceptible to the effects of dehydration because of diabetes and decreased renal or adrenal function. The decision of type and amount of contrast media used for the geriatric patient usually follows some sort of routine protocol. Assessment for contrast agent administration accomplished by the imaging technologist must include age; history of liver, kidney, or thyroid disease; history of hypersensitivity reactions and previous reactions to medications or contrast agents; sensitivity to aspirin; over-the-counter and prescription drug history including the use of acetaminophen (Tylenol); and history of diabetes and hypertension.[5]

The imaging technologist must be selective in locating an appropriate vein for contrast agent administration on the older adult patient. The technologist should consider the location and condition of the vein, decreased integrity of the skin, and duration of the therapy. Thin superficial veins, repeatedly used veins, and veins located in areas where the skin is bruised or scarred should be avoided. The patient should be assessed for any swallowing impairments, which could lead to difficulties with drinking liquid contrast agents. The patient should be instructed to drink slowly to avoid choking, and an upright position helps prevent aspiration.

JOINT COMMISSION CRITERIA

The Joint Commission is the accrediting and standards-setting body for hospitals, clinics, and other health care organizations in the United States. Employees in institutions accredited by the Joint Commission must demonstrate age-based communication competencies, which include the older adult. The standards were adopted as a means of demonstrating competence in meeting the physiologic and psychological needs of patients in special populations. These populations include infants, children, adolescents, and older adults.

Age-related competencies

Standard HR 01.05.03 of the Human Resources section of the Joint Commission manual states: "When appropriate, the hospital considers special needs and behaviors of specific age groups in defining qualifications, duties, and responsibilities of staff members who do not have clinical privileges but who have regular clinical contact with patients (e.g., radiologic technologists and mental health technicians)." The intent of the standard is to ensure age-specific competency in technical and clinical matters but is not limited to equipment and technical performance. Age-specific competencies address the different needs people have at different ages. Examples of age-specific care for older adults may include the following: assessing visual or hearing impairments; assessing digestive and esophageal problems, such as reflux, bladder, and bowel problems; addressing grief concerns; providing warmth; and providing safety aids. Being able to apply age-specific care also includes the use of age-appropriate communication skills. Clear communication with the patient can be the key to providing age-specific care. Knowledge of age-related changes and disease processes assists all health care professionals, including those in the radiation sciences, in providing care that meets the needs of the older adult patient.

Performing the Radiographic Procedure
RADIOGRAPHER'S ROLE

The role of the radiographer is no different than that of all other health professionals. The whole person must be treated, not just the manifested symptoms of an illness or injury. Medical imaging and therapeutic procedures reflect the impact of ongoing systemic aging in documentable and visual forms. Adapting procedures to accommodate disabilities and diseases of geriatric patients is a crucial responsibility and a challenge based almost exclusively on the radiographer's knowledge, abilities, and skills. An understanding of the physiology and pathology of aging and an awareness of the social, psychological, cognitive, and economic aspects of aging are required to meet the needs of older adult patients. Conditions typically associated with older adult patients invariably require adaptations or modifications of routine imaging procedures. The radiographer must be able to differentiate between age-related changes and disease processes. Production of diagnostic images requiring professional decision making to compensate for physiologic changes, while maintaining the compliance, safety, and comfort of the patient, is the foundation of the contract between the older adult patient and the radiographer.

To know how to care for individuals with Alzheimer disease, it is important to become familiar with some simple facts about the disease and behaviors that are associated with it. Alzheimer disease is a progressive disease with no known cure. There are five stages: preclinical stage, mild cognitive impairment, mild dementia, moderate dementia, and severe dementia. The disease is often diagnosed in the mild stage of dementia. Table 23.1 lists these stages and a brief description of each.

The rate of progression of Alzheimer disease varies widely. On average people with this disease live 8 to 10 years after diagnosis; however, some will live as long as 25 years after diagnosis. Pneumonia is a common cause of death because impaired swallowing allows food or beverages to enter the lungs, where an infection can begin. Other common causes of death include complications from urinary tract infections and falls.

It is important that the radiologic technologist becomes aware of and understands the various types of physical and cognitive impairments associated with Alzheimer disease. It requires patience and compassion and attentiveness when dealing with this patient group. Patients who are at risk of falling must never be left alone whether in the radiology waiting room or in the examination room. Caregivers should be encouraged to accompany the patient to appointments whenever possible. It is sometimes more comforting to the patient to have a familiar person with him or her in an unfamiliar setting. In addition, depending on the stage of the disease, some patients may tend to wander, often wanting to "go home." Home sometimes is their native town, state, or even country. So they can travel considerable distances before they are found. There have been cases where patients have wandered off, never to be found, or never to be found alive. For that reason the patient should never be left alone. Whenever possible, and whenever a caregiver has not accompanied the patient, a two-technologist team should be available to care for the patient while in the diagnostic radiology suite—one acquiring the images and one in the role of companion to the patient while the images are being processed and reviewed. The patient should be then handed off to the unit or responsible party upon completion of the exam.

It is not uncommon for Alzheimer's patients to ask repetitive questions or to become accusatory. The technologist should exercise a great deal of patience and use distraction techniques to eliminate the frustration this may cause. Simply changing the subject or asking an unrelated question may reduce the repetitive questioning or conversation. There may be occasions when the patient will require restraints to complete the exam. Note, however, that restraints should only be applied in cases where the patient can potentially cause harm to himself or to others.

Working quietly and smoothly around the patient and maintaining calm, relaxing, and noise-free surroundings is the preferred situation for Alzheimer's patients in the radiology department. The music, if any, should be soothing and relaxing. This will potentially benefit all types of patients.

Radiographic Positioning for Geriatric Patients

The preceding discussions and understanding of the physical, cognitive, and psychosocial effects of aging can help radiographers adapt to the positioning challenges of the geriatric patient. In some cases, routine examinations need to be modified to accommodate the limitations, safety, and comfort of the patient. Communicating clear instructions with the patient is important. The following discussion addresses positioning suggestions for various structures.

CHEST

The position of choice for the chest radiograph is the upright position; however, an older adult patient may be unable to stand without assistance for this examination. The traditional PA position is to have the "backs of hands on hips." This may be difficult for someone with impaired balance and flexibility. The radiographer can allow the patient to wrap his or her arms around the chest stand as a means of support and security (Fig. 23.12). The patient may not be able to maintain his or her arms over the head for the lateral projection of the chest. The radiographer should provide extra security and stability while the patient is moving the arms up and forward (Fig. 23.13).

TABLE 23.1
Stages and symptoms of Alzheimer disease

Stages of Alzheimer disease	Description of behaviors/symptoms
Preclinical stage	Symptoms usually go unnoticed during this stage. This stage of Alzheimer disease can last for years, possibly even decades. Diagnostic imaging technologies can now identify deposits of the amyloidal beta substance that have been associated with Alzheimer disease.
Mild cognitive impairment	Memory lapses, interrupted thought processes. Trouble with time management. Trouble making sound decisions.
Mild dementia	Memory loss of recent events. Difficulty with problem solving. Difficulty completing complex tasks and making sound judgments. Changes in personality—may become subdued, or withdraw from certain social situations. Difficulty organizing or expressing thoughts. Gets lost or wanders away from home. Misplaces belongings.
Moderate dementia	Displays increasingly poor judgment. Confusion deepens. Memory loss increases. Needs assistance with daily routine activities. Becomes suspicious or paranoid and accusatory to caregivers or family members. Rummaging, tapping feet, rubbing hands, banging. Outbursts of physical aggression.
Severe dementia (late stage)	Inability to hold coherent conversations. Inability to recognize some or all family members. Requires assistance with personal care. Decline in physical abilities—needs assistance walking or may experience uncontrollable bladder and bowel functions. Inability to swallow; rigid muscles; abnormal reflexes.

When the patient cannot stand, the examination may be done seated in a wheelchair or stretcher, but some issues affect the radiographic quality. First, the radiologist needs to be aware that the radiograph is an AP instead of a PA projection, which may make comparison difficult. Hyperkyphosis can result in the lung apices being obscured, and the abdomen may obscure the lung bases. In a sitting position, respiration may be compromised, and the patient should be instructed on the importance of a deep inspiration. Whenever anything other than the normal is done (e.g., AP in lieu of PA), this should be annotated on the radiograph as well as a computerized note for the radiologist.

Positioning of the image receptor (IR) for a kyphotic patient should be higher than normal because the shoulders and apices are in a higher position. Radiographic landmarks may change with age, and the centering may need to be lower if the patient is extremely kyphotic. When positioning the patient for the sitting lateral chest projection, the radiographer should place a large sponge behind the patient to lean him or her forward (Fig. 23.14).

SPINE

Radiographic spine examinations may be painful for a patient with osteoporosis who is lying on the x-ray table. Positioning aids such as radiolucent sponges, sandbags, and a mattress may be used as long as the quality of the image is not compromised (Fig. 23.15). Performing upright radiographic examinations may also be appropriate if a patient can safely tolerate this position. The combination of cervical lordosis and thoracic kyphosis can make positioning and visualization of the cervical and thoracic spine difficult. Lateral cervical projections can be done with the patient standing, sitting, or lying supine. The AP projection in the sitting position may not visualize the upper cervical vertebrae because the chin may obscure this anatomy. In the supine position, the head may not reach the table and result in magnification. The AP and open-mouth projections are difficult to do in a wheelchair.

Fig. 23.12 Radiographer positioning patient's arms around the chest stand for a PA chest radiograph. Having the patient hold on in this way provides stability.

Fig. 23.14 Positioning sponges and sandbags are commonly used as immobilization devices.

Fig. 23.13 Radiographer placing the IR behind a patient who is unable to stand. With careful positioning of the IR and x-ray tube, a quality image of the chest can be obtained.

Fig. 23.15 Recumbent lateral thoracic spine. Support placed under lower thoracic region; perpendicular central ray.

The thoracic and lumbar spines are sites for compression fractures. The use of positioning blocks may be necessary to help the patient remain in position. For the lateral projection, a lead blocker or shield behind the spine should be used to absorb as much scatter radiation as possible (see Fig. 23.15).

PELVIS AND HIP

Osteoarthritis, osteoporosis, and injuries as the result of falls contribute to hip pathologies. A common fracture in older adults is to the femoral neck. An AP projection of the pelvis should be done to examine the hip. If the indication is trauma, the radiographer should *not attempt to rotate the limbs*. The second view taken should be a cross-table lateral of the affected hip. If hip pain is the indication, assist the patient to internal rotation of the legs with the use of sandbags if necessary (Figs. 23.16 and 23.17).

Fig. 23.16 Legs inverted for AP projection of the pelvis. Wrapping flexible sandbags around the feet can help the geriatric patient hold his or her legs in this position.

Fig. 23.17 An older adult patient with Alzheimer disease was brought to the emergency department because he could not walk. The patient did not complain of pain. Note fracture of the right hip. Trauma radiograph was made with patient's pants on and the zipper is shown.

UPPER EXTREMITY

Positioning the geriatric patient for projections of the upper extremities can present its own challenges. Often the upper extremities have limited flexibility and mobility. A cerebrovascular accident or stroke may cause contractures of the affected limb. Contracted limbs cannot be forced into position, and cross-table views may need to be done. The inability of the patient to move his or her limb should not be interpreted as a lack of cooperation. Supination is often a problem in patients with contractures, fractures, and paralysis. The routine AP and lateral projections can be supported with the use of sponges, sandbags, and blocks to raise and support the extremity being imaged. The shoulder is also a site of decreased mobility, dislocation, and fractures. The therapist should assess how much movement the patient can do before attempting to move the arm. The use of finger sponges may also help with the contractures of the fingers (Fig. 23.18).

Fig. 23.18 Most projections of the upper limb can be obtained with the patient in a wheelchair and with some creativity. (A) Patient being positioned for an AP hand radiograph. Note use of a 4-inch sponge to raise the IR. (B) Patient being positioned for a lateral wrist radiograph. A hospital food tray table provides a base for IR and for ease of positioning.

LOWER EXTREMITY

The lower extremities may have limited flexibility and mobility. The ability to dorsiflex the ankle may be reduced as a result of neurologic disorders. Imaging on the x-ray table may need to be modified when a patient cannot turn on his or her side. Flexion of the knee may be impaired and require a cross-table lateral projection. If a tangential projection of the patella, such as the Settegast method, is necessary, and the patient can turn on his or her side, the radiographer can place the IR superior to the knee and direct the central ray perpendicular through the patellofemoral joint. Projections of the feet and ankles may be obtained with the patient sitting in the wheelchair. Positioning sponges and sandbags support and maintain the position of the body part being imaged (Fig. 23.19). Whenever possible, the technologist should keep the patient in the wheelchair or stretcher to perform upper and lower extremity exams. This will minimize the stress (to both patient and technologist) of transferring the patient to and from the examination table.

TECHNICAL FACTORS

Exposure factors also need to be taken into consideration when imaging the geriatric patient. The loss of bone mass and atrophy of tissues often require a lower kilovoltage (kVp) to maintain sufficient contrast. kVp is also a factor in chest radiographs when there may be a large heart and pleural fluid to penetrate. Patients with emphysema require a reduction in technical factors to prevent overexposure of the lung field. Patient assessment can help with the appropriate exposure adjustments.

Time may also be a major factor. Geriatric patients may have problems maintaining the positions necessary for the examinations. A short exposure time helps reduce voluntary and involuntary motion and breathing. The radiographer needs to ensure that the geriatric patient clearly hears and understands the breathing instructions.

Fig. 23.19 Projections of the lower limb, especially from the knee and lower, can be obtained with the patient in a wheelchair. (A) AP projection of the ankle with the patient's leg and foot resting on a chair. (B) Lateral projection of the ankle performed by using a chair as a rest and a sponge to raise the IR.

Conclusion

Imaging professionals will continue to see a change in the health care delivery system with the dramatic shift in the population of people older than age 65. This shift in the general population is resulting in an ongoing increase in the number of medical imaging procedures performed on older adult patients. Demographic and social effects of aging determine the way in which older adults adapt to and view the process of aging. An individual's family size and perceptions of aging, economic resources, gender, race, ethnicity, social class, and availability and delivery of health care affect the quality of the aging experience. Biologic age is much more critical than chronologic age when determining the health status of the older adult.

Healthier lifestyles and advancements in medical treatment are creating a generation of successfully aging adults, which should decrease the negative stereotyping of older adults. Attitudes of all health care professionals, whether positive or negative, affect the care provided to the growing older adult population. Education about the mental and physiologic alterations associated with aging, along with the cultural, economic, and social influences accompanying aging, enables the radiographer to adapt imaging and therapeutic procedures to the older adult patient's disabilities resulting from age-related changes.

The human body undergoes a multiplicity of physiologic changes and failure in all organ systems. The aging experience is affected by heredity, lifestyle choices, physical health, and attitude, making it highly individualized. No individual's aging process is predictable and is never exactly the same as that of any other individual. Radiologic technologists must use their knowledge, abilities, and skills to adjust imaging procedures to accommodate for disabilities and diseases encountered with geriatric patients. Safety and comfort of the patient are essential in maintaining compliance throughout imaging procedures. Communication, listening, sensitivity, and empathy lead to patient compliance. The Joint Commission, recognizing the importance of age-based communication competencies for older adults, requires the employees of accredited health care organizations to document their achievement of these skills. Knowledge of age-related changes and disease processes enhances the radiographer's ability to provide care that meets the needs of the increasing older adult patient population.

References

1. Rarey LK: Radiologic technologists' responses to elderly patients, *Radiol Technol* 69(6):566–572, 1998.
2. Boswell SS: Predicting trainee ageism using knowledge, anxiety, compassion, and contact with older adults, *Educ Gerontol* 38(11):733–741, 2012.
3. Rowe JW, Kahn RL: *Successful aging*, New York, 1999, Dell.
4. Chop WC, Robnett RH: *Gerontology for the health care professional*, ed 2, Philadelphia, 2009, FA Davis.
5. Norris TG: Special needs of geriatric patients. *ASRT Homestudy Series* 4(5), 1999.

Selected bibliography

Administration for Community Living (ACL): What is elder abuse? (Website). 2016. Available at https://www.acl.gov/programs/elder-justice/what-elder-abuse. (Accessed November 2017).

Alzheimer's Association: Early-stage caregiving. (Website). 2017. Available at http://www.alz.org/care/alzheimers-early-mild-stage-caregiving.asp. (Accessed November 2017).

Alzheimer's Association: Research center: the search for Alzheimer's causes and risk factors. (Website). 2017. Available at http://www.alz.org/research/science/alzheimers_disease_causes.asp#age. (Accessed November 2017).

Campbell PR: *U.S. population projections by age, sex, race and hispanic origin: 1995 to 2025*, Washington, DC, 1996, U.S. Bureau of the Census, Population Division. PPL-47.

Chop WC, Robnett RH: *Gerontology for the health care professional*, ed 2, Philadelphia, 2009, Davis.

Damjanov I: *Pathology for the health professions*, 5th ed, St. Louis, 2017, Elsevier.

Ferrara MH: *Alzheimer's disease: human diseases and conditions*, ed 2, vol 1, Detroit, 2010, Charles Scribner's Sons, pp 70–76.

Garfein AJ, Herzog AR: Robust aging among the young-old, old-old, and oldest-old, *J Gerontol Soc Sci* 50B(Suppl):S77, 1995.

Health professions in service to the nation, San Francisco, 1993, Pew Health Professions Commission.

Hobbs FB, Danion BL: 65+ in the United States, 1996, Washington, DC, U.S. Department of Commerce and U.S. Department of Health and Human Service, pp 23–190.

Kudlas M, Odle T, Kisner L: The state of forensic radiography in the United States American Society of Radiographic Technicians (ASRT), 2010. https://www.asrt.org/docs/default-source/publications/whitepapers/forensic_radiography_white_paperfin.pdf. (Accessed September 2018).

Mayo Clinic: Alzheimer's stages: how the disease progresses. (Website). 2015. Available at https://www.mayoclinic.org/diseases-conditions/alzheimers-disease/in-depth/alzheimers-stages/art-20048448. (Accessed November 2017).

Mazess RB: On aging bone loss, *Clin Orthop Relat Res* 165:239–252, 1982.

National Committee for the Prevention of Elder Abuse (NCPEA): What role do health and medical professionals play in elder abuse prevention? (Website). 2008. Available at http://www.preventelderabuse.org/elderabuse/professionals/medical.html. (Accessed November 2017).

Norris T: Special needs of geriatric patients, American society of radiologic technologists homestudy series, vol 4, no 5, 1999.

Park A: Alzheimer's unlocked, *Time [serial online]* 176:53–59, 2010.

Rarey LK: Radiologic technologists' responses to elderly patients, *Radiol Technol* 69:566–572, 1996.

Rimer BK, Resch N, King E, et al: Multistrategy health education program to increase mammography use among women ages 65 and older, *Public Health Rep* 107:369–380, 1992.

Spencer G: *What are the demographic implications of an aging U.S. population from 1990 to 2030?*, Washington, DC, 1993, American Association of Retired Persons and Resources for the Future.

Thali MJ, Viner MD, Brogdon BG: *Brogdon's forensic radiology*, ed 2, Boca Raton, FL, 2011, CRC Press, pp 287–288.

Thibodeau GA, Patton KT: *Anatomy & physiology*, ed 8, St. Louis, 2013, Elsevier.

Turkington C, Harris JR: Alzheimer's disease. In *The encyclopedia of the brain and brain disorders*, 3rd ed, New York, 2010, Facts on File, pp 16–22.

University of Pittsburgh Schools of the Health Sciences: New compound identifies Alzheimer's disease brain toxins, study shows, *Science Daily* 2008. http://www.sciencedaily.com. (Retrieved 7 November, 2012).

U.S. Department of Commerce, Economics and Statistics Administration: *65+ in the United States*, Washington, DC, 2000, U.S. Bureau of the Census.

VanMeter KC, Hubert RJ: *Gould's pathophysiology for the health professions*, 5th ed, St. Louis, 2014, Elsevier.

24

SECTIONAL ANATOMY FOR RADIOGRAPHERS

REX T. CHRISTENSEN

Overview

Imaging modalities, such as computed tomography (CT), magnetic resonance imaging (MRI), and diagnostic medical sonography, require the technologist to look at anatomy images in a totally different way than they are used to with general radiographs. These technologies create cross-sectional imaging planes, in effect visualizing a slice through the body. The advantage of visualizing cross-sectional anatomic structures is that images can be viewed without the confusing superimposition of other anatomic parts. Images are generated in various orientations, such as axial, sagittal, coronal, and oblique planes. These planes make it crucial for the technologists working within these modalities to have a clear and complete understanding of general anatomic principles. Without a clear understanding of general anatomy, it is difficult to feel confident identifying normal and abnormal structures in cross section. This chapter provides the radiographer who possesses a background in general anatomy with an orientation to sectional anatomy and correlates that anatomy with structures shown on images from the various computer-generated imaging modalities.

There are three major imaging planes: axial, sagittal, and coronal. Images that are off-axis from these planes are termed oblique. Axial planes (sometimes referred to as *transverse planes* or *transaxial*) transect the body from anterior to posterior and from side to side. In effect, this type of horizontal plane divides the body into superior and inferior portions. Most images generated by CT are examples of axial or transverse planes. When looking at an axial image, it is helpful to imagine standing at the patient's feet and looking up toward the head. With this orientation, the patient's right side is to the viewer's left and vice versa. The anterior aspect of the patient is usually at the top of the image. Coronal planes divide the body into anterior and posterior portions. Coronal planes pass from superior to inferior and from side to side. Images viewed in the coronal plane are similar to radiographs in that the patient's right side is on the technologist's left (one can imagine facing the patient while viewing this type of image). Sagittal planes divide the body into right and left portions. These planes pass from superior to inferior and from anterior to posterior. MR images frequently use the coronal and sagittal planes to present the desired anatomy. CT images may be obtained in the coronal or sagittal planes, or the computer may reformat information from axial images to obtain images in these planes. Imaging planes that are generated from a single source are termed multiplanar reformat (MPR) images. Any plane that does not fit the previous descriptions is referred to as an *oblique plane*. Oblique planes are useful when imaging complicated structures, such as the heart. Source images obtained from the imaging modality can be compiled to produce not only MPR images, but also three-dimensional images (Fig. 24.1). The CT three-dimensional images displayed in Fig. 24.1 help the physician with surgical and oncology treatment planning, and patient instruction and education.

Fig. 24.1 Three-dimensional reconstructed CT image of the head.

CT uses x-rays to generate images, so the various shades on the images correspond to the gray scale that radiographers are accustomed to seeing. Bones and other dense materials are white, whereas air and lower density materials are closer to black. Fat, muscle, and organs are represented with various shades of gray. Hounsfield units or CT numbers represent the scale of white to black that is used in CT imaging. Lower numbers represent anatomic structures that are more easily penetrated by the x-ray and appear closer to black on the image. Higher numbers are related to more radiopaque structures and are lighter gray or white on the image. Similar to routine radiographs, blood vessels and organs of the digestive system are not easily distinguishable from other structures. Tissue contrast limitations require these structures to be identified more accurately; therefore patients are frequently given a radiopaque contrast medium. Intravascular contrast medium highlights vessels, making them appear radiopaque and whiter on the image. To visualize the gastrointestinal system, patients may be given a contrast agent by mouth or via the rectum. A full description of CT fundamentals is presented in Chapter 25.

MRI uses magnetic fields and radiofrequencies to generate images. Anatomic structures are represented on the image with regard to the signal generated from their protons. Structures that produce a strong signal are generally lighter gray or white on the image, and structures that do not generate a strong signal tend to be darker on the image. The signal generated by these structures depends on many things, including the strength of the magnetic fields, relaxation times of tissues, and the radiofrequency characteristics of anatomical structures. Contrast medium may also be used when performing MRI to change the signal intensity of particular anatomic structures. Gadolinium, air, and fluid may be used as contrast agents, depending on the organ of interest and the imaging sequences employed. MRI is discussed in depth in Chapter 26.

The cadaveric sections depicted in this chapter are representative of major organ structures for each of the body regions, and they *are depicted from the inferior surface to correspond to the images.* All relational terms are used in relation to the body in anatomic position. (When a structure is described as being to the right of something, this refers to the *patient's* right, not the *viewer's* right.) The major anatomic structures normally seen when using current imaging modalities are labeled. For each region of the body, a cadaveric section is presented, and representative images are included to provide an orientation to anatomic structures normally seen using the available imaging modalities. The cadaveric sections and diagnostic images do not match exactly; some structures are seen on only one of the illustrations for each body region. Major anatomic structures in each region of the body are reviewed in the following sections to make it easier to identify the images provided. Systematic review of the bones, vessels, major organs, and muscles begin each section. Selected images are presented in axial, sagittal, and coronal planes to show these structures. In practice, images should be examined collectively because the size, shape, and placement of these structures vary from slice to slice. Scrolling through the various slices of a structure is frequently the ideal way to identify the size and characteristics of that structure.

Cranial Region

Fig. 24.2 is a cadaveric image that can be used to distinguish bone, muscle, and other soft tissue structures. Referring to this image is helpful in identifying the sometimes confusing shadows on the images. The head can be thought of systematically as being composed of the skull, central nervous system structures, various sensory organs, cranial blood supply, and associated cranial and facial muscles. The bones of the skull are categorized as the 8 cranial bones and the 14 facial bones. The cranial bones include the frontal, occipital, and two parietal bones that surround and protect the external surface of the brain. The other four cranial bones include the ethmoid, sphenoid, and two temporal bones. The frontal bone forms the anterior surface of the skull, with a vertical portion that corresponds to the forehead and a horizontal portion that forms the roof of the orbits. Between the inner and outer layers of the vertical portion of the frontal bone, just superior to the level of the eyes, are the paired frontal paranasal sinuses. The vertex is the most superior portion of the skull and is formed by the paired parietal bones. These roughly square-shaped bones articulate with the frontal bone at the coronal suture, with the temporal bones at the squamosal sutures, with the occipital bone at the lambdoidal suture, and with each other at the sagittal suture.

The posterior aspect of the skull is formed by the occipital bone, which is composed of a squamous (vertical) portion and a basilar portion. The foramen magnum is a large opening within the squamous portion that allows passage of the spinal cord into the brain. The external occipital protuberance is a large prominence on the posterior surface of this bone. Roughly corresponding in position to this landmark is the internal occipital protuberance. The ethmoid bone is found within the cranium and forms the medial walls of the orbits and part of the lateral walls of the nasal cavity. The ethmoid bone is divided into a horizontal portion called the *cribriform plate* and vertical portions called the *perpendicular plate* and *two labyrinths* or *lateral masses.*

The cribriform plate lies between the orbital plates of the frontal bone and supports the olfactory bulbs (cranial nerve I). The cribriform plate is perforated by many small foramina, which transmit nerves from the nose to this cranial nerve. Projecting superiorly from the cribriform plate is a small ridge of bone called the *crista galli,* which serves as the anterior attachment for the falx cerebri. Projecting inferiorly from the center of the cribriform plate is the perpendicular plate. This thin strip of bone forms the superior part of the bony nasal septum. Extending inferiorly from the lateral edges of the cribriform plate are the labyrinths or lateral masses. These are perforated by multiple air spaces, which are collectively called the *ethmoidal paranasal sinuses.* From the medial surface of each labyrinth, two scroll-shaped ridges of bone project into the nasal cavity. These are the superior and middle nasal conchae.

In the center of the base of the skull is the sphenoid bone. This bone is sometimes referred to as the *anchor bone of the cranium* because it articulates with all of

Fig. 24.2 (A) Line drawing of gross anatomic section. (B) Cadaveric image of skull.

the cranial bones. Thinking of this bone as being composed of a body, two sets of wings, and a pterygoid portion is helpful. The body is the central portion of the bone and contains the easily identifiable landmark known as the *sella turcica*. The sella turcica forms a cup-shaped depression that surrounds and protects the pituitary gland. The anterior surface of the sella is called the *tuberculum sellae*, and the posterior portion is called the *dorsum sellae*. Two posterior clinoid processes project from the superior edge of the dorsum sellae and are attachments for dura mater partitions. Within the body of the sphenoid and inferior to the sella turcica are the paired sphenoidal paranasal sinuses. The lesser wings of the sphenoid are triangular ridges of bone found posterior to the orbital plates of the frontal bone. Directly inferior to the medial edge of each lesser wing is the optic canal, which transmits the optic nerve (cranial nerve II). The larger, greater wings support the temporal lobes of the cerebrum and extend from the body to the external surface of the skull. The pterygoid processes project inferiorly from the body of the sphenoid and form the posterior walls of the nasal cavity.

The temporal bones form part of the lateral walls of the cranium and extend internally to meet the sphenoid and the basilar portion of the occipital bone. Parts of the temporal bone include the squamous, tympanic, mastoid, and petrous portions. The squamous portion is the thin, fan-shaped external part of the bone superior to the external ear. It articulates with the parietal and several other cranial bones. Its articulation with the parietal bone is called the *squamous suture*. The tympanic portion is the area of the bone surrounding the external ear canal. The zygomatic process arches anteriorly from just superior to the external ear canal. Just inferior to the origin of the zygomatic process is the mandibular fossa, in which the condyle of the mandible is found. On the inferior surface of the tympanic portion of the bone is the styloid process, which serves as an attachment for muscles. Posterior to the ear is the mastoid portion, which is perforated by many small, air-filled cavities. The mastoid portion extends inferiorly to form the cone-shaped mastoid process. The petrous portion of the bone lies within the cranium, normally forming an angle of approximately 45 degrees to the median sagittal plane. This dense ridge of bone surrounds and protects the organs

of hearing and balance, the facial and vestibulocochlear nerves, and the internal carotid artery.

The organs associated with the face are surrounded and protected by 14 bones. Each of these bones is paired with the exception of the vomer and the mandible. The lacrimal bones are about the size of a fingernail, and are found in the medial wall of the orbit between the maxilla and the labyrinth of the ethmoid bones. The nasal bones form the bridge of the nose and articulate superiorly with the frontal bone, laterally with the maxilla, and with each other in the midline. The zygomatic bones form the inferolateral walls of the orbits. Each of these bones articulates superiorly with the frontal bone, medially with the maxilla, and laterally with the zygomatic process of the temporal bone. The maxilla originates as two separate bones, which ultimately fuse along the midsagittal plane. This large bone forms the inferior surface of each orbit, the lateral walls of the nasal cavity, and the anterior portion of the roof of the mouth. On either side of the nasal cavity, large air-filled maxillary paranasal sinuses are embedded within the bone. The upper teeth are rooted within the alveolar process at the anteroinferior surface of the bone. The maxilla articulates with the nasal bones, the lacrimal bones, the frontal bone, the zygomatic bones, and the palatine bones. The inferior nasal conchae are scroll-shaped facial bones found in the nasal cavity, just inferior to the middle nasal conchae of the ethmoid bone. The L-shaped palatine bones form the posterior portion of the hard palate. The vertical portions of the palatines extend superiorly along the posterior nasal cavity to form a small part of the posterior orbit.

The vomer is an unpaired facial bone that rests on the hard palate and articulates with the inferior surface of the perpendicular plate of the ethmoid. It forms the inferior portion of the bony nasal septum. The mandible, which is also an unpaired facial bone, is formed by a body and two rami. The body comprises the anterior portion of the bone and presents an alveolar ridge in which the lower teeth are embedded. The rami extend superiorly from the body and end in anterior and posterior bony processes. The anterior process at the superior end of the ramus is the coronoid process, where muscles of mastication attach. The posterior process is the condyloid process, which rests in

the mandibular fossa of the temporal bone. This articulation, the temporomandibular joint, is the only movable articulation associated with the skull. (Refer to Chapter 11 for review of skull anatomy.)

The brain is surrounded by three layers of protective membranes called the *meninges*. From internal to external, they are the pia mater, arachnoid, and dura mater. The pia mater adheres directly to the brain and is composed of a fine network of capillaries and supporting tissue. The arachnoid is a delicate membrane that resembles a cobweb. The subarachnoid space lies between the arachnoid and pia mater. Cerebrospinal fluid (CSF) circulates in this space. The arachnoid does not closely adhere to cerebral structures. As it bridges the gap between various parts of the brain, enlarged regions or cisterns are formed in the subarachnoid space. Some of the more crucial cisterns include the cisterna magna, pontine, interpeduncular, and superior or *quadrigeminal cistern*. The cisterna magna is the largest of these and is found just inside the foramen magnum, between the cerebellum and the medulla oblongata. This cistern receives CSF from the fourth ventricle. The pontine cistern lies anterior to the pons and contains the basilar artery. The interpeduncular cistern is anterior to the midbrain. The infundibulum (stalk) of the pituitary and the vessels of the circle of Willis are seen here. The cistern found posterior to the midbrain is the superior cistern. It surrounds the pineal gland and the great cerebral vein. Ambient cisterns communicate with the superior cistern and extend laterally around the midbrain. The most external of the meninges is the double-layered dura mater. The outer layer of dura is attached to the inner surface of the cranial bones. The inner layer can be seen between cerebral structures and in large fissures. Dural sinuses are venous drainage channels formed where the inner dural layers separate from the outer layer. One of the largest dural flaps, the falx cerebri, is found in the longitudinal fissure between the cerebral hemispheres. It extends from the crista galli of the ethmoid to the occipital bone. The tentorium cerebelli extends between the cerebrum and the cerebellum. It attaches to the sella turcica and the internal surface of the occipital bones.

The structures of the central nervous system within the skull include the cerebrum, brain stem, and cerebellum. The cerebrum is the largest of these structures and is divided by the longitudinal fissure into two hemispheres. The hemispheres are connected to each other via a white matter tract called the *corpus callosum.* This arch-shaped structure is divided into the anterior genu, central body, and posterior splenium. Each cerebral hemisphere is divided into lobes that are named for the most adjacent cranial bone: frontal, parietal, temporal, and occipital. An additional lobe called the insula is buried deep to the temporal lobe. The cerebrum is thrown into numerous folds called *gyri,* which are separated by small fissures called *sulci.* The outer surface of the cerebrum consists of a thin layer of gray matter. The central portion of this part of the brain is mainly white matter (formed by myelinated nerve fibers). These fibers, referred to as the *corona radiata,* connect the gray matter of the cortex to deeper gray matter nuclei deep within each hemisphere. The buried gray matter centers are called *basal nuclei* or *basal ganglia* and include the claustrum, putamen, globus pallidus, and caudate nucleus. White matter tracts, or capsules, are found between these gray matter structures. Other gray matter structures found within the central cerebrum include the thalamus and hypothalamus. These form the walls of the third ventricle. Many of these gray and white matter structures are seen on the cadaveric section in Fig. 24.2.

The brain stem is formed by the midbrain, pons, and medulla oblongata. It lies between the cerebrum and cerebellum and serves as a relay for nerve impulses between the spinal cord and these two structures. The midbrain is the most superior of the three. White matter tracts called the cerebral peduncles extend from the anterior midbrain to the cerebrum. Toward the posterior aspect of the midbrain are the corpora quadrigemina, which are formed by two superior and two inferior colliculi that lie just inferior to the splenium of the corpus callosum. The cerebral aqueduct drains cerebrospinal (CSF) from the third ventricle to the fourth ventricle and passes through the posterior portion of the midbrain. The central portion of the brain stem is formed by the pons. It communicates with the medulla, with the midbrain, and via white matter cerebellar peduncles to the cerebellum. The most inferior of the brain stem structures is the medulla oblongata, which is continuous with the spinal cord as it passes through the foramen magnum.

The cerebellum lies in the posteroinferior region of the cranium. Although smaller in size, it is similar in composition to the cerebrum. A midline fissure divides the cerebellum into hemispheres that are connected by a midline vermis. It is also thrown into numerous small folds, here called folia, which are separated by numerous small fissures. The outer surface of the cerebellum is composed of gray matter, with white matter constituting most of the central portion of this part of the brain. Gray matter nuclei can be found here also, although they are difficult to distinguish on images and are not discussed in this chapter.

Four large cavities called *ventricles* are found in the brain. The ventricles' major function is to produce and store CSF; this is accomplished as blood is filtered through capillary networks called *choroid plexuses* in each of the ventricles. The largest of these chambers are the lateral ventricles, one of which is found in each cerebral hemisphere. The lateral ventricles are divided into a body and anterior, posterior, and inferior horns. CSF from these chambers passes into the midline third ventricle through the interventricular foramina. The third ventricle is found between the cerebral hemispheres inferior to the lateral ventricles. The cerebral aqueduct drains CSF from the third ventricle to the fourth ventricle. The fourth ventricle is found between the cerebellum and the brain stem. Its walls are formed by white matter tracts called *cerebellar peduncles,* which connect the brain stem and cerebellum. A central aperture and two lateral apertures allow CSF to pass from the fourth ventricle into the subarachnoid space.

The brain is a highly metabolic organ, and to function well it needs a rich blood supply. Four major arteries supply the brain and its related structures: the two internal carotid arteries and the two vertebral arteries. The internal carotid arteries supply the anterior structures of the brain. After passing superiorly through the neck, these arteries enter the skull via the carotid canals in the petrous portion of the temporal bones. After exiting the petrous portion, the internal carotid arteries pass along the lateral aspect of the sella turcica, ultimately dividing into the anterior and middle cerebral arteries. The posterior communicating artery arises from the internal carotid just before this bifurcation. The anterior cerebral arteries pass anteriorly and superiorly to the longitudinal fissure, where they curl around the external aspect of the corpus callosum and supply the anterior portion of the brain. The middle cerebral arteries pass laterally to the lateral fissures, where their branches supply the middle portion of the brain. The posterior communicating arteries pass posteriorly to join with the branches from the vertebrobasilar arterial system. The vertebral arteries traverse the neck in the transverse foramina of the cervical spine and enter the posterior skull via the foramen magnum. These arteries pass superiorly along the anterior aspect of the medulla and at the base of the pons join to form the basilar artery. At the superior aspect of the pons, the basilar artery splits to form the posterior cerebral arteries. A unique arterial anastomosis exists in the brain to protect it from sudden loss of blood supply. This vascular connection is called the *circle of Willis.* The blood supply to the anterior brain is connected to the blood supply for the posterior brain as the posterior communicating arteries extend from the internal carotid arteries to the posterior cerebral arteries. This communication lies in the interpeduncular cistern, just anterior to the midbrain.

Venous drainage in the cranium is accomplished by two systems: cerebral veins and dural venous sinuses. The dural sinuses are created by gaps formed between the inner and outer layers of the dura mater. These gaps are found in the areas where the dura invaginates between the various structures of the brain. The superior sagittal sinus is found in the superior border of the falx cerebri, and the inferior sagittal sinus is found in its inferior margin. The channel formed where the falx cerebri meets the tentorium cerebelli is the straight sinus (Fig. 24.3). This sinus is a continuation of the inferior sagittal sinus as it joins with the great cerebral vein. The great cerebral vein, also known as the vein of Galen, continues under the corpus callosum to form the internal cerebral vein. The transverse or lateral sinuses are found along the lateral aspect of the tentorium cerebelli as it meets the occipital bone. At the level of the petrous portions of the temporal bones, the transverse sinuses curl medially and inferiorly and become known as the *sigmoid sinuses.* As the sigmoid sinuses pass out of the cranium via the jugular foramina, these vessels change names again and become the internal jugular veins. One of the major veins within the skull is the great cerebral vein. This large venous structure is found in the superior cistern, and there it joins the inferior sagittal sinus to form the straight sinus.

Many muscles are associated with the face, only a few of which are referred to in the following sections. The temporalis muscle is found on the external surface of the squamous portion of the temporal bone. Its inferior attachment is to the coronoid process of the mandible. On the external surface of the mandibular rami are the masseter muscles, and on the internal surface of the rami are the pterygoid muscles. These muscles all are associated with moving the mandible and with swallowing (Fig. 24.4).

Superior Sagittal Sinus

Great Cerebral Vein

Internal Cerebral Vein

Straight Sinus

Fig. 24.3 Midsagittal contrast enhanced MR image of the brain.

Temporalis Muscle

Masseter Muscle

Lateral Pterygoid Muscle

Fig. 24.4 Axial T1-weighted MR image of the brain.

A lateral skull radiograph is used here for localization of the imaging plane in this section (Fig. 24.5A), and a sagittal MR image (see Fig. 24.5B) is used for localization of MRI cross sections of the brain. CT imaging for the cranium may be performed with the gantry parallel to or angled 15 to 20 degrees to the orbitomeatal line. Angling the gantry of the CT scanner allows for imaging of the brain without excess radiation to the eyes. MRI of the cranium generally results in images that are parallel to the orbitomeatal or infraorbitomeatal plane. More details on patient positioning for CT are provided in Chapter 25, and information on patient positioning for MRI is provided in Chapter 26. Because the imaging planes may be different for CT and MRI, some variation exists in the anatomic structures visualized on corresponding illustrations in this section. Seven identifying lines represent the approximate levels for each of the labeled images for this region.

The cranial CT image seen in Fig. 24.6 represents a CT slice obtained through the frontal and parietal bones, and Fig. 24.7 is a corresponding T2-weighted MR image. The *cortex*, or outer layer of gray matter, can be differentiated from the deeper *white matter*. The numerous *gyri*, or *convolutions*, and *sulci* are shown and are surrounded by the darker appearing CSF in the subarachnoid space. The *cerebral hemispheres* are separated by the *longitudinal cerebral fissure*. Invaginated in this fissure is a fold of *dura mater* called the *falx cerebri*. The *superior sagittal sinus*, which passes through the superior margin of the falx cerebri, follows the contour of the superior skull margin. In cross section, the anterior and posterior aspects of this sinus can normally be seen in the midline deep to the bony plates when the patient has been given an intravenous contrast agent, and appear as triangular expansions near the bones easily seen on both the CT and MR images. Two of the five *cerebral*

Fig. 24.5 (A) CT localizer (scout) image of skull. (B) Sagittal localizer for MRI of the brain.

Fig. 24.6 (A) Line drawing of CT section. (B) CT image representing anatomic structures located at level *A* in Fig. 24.5A.

lobes are seen (frontal and parietal). The *corona radiata* is the central tract of white matter in the cerebrum and is darker than the cortex on the CT image; the white matter is lighter than the gray matter on the MR image. These sections were obtained at a level that passes through the superiormost portion of the *corpus callosum*, which separates the anterior and posterior portions of the falx cerebri.

Fig. 24.8 is an axial CT slice through the superior portions of the lateral ventricles; Fig. 24.9 is the corresponding T1-weighted MR image. Visualized bony structures on the CT scan include the *frontal bone* and the two *parietal bones*. The falx cerebri is seen within the *longitudinal fissure*. The *frontal lobes* and *parietal lobes* of the cerebrum are shown. In the center of each image, the *lateral ventricles* are easily seen because of the dark appearance of the CSF circulating within each. In the posterior portions of the ventricles, the contrast-filled capillary network of the *choroid plexuses* also is visualized. A thin membrane called the *septum pellucidum* can be seen separating the ventricles. The corpus callosum is an arch-shaped structure; in cross section at this level, only the anterior *genu* and the posterior *splenium* can be seen. The *caudate nuclei* lie along the lateral surfaces of the ventricles and tend to follow their curves. Because these nuclei are composed of gray matter, they are the same shade of gray as the cortex on MR images (see Fig. 24.9). Several

Fig. 24.7 MRI corresponding to level *A* in Fig. 24.5B.

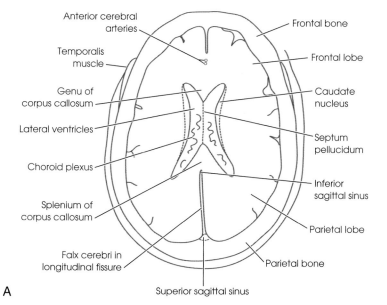

Anterior cerebral arteries
Temporalis muscle
Genu of corpus callosum
Lateral ventricles
Choroid plexus
Splenium of corpus callosum
Falx cerebri in longitudinal fissure
Superior sagittal sinus

Frontal bone
Frontal lobe
Caudate nucleus
Septum pellucidum
Inferior sagittal sinus
Parietal lobe
Parietal bone

A

B

Fig. 24.8 (A) Line drawing of CT section. (B) CT image representing structures located at level *B* in Fig. 24.5A.

Fig. 24.9 MRI corresponding to level *B* in Fig. 24.5B.

contrast-filled vascular structures are visible. The *anterior cerebral arteries* lie within the longitudinal fissure just anterior to the genu of the corpus callosum. A few branches of the *middle cerebral arteries* are seen near the lateral aspect of the skull on the CT scan. The anterior and posterior portions of the superior sagittal sinus are seen in the periphery of the falx cerebri. The *inferior sagittal sinus* lies in the internal edges of the falx. The thin strips of muscle seen on the external surface of the frontal bone correspond to the superior edges of the *temporalis muscles*.

The axial sections through the midportion of the cerebrum show many of the central structures of the cerebral hemispheres. (Fig. 24.10 is a CT image, and Fig. 24.11 is a T1-weighted MR image.) Images at this level pass through the frontal bone, greater wing of the *sphenoid*, and squamous portion of the *temporal bones*. The posterior portion of the skull comprises the top portion (squamous portion) of the *occipital bone* at this level. The falx cerebri is shown within the longitudinal fissure, with the superior sagittal sinus best shown in the midline of

the anterior and posterior margins of this membrane. In the CT image, the genu of the corpus callosum is found between the anterior horns of the lateral ventricles; however, the posterior portion of this slice is inferior to the level of the splenium. The MR image shows the genu and the splenium. At this level, the MR image shows the *frontal, temporal,* and *occipital lobes* along with the *insula* (fifth lobe or island of Reil), which is deep to the temporal lobe at the lateral fissure. Because of its orientation, the CT image shows the insula, frontal, and temporal lobes; the

Fig. 24.10 (A) Line drawing of CT section. (B) CT image representing anatomic structures located at level *C* in Fig. 24.5A.

Fig. 24.11 MRI representing anatomic structures located at level *C* in Fig. 24.5B.

cerebellum occupies the posterior aspect of the skull in this image.

The anterior and temporal horns of the lateral ventricles are seen on the CT scan, whereas the anterior and posterior horns are visible on the MR image. Within each posterior horn is a portion of the choroid plexus, which appears bright owing to the presence of contrast medium in the capillaries. The heads of the caudate nuclei lie along the external surfaces of the anterior horns of each lateral ventricle. Several areas of gray matter can be seen faintly on the CT image deep within the white matter of the cerebrum and constitute the basal nuclei. The MR image contrast has been enhanced so that the deep gray matter structures can be seen. The major components of the basal nuclei seen at this level are (from lateral to medial) the *claustrum*, *lentiform nucleus* (composed of the putamen and globus pallidus), and *caudate nucleus*. The lentiform nucleus is separated from the caudate nucleus and thalamus by a tract of white matter known as the *internal capsule*. These sections pass through the superior portion of the midline *third ventricle*. The *thalamus*, which serves as a central relay station for sensory impulses to the cerebral cortex, forms its lateral walls. The plane of the CT image passes through the structures of the midbrain. The anterior portions of the midbrain include the cerebral peduncles (white matter tracts that connect the cerebrum and the midbrain). The dark circular area at the posterior edge of the midbrain is the CSF-filled cerebral aqueduct. This passage connects the third and fourth ventricles and allows the circulation of CSF. A contrast-enhanced vessel, the great cerebral vein, is found just posterior to the third ventricle and the splenium of the corpus callosum on the MR image. It passes through the upper portion of the *superior cistern*. The pineal gland is also found in this cistern but is not clearly visualized in either image. This is an important radiographic landmark because of its tendency to calcify in adults. Branches of the middle cerebral artery are visible within the lateral fissures, and the anterior cerebral arteries can be seen in the anterior portion of the longitudinal fissure on the MR image.

Fig. 24.12 is a CT image that passes through the frontal lobe, pons, and cerebellum; Fig. 24.13 is the T2-weighted MR

Fig. 24.12 (A) Line drawing of CT section. (B) CT image representing anatomic structures located at level *D* in Fig. 24.5A.

Fig. 24.13 MRI through circle of Willis corresponding to level *D* in Fig. 24.5B.

image, which passes through the orbits, the midbrain, and the occipital lobes. Bony structures visible in the CT image include the frontal bone, the temporal bones, and the occipital bone. Within the temporal bones, the black air-filled structures represent the mastoid air cells. The internal protrusion of bone in the center of the occipital bone is the internal occipital protuberance. The darker area between the eyes on the MR image corresponds to the lower portion of the frontal sinuses. Frontal and temporal lobes of the cerebrum are shown on the CT image, whereas the frontal, temporal, and occipital lobes of the cerebrum are shown on the MR image. The CT scan passes just inferior to the midbrain, and the MR image passes through the level of the midbrain. The large dark area in the center of the CT image is the interpeduncular cistern. This is an enlarged area in the subarachnoid space containing CSF. The optic chiasm and the circle of Willis normally lie within the interpeduncular cistern. The pituitary stalk and some of the vessels that contribute to the circle of Willis are visible on this image. The pons lies posterior to the cistern. The cerebellum lies within the posterior fossa of the skull between the pons and the occipital bone. The large dark region between the pons and cerebellum is the CSF-filled fourth ventricle. The temporalis muscles are seen on the external surfaces on either side of the cranium. On the MR image, the *cerebral peduncles* form the anterior portions of the midbrain, and the *corpora quadrigemina* forms the posterior portion. The small light gray circle anterior to the colliculi is the CSF-filled *cerebral aqueduct*. Posterior to the midbrain is the *cerebellum*, which is surrounded by the *tentorium cerebelli*. The dark region anterior to the midbrain is the *interpeduncular cistern*, and the region posterior to the midbrain is the superior cistern. On the MR image, within and around the interpeduncular cistern the *optic tracts* are visualized, along with the *hypothalamus*, the inferior portion of the third ventricle, and *mammillary bodies*.

The CT image is just superior to the internal carotid arteries and shows the origins of the left anterior and middle cerebral arteries, at the anterior edge of the interpeduncular cistern. The anterior cerebral arteries pass from their origin toward the longitudinal fissure in the midline of the brain; the middle cerebral arteries course from their origins toward the lateral fissures. The CT image also shows the bifurcation of the basilar artery into the two posterior cerebral arteries. These vessels can be seen just anterior to the pons. The MR image shows the posterior portion of the superior sagittal sinus located near the internal occipital protuberance; the *straight sinus* can be seen in the edge of the tentorium cerebelli, just posterior to the cerebellum on the MR image.

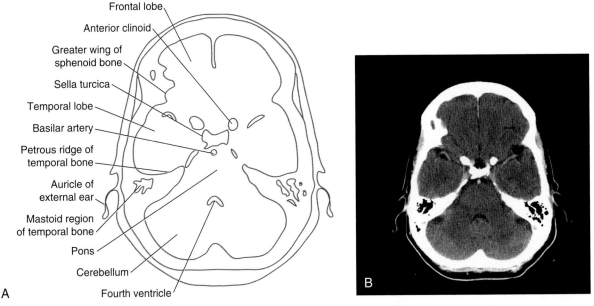

Frontal lobe
Anterior clinoid
Greater wing of sphenoid bone
Sella turcica
Temporal lobe
Basilar artery
Petrous ridge of temporal bone
Auricle of external ear
Mastoid region of temporal bone
Pons
Cerebellum
Fourth ventricle

A

B

Fig. 24.14 (A) Line drawing of CT section. (B) CT image representing anatomic structures located at level *E* in Fig. 24.5A.

Fig. 24.14 is a CT image through the sella turcica and the posterior fossa. The T1-weighted MR image (Fig. 24.15) passes through the center of the orbits, the tops of the ears, the pituitary and center of the sella turcica, and the cerebellum. The MR image shows the *nasal bones*, visible in the anterior skull. Between the eyes the *ethmoidal sinuses* and the *cribriform plate* of the ethmoid bone is seen. The *sphenoidal sinuses* lie posterior to the ethmoidal sinuses. The *sella turcica* and *dorsum sellae* are seen surrounding the *pituitary gland.* Several cranial bones are visible on the CT scan. The anterior clinoids of the sella turcica and the greater wings of the sphenoid are seen. The roof of the sella is formed by the lesser wings, anterior clinoids, and posterior clinoids. The temporal bone constitutes most of the lateral portions of the skull, and the *petrous ridges* can be seen on the CT image extending toward the median sagittal plane. The black air spaces near the lateral aspect of the petrous portions of these bones correspond to *mastoid air cells*, and the air spaces farther medial are associated with the internal structures of the ear. On the CT image, the frontal and temporal lobes of the cerebrum are visible, along with the pons and cerebellum. The dark region between the sella turcica and the pons is the pontine cistern, filled with CSF. The lower region of the fourth ventricle is seen between the pons and the cerebellum. On the MR image, both *globes* are visible within the orbits. Rectus muscles lie along the medial and lateral walls of each. The *optic nerves* are seen in the centers of the posterior orbits passing from the eyes toward the brain via the optic canal. The temporal lobes are found lateral to the sella turcica, resting in the middle cranial fossa. The *pons* lies posterior to the sella, and the cerebellum is seen filling the posterior cranial fossa. The edges of the tentorium cerebelli can be seen faintly between the temporal lobes and the cerebellum. The dark region anterior to the pons corresponds to the CSF-filled *pontine cistern* in which the contrast-filled *basilar artery* is easily visualized on both the CT and MR images. The dark region between the pons and the cerebellum is the superior region of the *fourth ventricle*. On the CT image, the contrast-filled basilar artery lies between the sella and the pons. At this level in the MR image, the *internal carotid arteries* lie lateral to the body of the sphenoid bone in an almost horizontal orientation. The *confluence of sinuses* can be seen just anterior to the internal occipital protuberance on the MR image. The confluence is the region where the superior sagittal sinus and the straight sinus meet the transverse sinuses. The *transverse sinuses* are seen on the MR image at this level lying just internal to the occipital bone. On the external surface of the skull in both images, the temporalis muscles lie along the temporal bones. The *auricle*, or cartilaginous portion of each ear, lies external to the temporal bone.

Fig. 24.15 T2-weighted MRI corresponding to the level of *E* in Fig. 24.5B.

The sectional images through the lower cranium show the inferior portions of the cerebrum, brain stem, cerebellum, and associated major skeletal structures. (Fig. 24.16 is a CT image, and Fig. 24.17 is a T1-weighted MR image.) The CT image shows the frontal sinuses and the roofs of the orbits. The greater and lesser wings of the sphenoid bone are shown. The optic foramina (canals) can be seen between the greater and lesser wings. The optic chiasm and cavernous sinus can be seen posterior to the optic foramen. The petrous and mastoid portions of the temporal bones are shown dividing the middle and posterior cranial fossae. The maxilla,

maxillary sinuses, and nasal bones are seen in the anterior skull on the MR image (note the mass within the right maxillary sinus). The *zygomatic bones* form the lateral walls of the orbits, and the *maxillae* form the medial walls. The *perpendicular plate* and *vomer* form the bony nasal septum seen in the center of the nasal cavity. Posterior to the nasal cavity, the sphenoidal sinuses are seen between the lower aspects of the greater wings. Both petrous ridges extend toward the midline; these are seen as dark areas on the MR image because of the lack of signal from this dense region of bone. Extending into the right petrous ridge is the *external auditory canal*. Just anterior

to the canal is the *condyle of the mandible* resting in the mandibular fossa. Mastoid air cells lie posterior to the external acoustic meatus.

In the center of the skull, the greater wings of the sphenoid, petrous ridges, and basilar portion of the occipital bone meet. The CT image shows the lower portions of the frontal lobes and temporal lobes, along with the lower margin of the pons and the cerebellum. On the MR image, the most inferior folds of the temporal lobes are found in the middle cranial fossae resting on the greater wings of the sphenoid. The *medulla oblongata* lies posterior to the basilar portion of the occipital bone.

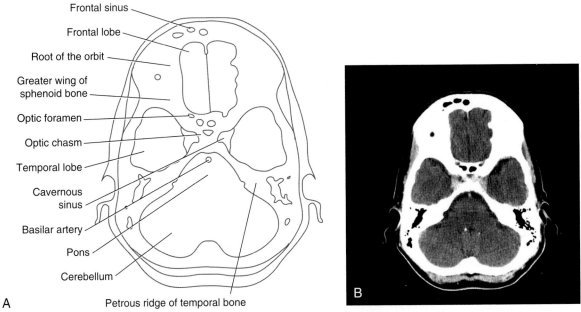

Fig. 24.16 (A) Line drawing of CT section. (B) CT image representing anatomic structures located at level *F* in Fig. 24.5A.

Fig. 24.17 MRI representing anatomic structures located at level *F* in Fig. 24.5B.

The cerebellum is seen within the posterior fossa. The small, dark space between the medulla and the cerebellum is the lower extent of the fourth ventricle. CSF in the *cisterna magna* circulates around the anterior and lateral reaches of the medulla. At the level of this image, the internal carotid arteries are found just posterior to the optic foramina, within the cavernous sinuses, on the CT scan; both are clearly visible as bright circles on the MR image. The *internal jugular veins* can also be seen on the MR image just posterior to the internal carotid arteries. The two *vertebral arteries* join, and lie anterior to the medulla on the MR image. The CT image is just superior to the junction of the vertebral arteries and shows the lower part of the basilar artery. The transverse venous sinuses have passed anteriorly to the level of the petrous ridges and are seen on the MR image. At this point, they change position and change names to become the *sigmoid sinuses.*

Fig. 24.18 is a CT image, and Fig. 24.19 is a T1-weighted MR image through the lower part of the skull. The plane of the CT image passes through the upper orbit, the sphenoidal sinuses, and the lower portion of the occipital bone. The frontal sinuses lie along the anterior skull. The crista galli is just posterior to these sinuses. This structure is a superior projection of bone from the cribriform plate of the ethmoid bone; it functions as an attachment for the falx cerebri. On either side of the crista galli, the lowermost portions of the frontal lobes can be seen resting on the cribriform plate. The sphenoidal sinuses lie posterior

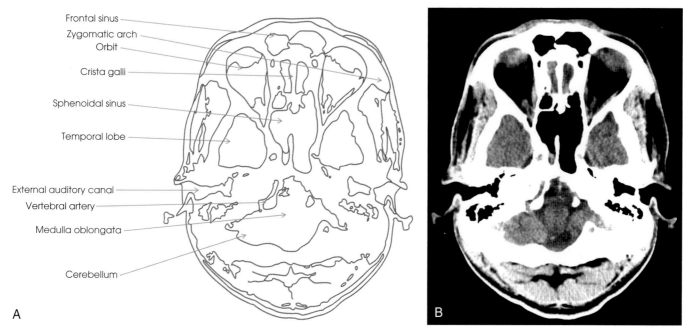

Frontal sinus
Zygomatic arch
Orbit
Crista galli
Sphenoidal sinus
Temporal lobe
External auditory canal
Vertebral artery
Medulla oblongata
Cerebellum

A

B

Fig. 24.18 (A) Line drawing of CT section. (B) CT image representing anatomic structures located at level *G* in Fig. 24.5A.

Inferior nasal concha
Mandibular ramus
Nasopharynx
Internal carotid artery
Vertebral artery

Fig. 24.19 MRI corresponding to level *G* in Fig. 24.5B.

to the crista galli, and the greater wings of the sphenoid extend laterally from the region of the sinuses. The external auditory canals extend into the petrous portions of the temporal bones, and mastoid air cells are visible posterior to the canals. The lower portion of the occipital bone forms the most posterior region of the skull on this image.

The MR image plane passes through the nose and the base of the skull. On the MR image, the large, air-filled maxillary sinuses lie on either side of the nose. The *inferior nasal conchae* and the vomer are seen within the nasal cavity. Posterior to the nasal cavity, the nasopharynx is seen on the MR image. Portions of the zygomatic arches are seen extending posteriorly from the sides of the sinuses on CT. The MR image is slightly inferior to the mandibular condyles and shows the rami of the mandible. The MR image passes through the mastoid processes and the top of the vertebral column. The CT shows the lower temporal lobes of the cerebrum, the *cerebellar tonsils*, and the medulla oblongata. The MR image shows the spinal cord because the structures in this image lie inferior to the foramen magnum. The contrast-filled internal carotid arteries lie anterior and lateral to the foramen magnum and spinal cord on the MR image but are not visible on the CT image. As the

sigmoid venous sinuses pass through the jugular foramina, they become the internal jugular veins. These veins are visible on the MR image posterior and lateral to the internal carotid arteries. The contrast-filled vertebral arteries are seen along the anterolateral aspects of the medulla and spinal cord. Muscular structures on the external surface of the mandible are the *masseters*, and the structures on the internal surface are the *pterygoids*.

Images in sagittal, coronal, and oblique planes are becoming increasingly more common. CT scanners have the capability to generate images in the axial and coronal planes and to reconstruct the information in alternate planes. Magnetic resonance is capable of direct axial, sagittal, oblique, and coronal imaging. Representative images have been selected in the sagittal and coronal planes to help interpret the anatomy shown.

Fig. 24.20 is a PA skull (Caldwell method) image used to represent the locations of the following sagittal images of the brain. Fig. 24.21 is a midsagittal T1-weighted MR image of the cranium. The relationship among the cerebral hemisphere, cerebellum, and brain stem is shown. In this image, the frontal, parietal, and occipital lobes of the cerebrum are seen and correspond to the cranial bones. The corpus callosum is a white matter

tract that connects the hemispheres and is found at the inferior aspect of the frontal and parietal lobes. CSF appears dark on this T1-weighted image, making it easy to trace the ventricular system. The anterior horn of the lateral ventricle is inferior to the genu of the corpus callosum. The third ventricle lies in the midline, between the two lateral ventricles. The lateral ventricles produce a great deal of CSF, which is transported to the third ventricle by way of the *intraventricular foramina (of Monro)*. The third ventricle is not optimally visualized in this image. What is seen is the thalamus, which forms the lateral wall of the third ventricle. CSF drains from the third ventricle via the *cerebral aqueduct (of Sylvius)*, which can be found within the midbrain (between the *corpora quadrigemina* and the *cerebral peduncles*). The *fourth ventricle* is also a triangular-shaped midline structure that is situated between the pons and cerebellum. The large air-filled sphenoidal sinus is located anterior to the pons. Superior to this sinus, the pituitary gland rests within hypophyseal fossa formed by the sella turcica. Directly superior to the pituitary gland is the optic chiasm.

Several vascular structures are well shown in Fig. 24.21. The basilar artery appears between the clivus and pons. Portions of the superior sagittal sinus can be

Fig. 24.20 PA projection of skull for localization of sagittal images.

seen between the cerebrum and the cranial bones. Between the cerebrum and cerebellum, the *straight sinus* (one of the dural venous sinuses) is noted within the tentorium cerebelli. This vessel is formed by the junction of the inferior sagittal sinus and the great cerebral vein (of Galen).

Fig. 24.22 is a sagittal T2-weighted MR image through the medial wall of the orbit.

The bright, fluid-filled lateral ventricle is seen in the center of the cerebral hemisphere. Just inferior to it are the caudate nucleus and the thalamus. Because this image was obtained in a plane lateral to the midline, one of the cerebral peduncles is seen at the inferior border of the thalamus, and one of the cerebellar peduncles

can be seen connecting the pons to the cerebellum. At the floor of the cranium, a dark circle is seen that represents the internal carotid artery. Cerebral vertebral bodies and arches can be seen in the neck on either side of the vertebral canal. In the face, the ethmoid sinus and tongue can be easily identified.

Fig. 24.21 (A) Line drawing of MRI section. (B) MRI through midsagittal plane, corresponding to level *A* in Fig. 24.20.

Fig. 24.22 (A) Line drawing of MRI section. (B) Sagittal MRI through medial wall of orbit corresponding to level *B* in Fig. 24.20.

Fig. 24.23 (A) Line drawing of MRI section. (B) Sagittal MRI through midorbit corresponding to level *C* in Fig. 24.20.

The sagittal T2-weighted MR image in Fig. 24.23 is sectioned through the center of the orbit. The frontal, parietal, occipital, and temporal lobes of the cerebrum all are visible. Within the cerebrum, CSF is seen within the temporal and posterior horns of the lateral ventricle (the fluid appears bright on this T2-weighted image). The cerebellum lies within the posterior fossa and is separated from the cerebrum by the tentorium cerebelli. Anterior to the cerebellum, the lateral aspect of the fourth ventricle can be seen. Within the orbit, several structures associated with the eye can be seen: the globe and the inferior rectus muscle. The dark area inferior to the orbit is the air-filled maxillary sinus. The medial pterygoid muscle, which lies on the internal aspect of the mandibular ramus, is visible inferior and posterior to the maxillary sinus.

A CT localizer, or scout, image (Fig. 24.24) is included as a reference for the next three coronal images. Fig. 24.25 is a coronal T2-weighted MR image through the anterior horns of the lateral ventricles and the pharyngeal structures. The anterior portions of the cerebral hemispheres are joined by the corpus callosum, which is immediately superior to the lateral ventricles. The membrane between the anterior horns of the lateral ventricles is the *septum pellucidum.* On the lateral aspect

Fig. 24.24 CT localizer (scout) image of skull.

of each cerebral hemisphere is the *lateral fissure*, which divides the frontal lobe from the temporal lobe. The insula lies deep to this fissure.

Structures of the basal nuclei can be faintly identified. The caudate nucleus is lateral to the anterior horns. Inferolateral to the caudate nuclei are the internal capsules—white matter tracts that connect the cortex to deeper gray matter structures. The anterior portion of the third ventricle is found in the midline inferior to the lateral ventricles. Inferior to the third ventricle are the optic chiasm and pituitary gland (hypophysis cerebri). The *superior* and *inferior sagittal sinuses* occupy the margins of the falx cerebri in the longitudinal fissure between the hemispheres of the cerebrum. The internal carotid arteries occupy the *cavernous sinuses* along with several cranial nerves and are found lateral to the pituitary gland and sella turcica. Branches of the middle cerebral arteries occupy the lateral fissures of the cerebrum. Fig. 24.26 is a coronal MR image through the bodies of the lateral ventricles, the brain stem, and the bodies of the cervical vertebrae. The third ventricle is well shown and bordered laterally by the thalamus. The dark region (low signal return) medial to the external acoustic canal corresponds to the *petrous portion of the temporal bone*. The first

Fig. 24.25 (A) Line drawing of MRI section. (B) Coronal MRI corresponding to level *A* in Fig. 24.24.

Fig. 24.26 (A) Line drawing of MRI section. (B) Coronal MRI corresponding to level *B* in Fig. 24.24.

Fig. 24.27 (A) Line drawing of MRI section. (B) Coronal MRI corresponding to level *C* in Fig. 24.24.

two cervical vertebrae are detailed in this section with the *dens* of the *axis* (C2) seen between the lateral masses of the *atlas* (C1). The large, intermediate gray masses inferior to the external acoustic canals are the *parotid glands.*

Fig. 24.27 shows a coronal MR image through the lateral ventricles and cerebellum. The splenium of the corpus callosum is found between the lateral ventricles. Inferior to the splenium is the superior cistern. Portions of the cerebellum are visualized superior and inferior to the middle cerebellar peduncles. The large, bright area near the center of the cerebellum is the fourth ventricle. The bright line between the cerebellum and cerebrum represents the tentorium cerebelli. The large, dark areas (signal void) lateral to the cerebellum correspond to the bony mastoid portions of the temporal bone.

Thoracic Region

The thorax extends from the thoracic inlet to the diaphragm. The inlet is an imaginary plane through the first thoracic vertebra and the top of the manubrium. Sectional images of the thorax are obtained to include all structures between these boundaries. Two cadaveric images are included to assist in identifying some of the structures of the thorax. Fig. 24.28 is a cadaveric image that corresponds to a level just superior to the sternoclavicular joints. Fig. 24.33 (presented later) lies near the level of the sixth thoracic vertebra and shows the chambers of the heart and other surrounding structures.

The bones of the thorax include the thoracic vertebrae, ribs, sternum, clavicles, and scapulae. Each of the 12 thoracic vertebrae is subdivided into a body and a vertebral arch. The opening formed between these divisions is the vertebral foramen, through which the spinal cord travels. Two pedicles, two laminae, two transverse processes, and one spinous process constitute the arch. The pedicles are more anterior and unite with the body of the vertebra; the laminae form the posterior part of the arch and unite to give rise to the spinous process. Transverse processes arise from the lateral arch where pedicles and laminae meet. Two superior articular processes arise from the superior arch, and two inferior articular processes arise from the inferior arch. Superior and inferior articular processes from adjacent vertebrae articulate to form zygapophyseal joints. Notches between succeeding arches form the intervertebral foramina. These foramina transmit spinal nerves. Articular disks are found between the vertebral bodies. These disks are composed of a dense cartilaginous outer rim called the *annulus fibrosus* and a gelatinous central core called the *nucleus pulposus.* Twelve pairs of ribs curl around the lateral thorax to protect the lungs and heart. The head of each rib is posterior and articulates with the body of a thoracic vertebra. These joints are called *costovertebral joints.* Tubercles of the ribs are lateral to the heads and articulate with transverse processes of the vertebrae, forming costotransverse joints. Anteriorly, the first 10 pairs of ribs articulate with the sternum either directly or indirectly via costal cartilage. The sternum lies in the midline of the anterior chest wall. From superior to inferior, the parts are the manubrium, body, and xiphoid process. An indentation at the superior

Fig. 24.28 (A) Line drawing of gross anatomic section. (B) Cadaveric image of superior thorax.

edge of the sternum, the jugular or sternal notch, lies at the level of the interspace between the second and third thoracic vertebrae. The manubrium joins the body of the sternum at the sternal angle, which corresponds to the interspace between the fourth and fifth thoracic vertebrae. The xiphoid process lies at approximately the level of the 10th thoracic vertebra. Familiarity with these vertebral levels can be helpful in orienting oneself when looking at thoracic sectional images.

The clavicles are slender, S-shaped bones that extend across the upper anterior thorax. The medial end of each clavicle articulates with the superolateral edge of the manubrium to form sternoclavicular joints. Acromioclavicular joints are formed where the lateral extremity of the clavicle articulates with the acromion process of the scapula. The scapulae are triangular bones in the superior posterior thorax. Thinking of the scapula as having two surfaces (anterior and posterior), three borders (superior, medial, and lateral), and three angles (superior, lateral, and inferior) is helpful. The posterior surface is divided into a superior fossa and an inferior fossa by the scapular spine. This bony ridge extends laterally and superiorly to end as the acromion process. The coracoid process projects from the superoanterior surface near the glenoid. The lateral angle is formed by the glenoid cavity, which articulates with the humeral head. Many of these bony structures are identifiable on Fig. 24.28.

Major components of the respiratory system are seen in the thorax. The trachea originates at the level of the sixth cervical vertebra (near the bottom of the thyroid cartilage). The trachea is formed by incomplete cartilage rings, which are open along its posterior surface. The trachea passes into the thorax and bifurcates into the right and left main bronchi near the level of the sternal angle (T4-5). The carina is the last cartilage ring of the trachea. The main bronchi pass through the hila of the lungs and branch to secondary bronchi, one for each lobe. The lungs are triangular organs enclosed in the thoracic cavity by the double-walled pleural membrane. The portion of the lung that lies superior to the clavicle is the apex; the part that rests on the diaphragm is the base. The most inferior and posterior reaches of the base constitute a region called the *costophrenic angle*. The bronchi and vascular structures enter and exit the center of the medial aspect of the lung at the hilum. Each lung is divided into superior and inferior lobes by an oblique fissure. The upper lobe of the right lung is divided further by a horizontal fissure to form a middle lobe that lies lateral to the heart. The portion of the left lung that corresponds in position to the right middle lobe is called the *lingula.*

The area between the lungs is the mediastinum. Within this cavity are the heart, trachea and bronchi, esophagus, major blood vessels, nerves, and lymphatic structures. The heart lies obliquely oriented in the lower mediastinum, surrounded by a double-walled fibrous sac called the *pericardium.* It rests on the diaphragm between the sternum and the thoracic spine. The superior surface is the base, and the inferior portion is the apex. The heart is divided into four chambers: two atria and two ventricles. The atria receive blood, and the ventricles pump blood away from the heart. The right atrium forms the right border of the heart and receives blood from the superior vena cava, inferior vena cava, and coronary sinus (the venous drainage channel for the heart muscle). Blood passes from here through the tricuspid (right atrioventricular) valve into the right ventricle. This chamber forms most of the anterior surface of the heart. As this ventricle contracts, blood passes through the right ventricular outflow tract, through the pulmonary semilunar valve, and into the main pulmonary artery toward the lungs. The left atrium forms the posterior border of the heart and receives blood from four pulmonary veins. Blood passes through the mitral (bicuspid or left atrioventricular) valve into the left ventricle. The most muscular of the chambers, the left ventricle, forms the left side and inferiormost portion of the heart. Blood is pumped out of the left ventricle through the left ventricular outflow tract through the aortic semilunar valve and into the aorta. A muscular wall, the interventricular septum, can be seen between the ventricles. Chambers of the heart are seen in Fig. 24.29.

One portion of the digestive system is typically found in the thorax. The esophagus originates at the level of the sixth cervical vertebra as the posterior continuation of the pharynx. It continues into the thorax, at first posterior to the trachea, and then posterior to the left atrium and ventricle of the heart. At the lower thorax, the esophagus pierces the diaphragm to continue into the abdomen.

The vascular system in the upper thorax can be confusing. To identify these structures, one must clearly understand the vascular anatomy. Tracing the paths of vessels through the scan can help alleviate some of the confusion. This discussion follows the path of circulation through the vessels. The discussion of arterial structures starts at the heart and follows the vessels toward the periphery. Veins are discussed from their peripheral origins and followed as they travel toward the heart.

The aorta originates from the left ventricle of the heart. Just distal to the aortic semilunar valve are the origins of the right and left coronary arteries, which supply the heart muscle. The aorta ascends along the posterior sternum, arches posterior and toward the left behind the sternal angle, and turns inferiorly to become the descending aorta. The descending aorta passes down the posterior thorax, resting against the left anterolateral surfaces of the vertebral bodies. The major vessels that supply the head and upper limbs arise from the aortic arch. From anterior to posterior, these are the brachiocephalic, left common carotid, and left subclavian arteries. The brachiocephalic artery passes superiorly and bifurcates into the right subclavian and right common carotid arteries posterior to the sternoclavicular joint. The right and left common carotid arteries ascend the neck along the lateral surface of the trachea. At approximately the level of the third cervical vertebra, each common carotid artery exhibits a dilation called the *carotid sinus* just proximal to bifurcating into internal and external carotid arteries. The subclavian arteries pass laterally across the upper thorax, just deep to the clavicles. At the outer edges of the first ribs, the subclavian arteries become the axillary arteries.

Venous drainage from the head is mainly through the jugular veins. The internal jugular veins accompany the carotid arteries down through the neck, lateral to the trachea. The subclavian veins are continuations of the axillary veins draining the upper limbs. These veins pass toward the midline, deep to the clavicles. At the sternoclavicular joints, the internal jugular veins and the subclavian veins unite to form the brachiocephalic veins. The right brachiocephalic vein passes vertically downward; the left passes obliquely down, posterior to the manubrium. These two vessels unite to form the superior vena cava. The superior vena cava lies posterior to the right border of the sternum and enters the right atrium just below the level of the sternal angle. Venous drainage from the lower body is via the inferior vena cava. This vessel is found along the right anterior surface of the vertebral bodies and empties into the inferior aspect of the right atrium. The azygos vein is a small vessel that passes up the posterior thorax along the right anterior aspect of the vertebral bodies. It arches anteriorly (near the level of the aortic arch) to drain into the superior vena cava.

The pulmonary vascular system transports blood between the lungs and heart. The main pulmonary artery receives deoxygenated blood from the right ventricle. At the level of the sternal angle, this vessel gives rise to the right and left pulmonary arteries, which pass laterally toward the hila of the lungs. The bifurcation of the main pulmonary artery is just inferior to the aortic arch. Four pulmonary veins exit the hila, two from each lung, and pass medially to enter the superolateral aspect of the left atrium.

Many muscles can be seen in the thorax, especially in the shoulder region. The pectoralis major is a large, fan-shaped muscle superficially located along the anterior chest wall. The pectoralis minor lies just deep to the pectoralis major. The trapezius is the most superficial of the posterior thoracic muscles. The rhomboid major and minor muscles are deep to the trapezius and lie between the medial scapular borders and the spinous processes of the upper thoracic spine. The serratus anterior muscles attach to the medial side of the anterior scapula and blanket the external surface of the rib cage. Several muscles are associated with the scapula; many of these also attach to the humerus. The subscapularis muscle lines the anterior surface. Supraspinatus and infraspinatus muscles lie in the supraspinous and infraspinous fossae. The teres major and

teres minor also lie along the infraspinous fossa. Four of these muscles are collectively known as the rotator cuff: subscapularis, supraspinatus, infraspinatus, and teres minor.

The CT localizer, or scout, image represents an AP projection of the thoracic region with identifying lines (Fig. 24.30). These lines show the approximate levels for each of the labeled images for this region. Most of the images for this region are CT scans. When performing scans of the thorax, the patient's arms are extended above the head. This fact must be kept in mind when looking at upper thoracic scans because some anatomic structures do not correspond to the normal anatomic position. MR images are frequently degraded by motion artifact in the thorax, so only a few representative images are included.

Fig. 24.29 (A) Line drawing of gross anatomic section. (B) Cadaveric image of central thorax.

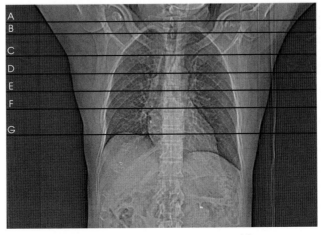

Fig. 24.30 CT localizer (scout) image of thorax.

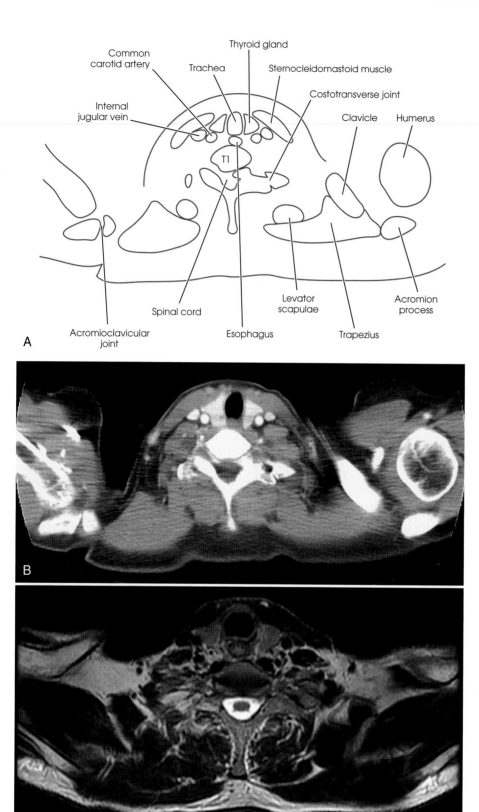

Common
carotid artery

Trachea

Thyroid gland

Sternocleidomastoid muscle

Costotransverse joint

Internal
jugular vein

Clavicle   Humerus

T1

Levator
scapulae

Acromion
process

Spinal cord

Acromioclavicular
joint

Esophagus

Trapezius

A

B

C

Fig. 24.31 (A) Line drawing of CT section. (B) CT image, and (C) MR image corresponding to level A in Fig. 24.30 through first thoracic vertebra.

Fig. 24.31B shows a CT and T2-weighted MR images at the level of T1 and show the relationship between the vertebral column, esophagus, and trachea. The body and *vertebral arch* of the first thoracic vertebra can be identified, and the spinal cord is seen in the vertebral foramen. The *costotransverse joint* between the first rib and the transverse process of the first thoracic vertebra is seen on the patient's left. Because the patient's arms are raised on the CT image, the scan passes through the surgical neck of the humerus. The inferior portion of the *thyroid gland*, which extends from C6 to T1, is positioned lateral to the *trachea*. The soft tissue shadow immediately posterior to the trachea is the *esophagus*. The outer esophageal lining is well demonstrated on the MR image. The *vertebral arteries* are positioned lateral to the vertebral column, and the *common carotid arteries* are found lateral to the trachea. At this level, the *internal jugular veins* are positioned to the lateral aspect of the carotid arteries. The CT image demonstrates the contrast-filled axillary arteries in the medial aspect of the arms. The *sternocleidomastoid muscles* are found lateral to the thyroid gland. The *trapezius* is the most superficial muscle of the posterior thorax, with the levator scapulae muscles lying just anterior.

Fig. 24.32 shows a CT and T2-weighted MR images through the lower edge of T2. These scans pass through the *jugular notch* of the sternum and are just superior to the sternoclavicular joints. The CT image demonstrates the costovertebral and costotransverse joints that are seen between the ribs and the spine. On the right, the glenoid portion and the acromion process of the scapula are seen. The humerus is visible where it articulates with the glenoid cavity. On the left, the spine and the body of the scapula are seen. Both images demonstrate the *trachea* and esophagus located anterior to the vertebral body. The major vessels of the superior thorax are visualized posterior to the clavicles. The right and left *brachiocephalic veins* are formed by the junction of the *subclavian veins* and the internal jugular veins. Because contrast medium was injected for the CT scan, the axillary and most of the right subclavian vein are filled with contrast medium. Posterior to the right clavicle, the right subclavian vein and internal jugular vein have joined. Because the CT image is slightly more inferior on the left, the image plane passes through the left brachiocephalic vein (below the junction of these two vessels). The brachiocephalic veins unite and form the *superior vena cava* at a more inferior level. The arterial branches to the head and upper limb are also well visualized on the CT image. From the patient's right to left, they are the *right subclavian artery*, *right common carotid artery*, *left common carotid artery*, and *left subclavian artery*. The brachiocephalic artery gives rise to the right subclavian and right common carotid arteries, and is inferior to this level. The *pectoralis major* and *pectoralis minor* lie along the anterior thoracic wall. The trapezius is the most superficial of the posterior muscles and is seen between the scapula and the spine on each side. The *subscapularis muscle* lines the left anterior scapula, the *infraspinatus* and *teres minor* line the posterior portion of this bone, and the *supraspinatus* is seen between the body and the scapular spine.

Fig. 24.32 (A) Line drawing of CT section. (B) CT image, and (C) MR image corresponding to level *B* in Fig. 24.30 through jugular notch.

Fig. 24.33 (A) Line drawing of CT section. (B) CT image corresponding to level *C* in Fig. 24.30 just superior to aortic arch.

Fig. 24.33 is a CT image through the level of T3. Bony structures depicted in this image include the *manubrium* and sternoclavicular joints anteriorly, the ribs laterally, and the scapulae and vertebra posteriorly. The spine and the body of the right scapula are visible at this level. Costovertebral and costotransverse joints are noted along the right side of the vertebra. Several vascular structures, highlighted with contrast medium, are visible posterior to the manubrium. The right and left brachiocephalic veins are seen just posterior to the right sternoclavicular joint. This level is just superior to where the vessels join to form the superior vena cava. The brachiocephalic artery, left common carotid artery, and left subclavian artery curl around the left side of the trachea. This scan is just superior to the arch of the aorta and visualizes the origins of these three vessels. Posterior to the vessels are the trachea and esophagus. The upper lobes of each lung lie lateral to the mediastinal structures. The pectoralis major and pectoralis minor lie external to the anterior ribs. Rotator cuff muscles (subscapularis, infraspinatus, and teres minor) are shown anterior and posterior to the scapulae. The trapezius and *rhomboid muscles* lie between the scapulae and the spinous process of the vertebra in this image.

Fig. 24.34 is a CT scan obtained through the lower edge of T4. At this level, the brachiocephalic veins have joined to form the *superior vena cava*. The large contrast-filled structure in the left anterolateral mediastinum is the *aortic arch*.

Fig. 24.35 is a CT image at the level of T5 and shows the great vessels superior to the heart. (The heart is normally positioned between T7 and T11, with most of the organ lying left of the midline.) The *ascending aorta* is found anteriorly in the midline; the *descending aorta* is related to the left anterolateral surface of the vertebral bodies. (This relationship between the descending aorta and vertebral column is continuous through the thorax and

A

B

Fig. 24.34 (A) Line drawing of CT section. (B) CT image corresponding to level *D* in Fig. 24.30 through aortic arch.

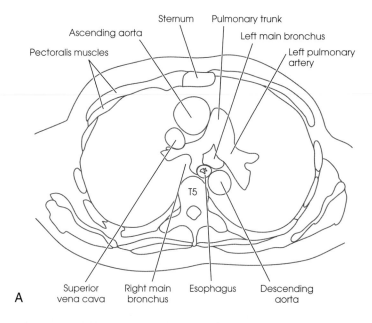

Pectoralis muscles

Ascending aorta

Sternum

Pulmonary trunk

Left main bronchus

Left pulmonary artery

T5

A

Superior vena cava

Right main bronchus

Esophagus

Descending aorta

B

Fig. 24.35 (A) Line drawing of CT section. (B) CT image corresponding to level *E* in Fig. 24.30 through pulmonary trunk.

abdomen.) Note the normal difference in caliber between the ascending and descending aorta. The superior vena cava is located to the right of the ascending aorta, and the pulmonary trunk and left and right pulmonary arteries are located to the left of the ascending aorta at this level. The *pulmonary trunk* originates from the right ventricle of the heart and divides into the right and left *pulmonary arteries*, which carry deoxygenated blood to the lungs. The left pulmonary artery is seen bifurcating into the two lobar branches at the hilum of the left lung. Near the T5 level the trachea divides into the left and right *primary bronchi.* The esophagus (in which a small amount of air is seen) is found just posterior to the left main bronchus. Fig. 24.36 is a T2-weighted MR image that corresponds in position to the previous CT image. The main pulmonary artery and the left pulmonary artery are seen on this image, although the right pulmonary artery is not visible. Muscular structures are easily differentiated. The spinal cord is seen within the vertebral canal, where it is surrounded by CSF.

Fig. 24.36 MRI corresponding to level *E* in Fig. 24.30.

A

B

Fig. 24.37 (A) Line drawing of CT section. (B) CT image corresponding to level *F* in Fig. 24.30 through base of the heart.

The CT image depicted in Fig. 24.37 shows the *lungs* and the base of the *heart*. In general, when the heart is imaged in cross section, the *left atrium* is the superiormost structure encountered, and the *pulmonary veins* are seen emptying into it (one of the right pulmonary veins can be seen here). The *right atrium* is seen lying the farthest toward the right side of the body, anterior and inferior to the left atrium. The superior vena cava may be seen at this level as it enters the right atrium. The *right ventricle* lies to the left of the right atrium and anterior to the more muscular *left ventricle*. Contrast-enhanced blood is seen here as blood exits the left ventricle to enter the root of the aorta. The *interventricular septum* can be seen between the ventricles.

The lungs are divided into superior and inferior lobes by the diagonally oriented *oblique fissure*. The *superior lobes* lie superior and anterior to the inferior lobes. The *superior lobe* of the right lung is divided further by the *horizontal fissure*, with the lower portion termed the *middle lobe*. The left lung has no horizontal fissure. The inferior and anterior portion of the left lung (corresponding to the right middle lobe) is termed the *lingula*. Although the fissures are not seen, the approximate locations of these lobes are identified here.

Muscular structures that can be seen at this level include the inferior insertions of the trapezius, the *latissimus dorsi*, and the *serratus anterior muscles*. The esophagus lies between the left atrium and the vertebral column at this level.

Fig. 24.38 lies at approximately T9 and shows the lower sternum and ribs. The descending aorta normally lies along the left anterolateral surface of the vertebral column, and the *azygos vein* is normally on the right anterolateral surface. Because this scan is inferior to the right ventricle, the *inferior vena cava* is seen between the heart and the liver. The superior portion of the liver is bulging against the base of the right lung, and the most superior portion of the left hemidiaphragm is seen at the base of the left lung. The right and left ventricles of the heart and the interventricular septum can be seen surrounded by pericardium. The major muscle structures that are visible are the serratus anterior, latissimus dorsi, and the deep back muscles.

Fig. 24.39 is a frontal CT localizer image representing the sagittal levels of the thorax presented here. Fig. 24.40 is located near the median sagittal plane of the chest. In this image, the central portion of the manubrium can be seen in the anterior thorax. The sternal angle is represented as a dark line separating the manubrium and the body of the sternum. Thoracic vertebral bodies, spinous processes, zygapophyseal joints, and intervertebral foramina border the posterior thorax. Because the body has a slight degree of curvature in the spine, different structures are seen in the spinal column at different levels. Within the upper thorax, the cartilage rings of the trachea can be observed. The soft tissue structure posterior to the trachea is the esophagus. The heart and great vessels lie near the center of the thorax. In this image, the most superior vascular structure is the arch of the aorta. At this level, the origin of the left common carotid artery is present. The left ventricle is the largest chamber of the heart and is seen here filled with contrast medium. It also empties into the aorta. The origin and ascending aorta can be seen just superior to the left ventricle. The left pulmonary artery lies immediately inferior to the aortic arch. This vessel is a branch of the pulmonary artery and originates from the right ventricle of the heart, which is anterior to the left ventricle. The left atrium of the heart is the most posterior chamber and is seen here posterior to the pulmonary trunk and left ventricle. The diaphragm is located inferior to the heart and separates the thoracic cavity from the abdomen.

Fig. 24.41 is a CT image that passes just medial to the left sternoclavicular joint. In this image, the entire aorta is present, from the root, through the arch, and continuing as the descending portion. The origins of the left common carotid and the left subclavian arteries are seen at the superior border of the arch. The left common carotid artery courses from its origin superiorly into the neck near the trachea. The upper portion of the esophagus is posterior to the trachea. The left pulmonary artery is visible just inferior to the arch, and the air-filled structure posterior to this vessel is the left main bronchus.

Fig. 24.42 represents a sagittal section through the left sternoclavicular joint. Anteriorly, the bony structures include the clavicle, the upper-outer corner of the manubrium, and the costosternal articulations. The posterior bony anatomy includes the thoracic spine and the upper

Fig. 24.38 (A) Line drawing of CT section. (B) CT image corresponding to level *G* in Fig. 24.30 through right hemidiaphragm.

Fig. 24.39 CT localizer image representing levels of sagittal sections through thorax.

183

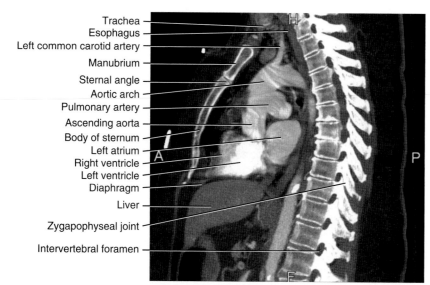

Trachea
Esophagus
Left common carotid artery
Manubrium
Sternal angle
Aortic arch
Pulmonary artery
Ascending aorta
Body of sternum
Left atrium
Right ventricle
Left ventricle
Diaphragm
Liver
Zygapophyseal joint
Intervertebral foramen

Fig. 24.40 Sagittal CT image of thorax corresponding to level *A* in Fig. 24.39.

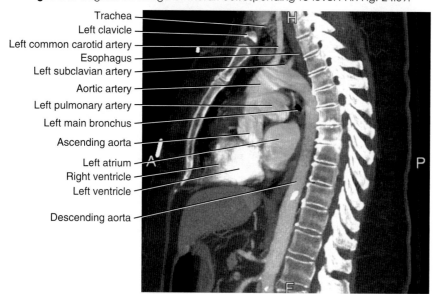

Trachea
Left clavicle
Left common carotid artery
Esophagus
Left subclavian artery
Aortic artery
Left pulmonary artery
Left main bronchus
Ascending aorta
Left atrium
Right ventricle
Left ventricle
Descending aorta

Fig. 24.41 Sagittal CT image of thorax corresponding to level *B* in Fig. 24.39.

Rib
Left clavicle
Left sternoclavicular joint
Manubrium
Left subclavian artery
Sternocostal joint
Pulmonary artery
Pulmonary veins
Left ventricle
Right ventricle
Left atrium

Fig. 24.42 Sagittal CT image of thorax corresponding to level *C* in Fig. 24.39.

ribs. Within the thorax, the arch and descending aorta are present. The left subclavian artery is the third branch from the aortic arch. This vessel passes superiorly to arch over the apex of the left lung. In this image, the proximal portion of this vessel is seen just superior to the aortic arch. In the anterior mediastinum, the contrast-filled right ventricle is pumping blood into the main pulmonary artery. The left pulmonary veins return blood from the lungs to the left atrium. The left ventricle lies between the right ventricle and the left atrium in this image.

Fig. 24.43 is a lateral chest x-ray to be used to localize the coronal sections of the thorax presented here. Fig. 24.44 is a coronal image passing through the anterior mediastinum. The clavicles, manubrium, and sternoclavicular joints are visible at the entrance into the thorax. Sections through the ribs line both lateral walls of the thoracic cavity. The setting for this image shows the lungs as black structures with a few vascular shadows visible within each. The mediastinum in the center of the thoracic cavity is occupied by the heart and great vessels. This scan passes through the anterior mediastinum, so the ascending portion of the aorta is visible. It lies between the pulmonary artery and the superior vena cava. In this slice, the superior vena cava is discernible at its entrance into the right atrium. The right ventricle is the most anterior chamber of the heart and is seen here lateral to the right atrium.

The coronal thoracic section seen in Fig. 24.45 passes through a plane near the median coronal plane of the thorax. Clavicles and ribs can be seen surrounding the superior and lateral thorax. The cartilage rings of the trachea lie in the median sagittal plane at the superior end of the thorax. The left lung is specked with several light gray vascular structures. The right lung shows infiltrates and central scar tissue from an old resection. This scan was performed with contrast enhancement, and the right axillary vein and superior vena cava are visible as bright white. The aortic arch gives rise to the vessels that supply the head and neck. In this image, the brachiocephalic artery and the origin of the left common carotid artery can be seen. The brachiocephalic veins are formed by the internal jugular and subclavian veins. The left brachiocephalic vein is located just to the left of the brachiocephalic artery and superior to the origin of the common carotid artery in this image.

The main pulmonary artery is visible inferior to the aorta. A small portion of the left atrium and the right atrium and ventricle can be seen.

Fig. 24.46 shows anatomy in a posterior plane through the mediastinum. Because of the curve of the spine, the lower cervical and thoracic vertebrae are visible, but most of the thoracic spine is posterior to this imaging plane. Near the level of the fourth or fifth thoracic vertebrae, the trachea bifurcates into the right and left main bronchi. In this image, the lower trachea, its bifurcation, and the main bronchi are visible. On the right, the main bronchus is dividing into lobar bronchi. The soft tissue structure detectable near the top of the visible portion of the trachea is the esophagus. On the left side of the esophagus, the left subclavian artery, filled with contrast medium, is seen as it starts its arch over the apex of the lung. The round contrast-filled vessels that lie on the left side of the trachea are the aortic arch (superior) and the left pulmonary artery (inferior). Inferior to the trachea, the left atrium is detectable, filled with contrast medium. One of the four pulmonary veins is visible, filled with contrast medium and to the right of the left atrium. Because this image is relatively posterior in the mediastinum, no other chambers of the heart can be seen; however, a section of the descending aorta, filled with contrast medium, lies inferior to the left atrium.

Fig. 24.44 Coronal CT image of thorax corresponding to level A in Fig. 24.43.

Fig. 24.45 Coronal CT image of thorax corresponding to level B in Fig. 24.43.

Fig. 24.43 Lateral chest x-ray representing levels of coronal sections through thorax.

Fig. 24.46 Coronal CT image of thorax corresponding to level C in Fig. 24.43.

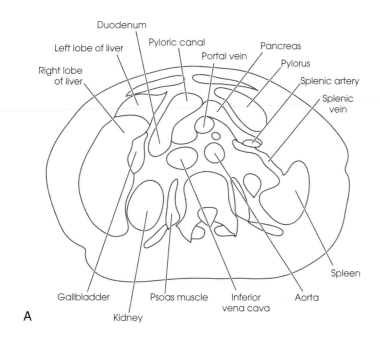

Duodenum

Left lobe of liver   Pyloric canal   Pancreas

Right lobe   Portal vein   Pylorus
of liver
Splenic artery

Splenic vein

Spleen

Gallbladder   Psoas muscle   Inferior   Aorta
vena cava
Kidney

A

B

Fig. 24.47 (A) Line drawing of gross anatomic section. (B) Cadaveric section through central abdomen at the level of L2.

Abdominopelvic Region

The abdominopelvic region includes the diaphragm and everything inferior to it. Fig. 24.47 is a cadaveric image at the level of the second lumbar vertebra. Major abdominal organs and vascular structures can be identified in this image. In the abdomen, five lumbar vertebrae are visible. Although these vertebrae are slightly larger than the vertebrae in the thorax, the anatomic components are roughly the same. In the pelvis, the lower spine and hip bones (os coxae or innominate) form an attachment for the lower limbs and support for the trunk. The lower spine comprises the sacrum and coccyx. These are triangular bones with their broad bases oriented superiorly. Each os coxae lies obliquely situated in the pelvis, articulating with the sacrum (sacroiliac joint) posteriorly and with the opposite os coxae anteriorly (symphysis pubis). At birth, this bone consists of three components: the ilium, ischium, and pubis. These three ultimately fuse at the acetabulum. The superior, wing-shaped portion of the os coxae is the ilium. The superior edge is the crest, which lies at the level of the lower fourth lumbar vertebra. The anterior superior and anterior inferior iliac spines lie along the anterior surface of the ilium. At the posterior ilium, posterior superior, and posterior inferior iliac spines are found at the top and bottom of the sacral articular surface. Below the posterior inferior iliac spine, the greater sciatic notch curves sharply toward the front of the bone. The inferior and anterior os coxae are composed of the pubis. The pubic bone extends from the acetabulum toward the midline and then curves inferiorly. The pubic bones articulate with each other at the symphysis pubis. The posterior inferior os coxae is formed by the ischium. This portion extends inferiorly from the acetabulum, and then curls forward to meet the lower part of the pubis. The obturator foramen is a circular opening formed by the junction of the pubis and ischium.

The abdominal cavity is lined by a double-walled membrane called the *peritoneum.* Some organs develop posterior to the peritoneum and are referred to as *retroperitoneal.* Others invaginate into the peritoneum and are referred to as *intraperitoneal.* Several large folds of the peritoneum are identifiable on sectional images because of the large amount of fat found within it. The greater omentum extends from the greater curvature of the stomach and the transverse colon to blanket the anterior surface of the abdominal organs, especially the digestive organs. The small intestines invaginate into the peritoneum as they develop, and a large flap of peritoneum—the mesentery—anchors this part of the digestive system to the posterior abdominal wall.

The spleen is an organ belonging to the lymphatic system. It lies inferior to the left hemidiaphragm and posterior to the fundus of the stomach. On the medial surface of the spleen, blood vessels enter and exit at the hilum.

The organs of the alimentary tract include the esophagus, stomach, small intestine, and large intestine. The esophagus lies anterior to the spine and passes through the diaphragm to enter the abdomen at about the level of T10. In the abdomen, it passes toward the left to enter the stomach. The opening into the stomach is the cardiac orifice, and the junction is the esophagogastric junction. The stomach is a J-shaped pouch in the left upper quadrant. The region above the level of the esophagogastric junction is the fundus, the central region is the body, and the distal part is the pyloric antrum. This last portion normally lies at about the level of the second lumbar vertebra. The medial and lateral borders are referred to as the *lesser and greater curvatures.* Internally, the stomach is thrown into multiple folds termed *rugae.* Food passes from the distal stomach through the pyloric canal into the small intestine. A muscle called the *pyloric sphincter* controls passage through the canal. The small intestine consists of the duodenum, jejunum, and ileum. The first portion or duodenum extends from the stomach laterally to the liver, where the remainder curls inferiorly and medially to form a C-shaped loop around the head of the pancreas. The duodenum is approximately 10 to 12 inches (24 to 30 cm) long, and at the ligament of Treitz it continues as the jejunum. The jejunum is approximately 8 ft (2.4 m) long and

mainly occupies the left upper abdomen. It continues as the ileum. This distalmost part of the small bowel is about 10 ft (3 m) long and occupies the right inferior abdominal cavity and the pelvis. The large intestine is about 6 ft (1.8 m) long. It frames the periphery of the abdominal cavity and comprises the cecum, colon (ascending, transverse, descending, and sigmoid portions), rectum, and anus. The ileum empties into the saclike cecum in the right lower quadrant via the ileocecal valve. The vermiform appendix frequently can be seen projecting off the cecum. From the cecum, the ascending portion of the colon passes superiorly. Just below the liver, this portion curves anteriorly and medially at the hepatic (right colic) flexure. The transverse portion passes from here across the anterior abdomen. This portion dips inferiorly into the abdomen to a variable degree depending on the body habitus of the patient. As the colon reaches the spleen, it turns posteriorly and inferiorly at the splenic (left colic) flexure to become the descending colon. This portion passes down the posterior aspect of the left side of the abdomen toward the pelvis, where it continues as the sigmoid colon. The sigmoid colon curls medially and posteriorly in the pelvis, and at the mid-sacrum it curves inferiorly as the rectum. The rectum lies anterior to and follows the curve of the sacrum to become the anal canal as the large intestine exits the pelvis.

Several accessory organs of the digestive system are located in the upper abdomen. The liver occupies most of the right upper quadrant. This triangular organ is divided anatomically into a large right lobe and a much smaller left lobe. The falciform ligament is located along the division between these lobes on the anterior surface, and the ligamentum venosum and ligamentum teres are found along the division on the posterior surface of the liver. On the posteroinferior surface of the right lobe are two smaller lobes: the caudate (superior) and the quadrate (inferior). These two lobes are separated by the porta hepatis (hilum) of the liver. The hepatic artery, portal vein, and hepatic bile ducts enter and exit the liver here. The gallbladder rests against the undersurface of the liver. This organ functions as a storage vessel for bile, which is produced in the liver. Bile drains from the liver through the right and left hepatic ducts. These ducts unite to form the common hepatic

duct, which meets the cystic duct from the gallbladder. Distal to this junction, the continuation of this duct is known as the *common bile duct.* Bile passes through this duct to empty into the second part of the duodenum at the hepatopancreatic ampulla (ampulla of Vater). The pancreas, which functions as an endocrine and exocrine gland, lies transversely across the abdomen near the level of the second lumbar vertebra. The divisions of this retroperitoneal organ, from right to left, are the head, neck, body, and tail. The head is the most inferior portion and is encircled by the duodenum. The tail is located near the hilum of the spleen. The pancreatic duct traverses the length of the organ and enters the second part of the duodenum at or near the common bile duct.

The urinary system includes the two kidneys and ureters, the bladder, and the urethra. The kidneys are retroperitoneal and lie between the 12th thoracic and 3rd lumbar vertebrae. The center or hilar region is normally near the interspace between L1 and L2. Suprarenal (adrenal) glands are perched on the upper surface of each kidney. The right adrenal gland can be seen between the liver and the right diaphragmatic crus, and the left lies between the left crus and the pancreatic tail and spleen. Each kidney is surrounded by a dense membrane, the renal fasciae, and a layer of fat, the perirenal fat. Urine is formed in the parenchyma of the kidney and collects in the calyceal system. The calyces unite to form the renal pelvis, which is continuous with the ureter. The ureters are musculomembranous tubes that extend down the posterior abdomen, resting along the anterior surface of the psoas muscles. They are difficult to visualize unless filled with radiopaque contrast medium. In the pelvis, the ureters empty into the posteroinferior region of the bladder. The bladder is a collapsible muscular sac that serves as a reservoir for urine until it is expelled from the body. The bladder rests on or near the pelvic floor, posterior to the symphysis pubis and anterior to the rectum in males or the vagina in females. The urethra is the muscular passageway that originates from the apex (inferior surface) of the bladder and by which urine is expelled. The urethra is relatively short in females, passing through the floor of the pelvis. The urethra is much longer in males because it passes through the prostate gland and the membranous and cavernous portions of the penis.

The internal organs of the male reproductive system include the ductus deferens, seminal vesicles, and prostate. Internal and external reproductive structures are connected by the spermatic cord, which includes the ductus deferens, testicular vessels, nerves, and lymphatic structures. The spermatic cord is seen anterior and medial to the femoral artery and vein, and anterior and lateral to the pubis. The ductus deferens enters the pelvis through the spermatic cord and then arches over the anterior and lateral aspect of the bladder. It passes down the posterior surface of the bladder and enters the superior prostate. The seminal vesicles are found on the posterior and inferior surface of the bladder near the insertion of the ureters. The prostate gland lies inferior to the bladder, between the symphysis pubis and the rectum. The prostatic portion of the urethra passes through the prostate.

The organs of the female reproductive system include the uterus, uterine (fallopian) tubes, ovaries, and vagina. The uterus, which normally lays superior and posterior to the urinary bladder, is divided into a fundus, body, isthmus, and cervix. The fundus is the upper, rounded portion of the organ, superior to the orifices of the uterine tubes. The central portion is the body, which narrows at its lower end to become the isthmus. The narrowed lower ¾ inch (2 cm) of the uterus is the cervix, which is continuous with the vagina. The uterus is suspended in the pelvis by folds of peritoneum called the *broad ligaments*. The ovaries lie lateral to the body of the uterus within the broad ligament. They are normally found near the lateral pelvic wall at or slightly below the level of the anterior superior iliac spine. Extending between the ovaries and uterus, in the superior rim of the broad ligament, are the uterine tubes. The medial ends open into the upper body of the uterus. The lateral end of each tube, the infundibulum, is expanded and terminates in multiple fingerlike projections called *fimbriae*. This end of the tube is superior to the ovary but not attached. The inferior-most part of the internal female reproductive system is the vagina. This muscular tube lies between the rectum and the bladder and opens to the external body surface posterior to the urethral meatus.

Three vascular systems can be described in the abdomen: arterial, venous, and portal. The descending, or abdominal, aorta is the main conduit for arterial blood and passes through the diaphragm at approximately the level of T11 and extends to the pelvis along the left anterolateral surface of the vertebral bodies. Just below the diaphragm, at approximately the level of the 12th thoracic vertebra, the celiac artery originates from the anterior aorta. This fairly short vessel divides into the splenic, common hepatic, and left gastric arteries. The splenic artery passes toward the left to enter the hilum of the spleen. The common hepatic artery extends to the right to the porta hepatis. The superior mesenteric artery arises from the left anterior aorta near the first lumbar vertebra. The origin of this vessel is posterior to the neck of the pancreas. It extends anteriorly for a short distance and then turns inferiorly as it sends its branches to supply the small intestine and the proximal half of the large intestine. Near the level of the second lumbar vertebra, the renal arteries arise from the lateral surface of the aorta. The renal arteries pass laterally to enter the hila of the kidneys. The right renal artery is longer than the left because it must cross the spine to reach the right kidney. The inferior mesenteric artery arises from the abdominal aorta at L3 and supplies the distal half of the large bowel. At the fourth lumbar vertebra, the abdominal aorta bifurcates to form the right and left common iliac arteries. Each common iliac artery divides into internal and external iliac arteries near the top of the sacrum. Internal iliac arteries divide rapidly as branches are sent to various structures within the pelvis. The external iliac arteries pass anteriorly and inferiorly through the pelvis. These vessels pass deep to the inguinal ligaments and become the femoral arteries.

The femoral veins carry venous blood from the lower limbs toward the pelvis. The femoral vein becomes the external iliac vein as it passes deep to the inguinal ligament. It is joined within the pelvis by the internal iliac vein to form the common iliac vein. The two common iliac veins unite at the level of the fifth lumbar vertebra to form the inferior vena cava. The inferior vena cava passes up the right anterolateral surface of the vertebral bodies, pierces the diaphragm, and empties into the inferior surface of the right atrium. The major tributaries of the inferior vena cava are the renal veins and the hepatic veins. The renal veins enter the lateral inferior vena cava near L2; the three hepatic veins enter near the top of the liver.

The vessels that drain the spleen and digestive system form the portal venous system. The major tributaries of this system are the superior and inferior mesenteric veins and the splenic vein. The inferior mesenteric vein empties into the splenic vein, which meets the superior mesenteric vein just posterior to the head of the pancreas. The junction of these

Fig. 24.48 CT localizer (scout) image of abdominopelvic region.

two vessels forms the portal vein. These vessels extend superiorly to enter the porta hepatis of the liver.

Fig. 24.48 is a CT localizer, or scout, image representing an AP projection of the abdominopelvic region. Fig. 24.48 has 11 identifying lines showing the levels for each of the labeled images for this region.

Fig. 24.49 represents structures seen at the T9 level. The tip of the xiphoid process and lower ribs are seen. The image shows the *right hemidiaphragm* surrounding the superior portion of the *liver* and the *left hemidiaphragm* encircling the pericardial fat surrounding the apex of the heart and the *fundus* of the stomach. A small amount of oral contrast agent can be seen in the dependent portion of the stomach in this image. The *esophagus*, posterior to the liver, has migrated toward the patient's left as it nears its entrance into the stomach. The lower lobes of each lung are seen external to the diaphragm. The *aorta* is in its normal position, anterior and slightly left of the vertebral body; the azygos vein lies to the right of the aorta. The inferior vena cava appears embedded within the liver. Three *hepatic veins* drain into the inferior vena cava at this level. Serratus anterior muscles are seen external to the lateral aspects of the ribs; latissimus dorsi muscles extend superficially across the posterior abdomen.

Fig. 24.50 is a CT image at the level of the 10th thoracic vertebra. It shows the aorta and inferior vena cava and contrast-enhanced vessels within the liver. These represent branches of the hepatic and portal venous circulation. The right, left, and *caudate lobes* of the liver are visible. On the patient's left, the contrast-filled body of the stomach and the *spleen* can be identified. This is normally the level at which the esophagus enters the cardiac portion of the stomach. The *greater omentum* (a large fold of peritoneum) lies along the greater curvature of the stomach. Fig. 24.50 shows the greater omentum anterior and lateral to the stomach. The inferior lobes of the lungs are seen posterior to the liver and the spleen. The *crura of the diaphragm* are the lower tendinous insertions of this muscle. They can be seen extending around the anterior aorta and the posterior liver and spleen. This scan shows the latissimus dorsi and the lower reaches of the serratus anterior. The upper portions of the anterior abdominal muscles (rectus abdominis, external oblique) can also be seen.

Fig. 24.49 (A) Line drawing of CT section. (B) CT image corresponding to level *A* in Fig. 24.48.

A

B

Fig. 24.50 (A) Line drawing of CT section. (B) CT image corresponding to level *B* in Fig. 24.48.

A CT image at the level of T11 (Fig. 24.51) shows the relationships among the liver, stomach, and spleen. The cardiac portion of the stomach is located at approximately the T10-11 level in the anterior aspect of the left upper quadrant, and the *pyloric portion* normally lies anterior to L2. This scan passes through the center or body of the stomach. An air-fluid level exists between the gas in the anterior stomach and the contrast medium in the posterior stomach. The spleen, located between the levels of T12 and L1, is in the posterolateral aspect of the left upper quadrant posterior to the fundus and body of the stomach. Contrast medium in the patient's colon is seen at the *splenic flexure*, seen here between the body of the stomach and the spleen. The liver is generally found between T11 and L3 and occupies the entire right upper quadrant. The right lobe of the liver has two small subdivisions, the caudate and *quadrate lobes*, which are bounded by the *gallbladder*, *ligamentum teres*, and inferior vena cava. The left lobe of the liver stretches across the midline and into the left upper quadrant. The *porta hepatis*, or hilum of the liver, is visible between the right and left lobes at this level. The inferior vena cava is found between the right and caudate lobes of the liver. In this image, it is nearly isodense with liver tissue. Large branches of the portal vein are seen at the porta hepatis.

Fig. 24.51 (A) Line drawing of CT section. (B) CT image corresponding to level *C* in Fig. 24.48.

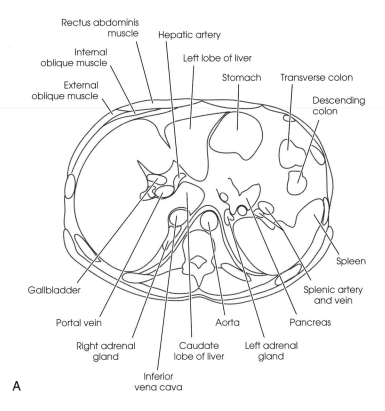

Rectus abdominis muscle
Internal oblique muscle
External oblique muscle
Hepatic artery
Left lobe of liver
Stomach
Transverse colon
Descending colon
Spleen
Splenic artery and vein
Pancreas
Gallbladder
Portal vein
Right adrenal gland
Caudate lobe of liver
Aorta
Left adrenal gland
Inferior vena cava

A

B

Fig. 24.52 (A) Line drawing of CT section. (B) CT image corresponding to level *D* in Fig. 24.48.

Fig. 24.52 lies at the inferior edge of T11. It shows the right, left, and caudate lobes of the liver and the porta hepatis. Anteriorly, the falciform ligament lies near the fissure between the right and left lobes (not seen on this image). The pyloric antrum of the stomach lies near the left lobe of the liver. This scan is inferior to the splenic flexure, so the *transverse and descending portions of the colon* can be differentiated. The spleen lies along the left posterior abdominal wall. This scan lies near the hilum, and vascular structures are seen in this region. The tail of the pancreas normally lies near the spleen and can be seen here between the stomach and spleen. The *suprarenal glands* are normally located superior to the kidney. The right suprarenal gland is found at this level between the liver and the right diaphragmatic crus. The left suprarenal gland is medial to the pancreas and spleen. The abdominal aorta is positioned anterior and to the left of the vertebral column; the inferior vena cava is between the right and caudate lobes of the liver. The portal vein is seen within the porta hepatis, along with branches of the hepatic artery. The splenic artery is normally tortuous and not seen in its entirety. At this level, the bright circles along the posterior pancreas most likely represent portions of the contrast-filled *splenic artery.*

The CT scan in Fig. 24.53 passes through the upper portion of T12. The difference in density between the liver tissue and the bile-filled *gallbladder* makes these organs easy to differentiate. The antrum of the stomach, pyloric canal, and bulb (first portion) of the *duodenum* are seen in the anterior abdomen. The neck of the pancreas is posterior to the pyloric canal of the stomach in this image. The transverse and descending colon lie in the anterior left abdomen. The spleen is posterior to the descending colon. Loops of *jejunum*, the second part of the small bowel, are posterior to the antrum of the stomach. The left adrenal gland is lateral to the aorta and left diaphragmatic crus. The right adrenal gland is posterior to the IVC. The three branches of the *celiac trunk* (hepatic, splenic, left gastric arteries) supply the liver, spleen, pancreas, and stomach with oxygen-rich blood. In this image, the celiac trunk is seen as it divides into the *common hepatic artery* and the splenic artery. The left gastric artery is not seen. The splenic artery runs a tortuous course and normally cannot be visualized in its entirety in axial sections. Here, branches of the splenic artery and vein lie in close proximity and are difficult to differentiate. The inferior vena cava can be seen in its normal position anterior and to the right of the vertebral column. The main portion of the portal vein is just posterior to the duodenal bulb.

A

B

Fig. 24.53 (A) Line drawing of CT section. (B) CT image corresponding to level *E* in Fig. 24.48.

Fig. 24.54 (A) Line drawing of CT section. (B) CT image corresponding to level *F* in Fig. 24.48.

The muscles of the abdomen are located between the lower rib cage and the iliac crests. This group of muscles includes the *external oblique, internal oblique,* and *transverse abdominal muscles.* The two *rectus abdominis muscles* are located on the anterior aspect of the abdomen on either side of the midline and extend from the *pubic symphysis* to the xiphoid process.

The CT image in Fig. 24.54 is through the level of the first lumbar vertebra. The lower right lobe of the liver lies along the right side of the abdomen. The hepatic (right colic) flexure lies just medial to the liver. The duodenum forms a C-shaped loop around the head of the pancreas. In this scan, the head of the pancreas is seen between the duodenum (second portion) and the superior mesenteric vein. On the left side of the abdomen, loops of small bowel and the transverse and descending colon are seen. Folds of *mesentery* can be seen connecting some of the small bowel loops. The most inferior edge of the spleen lies along the left posterior abdomen. The upper poles of the kidneys appear on either side of the vertebral body. At this level, the *superior mesenteric artery* is seen as it originates from the anterior aorta. The *left renal vein* can also be seen as it empties into the lateral aspect of the inferior vena cava.

Fig. 24.55 is a CT scan through the third lumbar vertebra. The ascending colon is found on the right side of the abdomen. In this image, most of the transverse colon can be seen across the anterior abdomen. The descending colon lies along the posterior left abdomen. Loops of small bowel are found in the central portion of the abdomen. Ileal loops are filled with contrast medium that has refluxed through the ileocecal valve from the colon. This level is just below the hila of the kidneys, and some of the central collecting system can be observed. The inferior vena cava and contrast-filled aorta lie anterior to the vertebral body. The rectus abdominis muscles lie on either side of the midline in the anterior abdomen. The three layers of the lateral abdominal muscles (external oblique, internal oblique, and transverse abdominis) are separated by fat and can plainly be seen in this scan. The *psoas muscles* originate from the body of T12 and the transverse processes of the lumbar vertebrae and descend the abdomen lateral to the vertebral bodies. The *quadratus lumborum muscles* are located posterolateral to the psoas muscles through the abdomen. These muscles can be seen on either side of the vertebra. The *spinal cord* normally terminates at the level of L1. Inferior to L1 the *spinal nerves*, known as *cauda equina*, are seen within the spinal canal.

Fig. 24.55 (A) Line drawing of CT section. (B) CT image corresponding to level G in Fig. 24.48.

Fig. 24.58 (A) Line drawing of CT section. (B) CT image of female pelvis corresponding to level *J* in Fig. 24.48.

Fig. 24.58 is a CT image obtained just superior to the level of the *acetabulum*. In this image, the inferior sacrum is visible, and the junction of the *ilium, ischium,* and *pubis* lies near the upper part of the acetabulum. Loops of ileum, filled with contrast medium, are seen in the anterior right pelvis. The *haustral folds* of the *sigmoid colon* are found in the center of the pelvis as this part of the large intestine curls toward the sacrum. A portion of the rectum is seen just anterior to the sacrum in this image. The fundus of the *uterus* lies medial to the right acetabulum and posterior to the ileal folds. The ureters are filled with contrast medium in this image and are easily identifiable in the posterior and lateral regions of the pelvic cavity. The external iliac arteries and veins run a diagonal course through the pelvis, lying near the sacrum in the upper part of the pelvis and passing anteriorly as they pass down through the pelvis toward the lower extremities. In this scan the external iliac vessels are seen just medial to the anterior edges of the acetabula. Multiple muscular structures are found at this level. The rectus abdominis muscles lie on either side of the midline in the anterior abdomen. The gluteal muscles (maximus, medius, and minimus) lie along the external surface of the posterior pelvis. Other muscles of the lower limbs are found just anterior to the acetabula. The large sciatic nerve can be plainly seen on the left between the gluteus maximus and medius muscles.

The CT scan in Fig. 24.59 is of a female patient and is at a level just superior to the pubic symphysis. The pubic bones, *ischia*, *acetabula*, *femoral heads*, and *greater trochanters* are visualized. The relationship between the *rectum*, *cervix*, and wall of the *bladder* is shown from posterior to anterior in the pelvic region. The ureters entered the bladder just superior to this scan and so are no longer visible. The external iliac vessels are now referred to as the *femoral vessels*, with the name change occurring at the inguinal ligament, which is found between the pubic symphysis and the anterior superior iliac spine. The *iliopsoas muscles* (formed by the junction of the psoas and iliacus muscles) are found anterior to the femoral heads; the *obturator internus muscle*, with its characteristic right-angle bend, is found medial to the acetabulum.

Fig. 24.59 (A) Line drawing of CT section. (B) CT image of female pelvis corresponding to level *K* in Fig. 24.48.

Fig. 24.60 (A) Line drawing of CT section. (B) CT image of male pelvis corresponding to level *K* in Fig. 24.48.

Fig. 24.60 is a CT scan through the lower pelvis of a male patient. This scan is at a slightly more inferior level than the previous scan. The symphysis pubis is seen here, along with the acetabula, *ischial spines*, and *femoral heads* and *greater trochanters*. The tip of the *coccyx* is visible in the posterior pelvis. In the male pelvis, the prostate gland lies inferior to the bladder and is traversed by the *urethra*. In this image, the prostate gland, seminal vesicles, and rectum occupy the pelvic cavity from anterior to posterior. The bright spot within the prostate gland is the contrast-filled urethra. The *spermatic cords* transmit the ductus deferens and vascular structures between the pelvis and the testicular structures, and are found on either side of the midline just anterior to the symphysis pubis.

Fig. 24.61 is a sagittal MR image of the female pelvis near the midline. The fourth and fifth lumbar vertebrae, the sacrum, and the coccyx are visualized. The cauda equina is seen descending the spinal canal. The areas of signal void anterior to the sacrum represent the rectum. The musculature and cavity of the uterus are visible anterior to the rectum. In the anterior pelvis, the bladder is seen posterior and superior to the symphysis pubis. Multiple loops of small bowel fill the upper anterior region of the pelvis but are blurry owing to peristaltic motion. The rectus abdominis muscle extends superiorly from the pubis in the anterior abdominal wall. Fig. 24.62 is a sagittal MR image of a male patient. Note the prostate gland lying inferior to the bladder. A portion of the urethra can be seen passing through the prostate in this image.

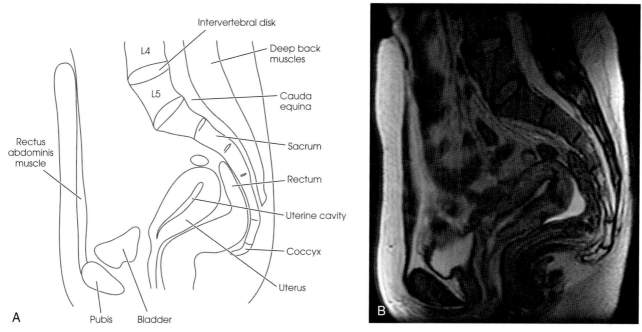

Fig. 24.61 (A) Line drawing of MRI section. (B) MRI of female abdominopelvic region at midsagittal plane.

Fig. 24.62 MRI of male abdominopelvic region at midsagittal plane.

Liver
Diaphragm
Gallbladder
Duodenal bulb
Hepatic flexure

Splenic flexure
Ascending colon

Small bowel

Bladder

Fig. 24.63 Coronal CT image through anterior abdomen.

Liver

Stomach

Portal vein
Splenic artery
Hepatic flexure
Common hepatic artery

Superior mesenteric artery
Inferior vena cava

Descending colon
Bifurcation of aorta

Psoas muscle

Ilium

Bladder

Fig. 24.64 Coronal CT image through central abdomen.

Fig. 24.63 is a coronal CT image through the abdomen and pelvis. The only bony structures visible are the lower ribs. At the top of the abdomen, the diaphragm separates the heart and lungs from the liver and gastrointestinal structures. The right lobe of the liver occupies most of the right upper quadrant. On the inferolateral surface of the liver is a fluid-filled circle, which represents the gallbladder. Several structures of the gastrointestinal system are visible in this image. Near the midline, inferior to the liver, are contrast-filled structures, which represent the proximal duodenum and the stomach. The right (hepatic) and left (splenic) flexures of the large intestine are visible. The hepatic flexure is just inferior to the liver and gallbladder; the splenic flexure is just inferior to the left hemidiaphragm. The ascending colon lies along the right lateral abdominal wall, and multiple loops of small bowel with and without contrast enhancement can be seen within the central portion of the abdomen. The urinary bladder occupies the center of the pelvis.

Fig. 24.64 lies near the median coronal plane. At this level, the right and left lobes of the liver and a small portion of the gallbladder are apparent. The porta hepatis is the region of the liver where vascular structures enter and leave the organ. It is sometimes referred to as the hilum of the liver and is seen here on the inferior surface near the center. The contrast-filled body of the stomach lies near the left lobe of the liver. Several loops of small bowel are visible in the central abdomen, and the hepatic flexure and descending portion of the colon are along the lateral walls. The aorta and inferior vena cava are found anterior to the vertebral column within the abdomen. The aorta lies on the left, and the vena cava lies on the right. Major visceral branches of the abdominal aorta are (from superior to inferior) the celiac artery (sometimes called the celiac trunk), which originates from the anterior aorta near the level of T12; the superior mesenteric artery, which originates from the anterior aorta near the level of L1; the right and left renal arteries, which originate from the lateral aorta near the level of L2; the inferior mesenteric artery, which originates between the lateral and anterior surface of the aorta near the level of L3; and the common iliac arteries, which result when the aorta bifurcates near the level of L4. In this image, the aorta is bright because of contrast enhancement. The celiac trunk is a short vessel that almost immediately bifurcates into the common hepatic, splenic, and left gastric arteries. This image shows the common hepatic artery, which passes right to supply the liver, and the splenic artery, which branches toward the left to supply the spleen. Just below these vessels, the origin of the superior mesenteric artery is also apparent. The image clearly shows the lower abdominal aorta, its bifurcation, and the common iliac arteries. The portal system drains blood from the digestive system and carries nutrients to the liver. The portal vein is formed by the junction of the superior mesenteric vein and the splenic vein, and can be seen within the porta hepatis.

Fig. 24.65 is a coronal CT image that represents a plane just posterior to the median coronal plane. Ribs are seen on the superior lateral aspect of the lower thorax and upper abdomen. Several lumbar vertebral bodies are visible in the center of the abdomen, and the iliac wings, acetabuli, femoral heads, and symphysis pubis are discernible in the pelvis. The right lobe of the liver lies in the right upper quadrant, and the spleen is found in the left upper quadrant where it is positioned lateral to the stomach and inferior to the diaphragm. The pancreas is a long, thin organ that lies horizontally across the center of the abdomen. In this scan, the tail of the pancreas can be found near the hilum of the spleen. The stomach, filled with contrast medium, rests inferior to the left hemidiaphragm, superior to the pancreatic tail, and between the liver and spleen. The right and left kidneys are retroperitoneal organs. Most of the right kidney is visible on this image; the anterior surface of the left kidney can also be seen. The central abdominal portions of the aorta and inferior vena cava are present in the center of the abdomen. The aorta is brighter, owing to contrast enhancement. The left renal artery is visible at its origin from the aorta, and a small segment of the right renal artery is seen near the hilum of the right kidney.

Fig. 24.65 Coronal CT image of abdomen posterior to midcoronal plane.

Selected bibliography

Anderson MW, Fox FG: *Sectional anatomy*, ed 4, St. Louis, 2016, Elsevier.

Applegate E: *The sectional anatomy learning system*, ed 3, Philadelphia, 2010, Saunders.

Bo WJ, et al: *Basic atlas of sectional anatomy*, ed 4, Philadelphia, 2007, Saunders.

El-Khoury GY, et al: *Sectional anatomy by MRI and CT*, ed 3, New York, 2007, Churchill Livingstone.

Ellis H, et al: *Human cross-sectional anatomy: atlas of body sections and CT images*, ed 3, London, 2009, Hodder Arnold.

Kelley LL, Petersen CM: *Sectional anatomy for imaging professionals*, ed 4, St Louis, 2018, Mosby.

Madden ME: *Introduction to sectional anatomy*, ed 3, Philadelphia, 2012, Lippincott Williams & Wilkins.

National Institutes of Health: The visible human project. Available at: www.nlm.nih.gov/research/visible/visible_human.html. (Accessed 1 September 2013).

Weber E, et al: *Netter's concise radiologic anatomy*, Philadelphia, 2009, Saunders.

Weir J, Abrahams PH: *Imaging atlas of human anatomy*, ed 5, London, 2016, Mosby.

25

COMPUTED TOMOGRAPHY

GAYLE K. WRIGHT • NANCY M. JOHNSON

Fundamentals of Computed Tomography

Computed tomography (CT) is the process of creating a cross-sectional tomographic plane of any part of the body (Fig. 25.1). For CT, a patient is scanned by an x-ray tube rotating around the body part being examined. A detector assembly measures the radiation exiting the patient and feeds back the information, referred to as primary data, to the host computer. After the computer has compiled and calculated the data according to a preselected *algorithm*, it assembles the data in a *matrix* to form an *axial* image. Each image, or *slice*, is displayed in a cross-sectional format.

In the early 1970s, CT scanning was used clinically only for imaging of the brain. The first CT scanners were capable of producing only axial images and were called *computed axial tomography (CAT)* units by the public; this term is no longer accurate because images can now be created in multiple planes. Dramatic technical advancements have led to the development of CT scanners that can be used to image virtually every structure within the human body. Improvements in scanner design and computer science have produced CT units with new imaging capabilities and reconstruction techniques. Three-dimensional reconstructions of images of the internal structures are used for surgical planning, CT angiography (CTA), radiation therapy planning, and virtual reality imaging.

Interventional procedures such as CT-guided biopsies and fluid drainage offer an alternative to surgery for some patients. Although these procedures are considered invasive, they offer shorter recovery periods, no exposure to anesthesia, and less risk of infection.

Computed Tomography and Conventional Radiography

When a conventional x-ray exposure is made, the radiation passes through the patient and produces an image of the body part. Frequently, body structures are superimposed (Fig. 25.2). Visualizing specific structures requires the use of contrast media, varied positions, and usually more than one exposure. Localization of masses or foreign bodies requires at least two exposures and a ruler calibrated for magnification.

During the CT examination, a tightly collimated x-ray beam is directed through the patient from many different angles, resulting in an image that represents a cross section of the area scanned. This imaging technique essentially eliminates the superimposition of body structures. The CT technologist controls the method of acquisition, the slice thickness, the reconstruction algorithm, and other factors related to image quality.

Fig. 25.1 CT scanner provides cross-sectional images by rotating around the patient.

Fig. 25.2 Conventional radiograph superimposes anatomy and yields one diagnostic image with fixed density and contrast.

The digital radiograph of the abdomen illustrated in Fig. 25.3 shows high-density bone and low-density gas, but many soft tissue structures, such as the kidneys and intestines, are not clearly identified. A contrast medium is needed to visualize these structures. A CT examination of the abdomen would show all of the structures that lie within the slice. In Fig. 25.4A, the liver, stomach, kidneys, spleen, and aorta can be identified. In addition to eliminating superimposition, CT is capable of differentiating among tissues with similar densities. This differentiation of densities is referred to as *contrast resolution*. The improved contrast resolution with CT compared with conventional radiography is due to a reduction in the amount of scattered radiation.

Fig. 25.4B is an axial image of the brain that differentiates the gray matter from the white matter and shows bony structures and cerebrospinal fluid within the ventricles. Because CT can show subtle differences in various tissues, radiologists are able to diagnose pathologic conditions more accurately than if they were to rely on radiographs alone. Because the image is digitized by the computer, numerous image manipulation techniques can be used to enhance and optimize the diagnostic information available to the physician (Fig. 25.5).

Fig. 25.3 Digital kidney, ureter, and bladder (KUB).

Fig. 25.4 (A) Axial image of abdomen showing liver (*L*), stomach (*ST*), spleen (*SP*), aorta (*A*), inferior vena cava (*IVC*), vertebral body of thoracic spine (*VB*), and kidney (*K*). (B) Axial CT scan of lateral ventricles–anterior horns (RightALV), posterior horns (LeftPLV), and third ventricle (3V).

(B, From Kelley LL, Peterson CM: *Sectional anatomy for imaging professionals*, ed 2, St Louis, 2007, Mosby.)

Fig. 25.5 Image manipulation techniques used to enhance diagnostic information in CT image. (A) Multiple imaging windows. (B) Image magnification. (C) Measurement of distances. (D) Superimposition of coordinates on the image. (E) Highlighting. (F) Histogram.

(Courtesy Siemens Medical Systems, Iselin, NJ.)

Historical Development

CT was first performed successfully in 1970 in England at the Central Research Laboratory of EMI, Ltd. Hounsfield, an engineer for EMI, and Cormack, a nuclear physicist from Johannesburg, South Africa, are generally given credit for the development of CT. For their research, they were awarded the Nobel Prize in medicine and physiology in 1979. After CT was shown to be a useful clinical imaging modality, the first full-scale commercial unit, referred to as a *brain tissue scanner*, was installed in Atkinson Morley's Hospital in 1971. An early dedicated head CT scanner is shown in Fig. 25.6. Physicians recognized its value for providing diagnostic neurologic information, and its use was accepted rapidly. The first CT scanners in the United States were installed in June 1973 at the Mayo Clinic, Rochester, Minnesota, and later that year at Massachusetts General Hospital, Boston. These early units were also dedicated head CT scanners. In 1974, Ledley at Georgetown University Medical Center, Washington, DC, developed the first whole-body scanner, which greatly expanded the diagnostic capabilities of CT.

After physicians accepted CT as a diagnostic modality, numerous companies in addition to EMI began manufacturing scanners. Although the units differed in design, the basic principles of operation were the same.

Computed Tomography Scanner Generation Classifications

CT scanners have historically been categorized by *generation*, which is a reference to the level of technologic advancement of the tube and detector assembly. The original "generation" classification of scanners was a clear distinction of tube movement versus detector rotational path. As scanner technology has progressed, the tube movement and detector rotation relationship has remained relatively constant, but the tube power source and the detector configurations have changed. Some authors have used slip ring or detector advancements to assign a generation number. These varied opinions and discussions have led to some confusion concerning scanner generation classifications. The following discussion of scanner generations follows the original standards of tube movement versus detector rotation.

The early units, referred to as *first-generation scanners*, worked by a process known as *translate/rotate*. The tube produced a finely collimated beam, or pencil beam. Depending on the manufacturer, one to three *detectors* were placed opposite the tube for radiation detection. The

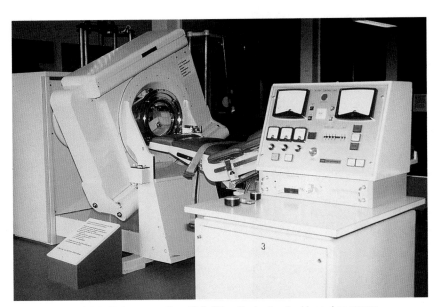

Fig. 25.6 First-generation EMI CT unit: dedicated head scanner.

(Photograph taken at Reöntgen Museum, Lennep, Germany.)

linear tube movement (translation) was followed by a rotation of 1 degree. Scan time was usually 3 to 5 minutes per scan, which required the patient to hold still for extended periods. Because of the slow scanning and reconstruction time, the use of CT was limited almost exclusively to neurologic examinations because of the aperture size and the water bag construction. A CT image from a first-generation scanner is shown in Fig. 25.7.

The *second-generation scanners* were considered a significant improvement over first-generation scanners. The x-ray tube emitted a fan-shaped beam that was measured by approximately 30 detectors placed closely together in a detector array. Tube and detector movement was still *translate/rotate*; however, the gantry rotated 10 degrees between each

translation. These changes improved overall image quality and decreased scan time to about 20 seconds for a single slice. The time required to complete one CT examination remained relatively long, however.

The *third-generation scanners* introduced a *rotate/rotate movement*, in which the x-ray tube and detector array rotate simultaneously around the patient. An increase in the number of detectors (>750) and their arrangement in a "curved" detector array considerably improved image quality (Fig. 25.8). Scan times were decreased to 0.35 to 1 second per slice, which made the CT examination much easier for patients and helped decrease motion artifact. Advancements in computer technology also decreased image reconstruction time, substantially

reducing examination time. Most current scanners are third-generation configurations with one of the following technical variations:

- *Helical CT, single-slice helical CT (SSHCT)*. Slip-ring technology allows 360-degree continuous rotation of tube and detector. Reduces scan times to subsecond per slice.
- *Multislice detectors (MSHCT or MDCT)*. Increase in number of detector rows allows multiple slices to be produced in one rotation. As detector rows increase, the fan beam geometry of the x-ray beam has been adapted, the beginning of cone-beam configuration. Began with two-slice scanners and quickly moved to four slices and more.
- *Volume CT (VCT)*. Multislice scanners with 64 detector rows or more. The

Fig. 25.7 Axial brain image from the first CT scanner in operation in the United States: Mayo Clinic, Rochester, Minnesota. The 80 × 80 matrix produced a noisy image. The examination was performed in July 1973.

Fig. 25.8 Rotate/rotate movement: tube and detector movement of a third-generation scanner.

x-ray beam geometry must be a cone-beam configuration to accommodate the increased length of the scanning field.

- *Flat-panel CT (FP-CT or FD-CT)*. A detector plate similar to plates used in digital radiography (DR) replaces the typical detector configuration. In dedicated breast units, the tube and detector travel a full 360 degrees. In other applications, interventional and intraoperative, the unit functions more like a C-arm fluoroscopy unit in which the tube and detector do not travel in a full 360 degrees. Scanners provide excellent spatial resolution but slightly lower contrast resolution.

The *fourth-generation scanners* introduced the *rotate-only movement* in which the tube rotates around the patient, but the detectors were in fixed positions, forming a complete circle within the gantry (Fig. 25.9). The use of stationary detectors required greater numbers of detectors to be installed in a scanner. Fourth-generation scanners tended to yield a higher patient dose per scan than previous generations of CT scanners because the CT tube is closer to the patient.

The *fifth-generation scanners* are classified as high-speed CT scanners because of millisecond acquisition times. These scanners are electron-beam scanners (EBCT) in which x-rays are produced from an electron beam in a fan beam configuration that strikes stationary tungsten target rings (Fig. 25.10). The detector rings are in a ±210-degree arc. These scanners were primarily used for cardiac studies because of the improved temporal resolution.

The *sixth-generation scanners* are dual-energy source (two x-ray tubes; DSCT, DE-CT) that have two sets of detectors that are offset by 90 degrees. These DSCT scanners provide improved temporal resolution needed for imaging moving structures such as the heart (Fig. 25.11). The latest dual source/dual detector (DSDD) CT scanners offer dual-energy capabilities, typically 80 and 120 kVp, between the two CT tubes. Using Flash Spiral scanning offered by Siemens, the dual source spiral scanning allows for gapless volume coverage using a pitch of 3.4, which increases the temporal resolution to one quarter of the rotation time. This technology allows a marked decrease in patient radiation dose as no overlapping scanning occurs.

Most scanners in use today are third-generation variations that have 4 to 320 rows of detectors in a single array. This increase in numbers of detector rows has increased the length of the scanning field, which requires the x-ray beam to be cone shaped to encompass the full detector

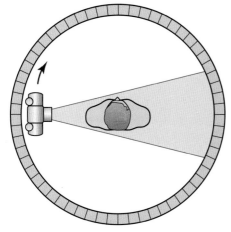

Fig. 25.9 Rotate-only movement: tube movement with stationary detectors of a fourth-generation scanner.

Fig. 25.10 Electron beam CT scanner configuration. X-rays, produced from electron beam, strike four target rings.

array. This is a change from the original third-generation fan beam. The flat panel detector also requires cone-beam geometry. The increased detector size and the cone-beam geometry pose various challenges in maintaining image quality, but this discussion is too involved for this chapter.

Technical Aspects

The axial images acquired by CT scanning provide information about the positional relationships and tissue characteristics of structures within the section of interest. The computer performs a series of steps to generate one axial image. With the patient and gantry perpendicular to each other, the tube rotates around the patient, irradiating the area of interest. For every position of the x-ray tube, the detectors measure the transmitted x-ray values, convert them into an electrical signal, and relay the signal to the computer. The measured x-ray transmission values are called *projections (scan profiles)* or *raw data*. When collected, the electrical signals are digitized, a process that assigns a whole number to each signal. The value of each number is directly proportional to the strength of the signal.

The digital image is an array of numbers arranged in a grid of rows and columns called a *matrix*. A single square, or picture element, within the matrix is called a *pixel*. The slice thickness gives the pixel an added dimension called the *volume element*, or *voxel*. Each pixel in the image corresponds to the volume of tissue in the body section being imaged. The voxel volume is a product of the pixel area and slice thickness (Fig. 25.12). The *field of view* (FOV) determines the amount of data to be displayed on the monitor.

Each pixel within the matrix is assigned a number that is related to the linear attenuation coefficient of the tissue within each voxel. These numbers are called *CT numbers* or *Hounsfield units*. CT numbers are defined as a relative comparison of x-ray attenuation of a voxel of tissue with an equal volume of water. Water is used as reference material because it is abundant in the body and has a uniform density; water is assigned an arbitrary value of 0. Tissues that are denser than water are given positive CT numbers, and tissues with less density than water are assigned negative CT numbers. The scale of CT numbers ranges from −1000 (air/gas) to −3000 (dense bone). Average CT numbers for various tissues are listed in Table 25.1.

For displaying the digital image, each pixel within the image is assigned a level of gray. The gray level assigned to each pixel corresponds to the CT number for that pixel. The bit depth determines the number of shades of gray that can be assigned to a pixel. A bit depth of 8 would have 256 shades of gray available, whereas a bit depth of 12 would have 4096 shades.

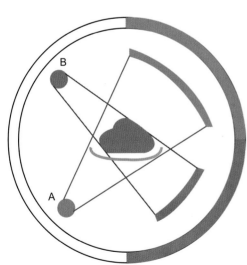

Fig. 25.11 Dual-source CT scanner (DSCT) configuration with tubes A and B rotating at a 90-degree relationship simultaneously. This is considered a sixth-generation scanner.

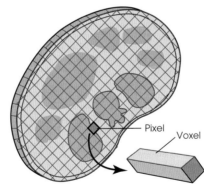

Fig. 25.12 CT image is composed of a matrix of pixels, with each pixel representing a volume of tissue (voxel).

TABLE 25.1

Average Hounsfield units (HU) for selected substances

Substance	HU
Air	−1000
Lungs	−250 to −850
Fat	−100
Orbit	−25
Water	0
Cyst	−5 to +10
Fluid	0 to +25
Tumor	+25 to +100
Blood (fluid)	+20 to +50
Blood (clotted)	+50 to +75
Blood (old)	+10 to +15
Brain	+20 to +40
Muscle	+35 to +50
Gallbladder	+5 to +30
Liver	+40 to +70
Aorta	+35 to +50
Bone	+150 to +1000
Metal	+2000 to +4000

System Components

The three major components of the CT scanner are shown in Fig. 25.13. Because each component has several subsystems, the following sections provide only a brief description of their main functions.

COMPUTER

The computer provides the link between the CT technologist and the other components of the imaging system. The computer system used in CT has four basic functions: control of data acquisition, image reconstruction, storage of image data, and image display.

Data acquisition is the method by which the patient is scanned. The technologist must select among numerous parameters, such as scanning in the conventional or helical mode, before the initiation of each scan. The *data acquisition system (DAS)* is involved in sequencing the generation of x-rays, turning the detectors on and off at appropriate intervals, transferring data, and monitoring the system operation.

The *reconstruction* of a CT image depends on the millions of mathematic operations required to digitize and reconstruct the raw data. This image reconstruction is accomplished using an array processor that acts as a specialized computer to perform mathematic calculations rapidly and efficiently, freeing the host computer for other activities. Currently CT units can acquire scans in less than 1 second and require only a few seconds more for image reconstruction.

The *host computer* in CT has limited storage capacity, so image data can be stored only temporarily. Other storage mechanisms are necessary to allow for long-term *data storage* and *retrieval*. After reconstruction, the CT image data can be transferred to another storage medium such as an optical disk. CT studies can be removed from the limited memory of the host computer and stored independently, a process termed *archiving*.

The reconstructed images are displayed on a monitor. At this point, the technologist or physician can communicate with the host computer to view specific images, post images on a scout, or implement image manipulation techniques such as zoom, control contrast and brightness, and image analysis techniques.

GANTRY AND TABLE

The *gantry* is a circular device that houses the x-ray tube, DAS, and detector array. Helical CT units also house the continuous *slip ring* and high-voltage generator in the gantry. The components housed in the gantry collect the necessary attenuation measurements to be sent to the computer for image reconstruction.

The x-ray tube used in CT is similar in design to the tubes used in conventional radiography, but it is specially designed to handle and dissipate excessive heat units created during a CT examination. The newest CT x-ray tubes use a rotating anode to increase heat dissipation, all metal larger anodes and a metal housing. Many CT x-ray tubes can handle around 8 million heat units (MHU), whereas advanced CT units can tolerate 20 MHU.

The detectors in CT function as image receptors. A detector measures the amount of radiation transmitted through the body and converts the measurement into an electrical signal proportional to the radiation intensity. Current detectors are gadolinium oxysulfide (GOS) ceramic scintillation (solid-state) detectors.

Fig. 25.13 Components of a CT scanner: *1,* Computer and operator's console; *2,* gantry; *3,* patient table.

(Courtesy GE Medical Systems, Waukesha, WI.)

The gantry can be tilted forward or backward up to 30 degrees to compensate for body part angulation. The opening within the center of the gantry is termed the *aperture*. Most apertures are about 28 inches (71.1 cm) wide to accommodate a variety of patient sizes as the patient table advances through it. To accommodate larger patients and for interventional applications, a 34-inch (85-cm) aperture is available.

For certain head studies, such as studies of facial bones, sinuses, or the sella turcica, a combination of patient positioning and gantry angulation results in a *direct coronal* image of the body part being scanned. Fig. 25.14 shows a typical direct coronal image of the paranasal sinuses.

The *table* is an automated device linked to the computer and gantry. It is designed to move in increments *(index)* according to the scan program. The table is an extremely important part of a CT scanner. Indexing must be accurate and reliable, especially when thin slices (1 or 2 mm) are taken through the area of interest. Most CT tables can be programmed to move in or out of the gantry, depending on the examination protocol and the patient.

CT tables are made of a low-density carbon fiber composite, both of which support the patient without causing image artifacts. The table must be very strong and rigid to handle patient weight and at the same time maintain consistent indexing. All CT tables have a maximum patient weight limit; this limit varies by manufacturer from 450 to 650 lb (204 to 255 kg). Exceeding the weight limit can cause inaccurate indexing, damage to the table motor, and even breakage of the tabletop, which could cause serious injury to the patient.

Accessory devices can be attached to the table for various uses. A special device called a *cradle* is used for head CT examinations. The head cradle helps hold the head still; because the device extends beyond the tabletop, it minimizes artifacts or attenuation from the table while the brain is being scanned. It can also be used in positioning the patient for direct coronal images.

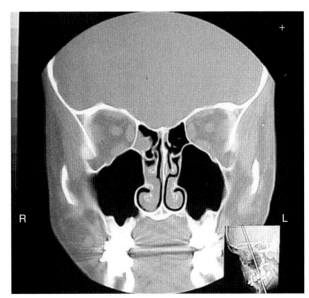

Fig. 25.14 Direct coronal of paranasal sinuses.

OPERATOR'S CONSOLE

The *operator's console* (Fig. 25.15) is the point from which the technologist controls the scanner. A typical console is equipped with a keyboard for entering patient data and a graphic monitor for viewing the images. Other input devices, such as a touch display screen and a computer mouse, may also be used. The operator's console allows the technologist to control and monitor numerous scan parameters. Imaging technique factors, slice thickness, table index, and reconstruction algorithm are some of the scan parameters that are selected at the operator's console.

Before starting an examination, the technologist must enter the patient information.

A keyboard is still necessary for some functions. Usually the first scan program selected is the scout program from which the radiographer plans the sequence of axial scans. An example of a typical scout image is shown in Fig. 25.3. The operator's console is also the location of the monitor, where image manipulation takes place. Most scanners display the image on the monitor in a 1024 matrix interpolated by the computer from the 512 reconstructed images.

One of the most important functions of the operator's console is to initiate the process to store or archive the images for future viewing. Most modern imaging departments now have picture archiving and communications systems (PACS) that are used to store and retrieve soft copy (digital) images.

OTHER COMPONENTS
Display monitor

For the CT image to be displayed on a monitor in a recognizable form, the digital CT data must be converted into a *grayscale image*. This process is achieved by the conversion of each digital CT number in the matrix to an analog voltage. The brightness values of the grayscale image correspond to the pixels and CT numbers of the digital data they represent.

Fig. 25.15 CT operator's console, workstation for three-dimensional image manipulation, and power injector control panel.

System Components

Because of the digital nature of the CT image data, image manipulation can be performed to enhance the appearance of the image. One of the most common image processing techniques is called *windowing*, or *gray-level mapping*. This technique allows the technologist to alter the contrast of the displayed image by adjusting the window width (WW) and window level (WL). The *window width* is the range of CT numbers that are used to map signals into shades of gray. Basically the window width determines the number of gray levels to be displayed in the image controlling contrast resolution. A narrow window width means that there are fewer shades of gray, resulting in higher contrast. Likewise, a wide window width results in more shades of gray in the image, or a longer gray scale. The *window level* determines the midpoint of the range of gray levels to be displayed on the monitor. It is used to set the center CT number within the range of gray levels being used to display the image and controls image brightness. The window level should be set to the CT number of the tissue of interest, and the window width should be set with a range of values that would optimize the contrast between the tissues in the image. Fig. 25.16 shows an axial image seen in two different windows: a standard abdomen window and a bone window adjusted for the spine.

The gray level of any image can be adjusted on the monitor to compensate for differences in patient size and tissue densities, or to display the image as desired for the examination protocol. Examples of typical window width and level settings are listed in Table 25.2. These settings are averages and usually vary by vendor and radiologist's preference. The level, although an average, is approximately the same as the CT numbers expected for the tissue densities.

TABLE 25.2
Typical window settings

CT examination	Width	Center (level)
Brain	190	50
Skull	3500	500
Orbits	1200	50
Abdomen	400	35
Liver	175	45
Mediastinum	325	50
Lung	2000	−500
Spinal cord	400	50
Spine	2200	400

Fig. 25.16 (A) Abdominal image, soft tissue window. (B) Abdominal image, bone window.

Workstation for image manipulation and multiplanar reconstruction

Another advantage of the digital nature of the CT image is the ability to reformat the image data into coronal, sagittal, or oblique body planes without additional radiation to the patient. Image reformation in various planes is accomplished by stacking multiple contiguous axial images, creating a volume of data. Because the CT numbers of the image data within the volume are already known, a sectional image can be generated in any desired plane by selecting a particular plane of data. This postprocessing technique is termed *multiplanar reconstruction* (MPR). A coronal reformation from image data is shown in Figs. 25.17 and 25.18. Fig. 25.17 shows a coronal image of the abdomen (note the liver lesion), and Fig. 25.18 shows coronal images of the lungs displayed with a lung window width and window level. MPRs may also be performed in what is referred to as *curved planar reformations* to visualize structures better. Fig. 25.19 shows an axial image and oblique reformation of the mandible from the axial images. Other postprocessing techniques used today are three-dimensional imaging, surface rendering, and volume rendering (VR).

Diagnostic Applications

The original CT studies were used primarily for diagnosing neurologic disorders. As scanner technology advanced, the range of applications was extended to other areas of the body. The most commonly requested procedures involve the head, chest, abdomen, and pelvis. CT is the examination of choice for head trauma; it clearly shows skull fractures

Fig. 25.17 Coronal reformatted image produced from axial images of abdomen and pelvis.

(Courtesy Philips Medical Systems.)

Fig. 25.18 Coronal reformatted images produced from axial low-dose lung nodule study of the chest. Scans produced with Philips Brilliance iCT.

(Courtesy Philips Medical Systems.)

Fig. 25.19 (A) Axial mandible showing reformatted planes. (B) Oblique MPR of left mandible (note fracture). (C) Oblique MPR of right mandible.

(Courtesy Philips Medical Systems.)

Fig. 25.20 Three-dimensional abdominal aortic aneurysm (AAA).

and associated subdural hematomas. CT examinations of the head are one of the first exams performed on patients being evaluated for stroke or cerebrovascular accident where evidence of hemorrhage must be ruled out. CT imaging of the central nervous system can show infarctions, hemorrhage, disk herniations, craniofacial and spinal fractures, tumors, and cancers. CT imaging of the body excels at differentiating or distinguishing soft tissue structures within the chest, abdomen, and pelvis. Among the abnormalities shown in this region are metastatic lesions, aneurysms (Fig. 25.20), abscesses, and fluid collections from blunt trauma.

CT is also used for numerous interventional procedures, such as abscess drainage, tissue biopsy (Fig. 25.21), and cyst aspiration. In addition, CT is used during radiofrequency ablations and cryoablations of tumors. Fig. 25.22 shows numerous structures and pathologic conditions identified by CT. Fig. 25.23 shows a liver lesion before radiofrequency ablation, during the procedure and after ablation.

For any procedure, a protocol is required to maximize the amount of diagnostic information available. Specific examination protocols vary according to the needs of different medical facilities and physicians.

Fig. 25.21 (A) Needle biopsy of orbital mass. (B) Needle biopsy of infectious spondylitis of lumbar vertebral body.

Fig. 25.22 (A) Abdominal image showing transverse colon *(TC)* with air-fluid levels; liver *(L)*, pancreas *(P)*, spleen *(SP)*, kidney *(K)*, portal vein *(PV)*, celiac trunk *(CT)*, and splenic veins *(SV)* are shown with contrast medium. Surgical clips are seen in posterior liver. (B) Abdominal image showing extremely large ovarian cyst *(arrows)*. (C) Brain image showing parietooccipital mass *(arrow)* with characteristic IV contrast ring enhancement *(arrowhead)*. (D) Image of L3 after myelography showing contrast material in thecal sac *(arrow)*.

Contrast Media

A contrast medium is used in CT examinations to help distinguish normal anatomy from pathology and to make various disease processes more visible. A contrast agent can be administered intravenously, orally, or rectally. In general, intravenous (IV) contrast media are the same as media used for excretory urograms. Most facilities use nonionic contrast material for these studies because of the low incidence of reaction and known safety factors associated with nonionic contrast material. IV contrast media are useful for demonstrating tumors within the head; Fig. 25.24 shows a brain scan with and without contrast media. The anterior lesion is evident in the unenhanced scan; in the enhanced scan, the tumor shows characteristic ring enhancement typical of specific tumors seen in CT scans. IV contrast media are also used to visualize vascular structures in the body.

Fig. 25.23 Low-dose axial CT images from radiofrequency ablation study. Scans are before study (A), during study (B), and after study (C).

(Courtesy Philips Medical Systems.)

Fig. 25.24 (A) Brain image without IV contrast agent showing a low-density lesion *(arrow)*. (B) Brain image with IV contrast agent demonstrating ring enhancement.

IV contrast media should be used only with the radiologist's approval and after careful consideration of the patient's medical and allergy history. The patient's renal function must be evaluated before iodinated contrast material is given. Creatinine (Cr) level and glomerular filtration rate (GFR) are the most common laboratory values used to determine renal function. Many CT examinations can be performed without IV contrast material, if necessary; however, the amount of diagnostic information available may be limited.

Oral contrast media must be used for imaging the abdomen. When given orally, the contrast material in the gastrointestinal tract helps differentiate between loops of bowel and other structures within the abdomen. An oral contrast medium is generally a 2% barium mixture. The low concentration prevents contrast artifacts but allows good visualization of the stomach and intestinal tract. An iodinated contrast material such as oral Hypaque can be used, but it must be mixed at low concentrations to prevent contrast artifacts. A rectal contrast medium is often requested as part of an abdominal or a pelvic protocol. Usually mixed in the same concentration as the oral contrast medium, the rectal contrast material is useful for showing the distal colon relative to the bladder and other structures of the pelvic cavity. Tap water may also be used as a contrast medium depending on the area of interest and pathologic indications.

POWER INJECTOR USE FOR ADMINISTERING INTRAVENOUS CONTRAST MEDIA

Power injector use in CT examinations became mandatory when the first helical CT scanners were introduced. Faster delivery of IV contrast media became necessary with the reduced scan times used in helical CT. The advantage of power injector use is that a bolus injection of contrast medium can be delivered quickly, which provides for better contrast enhancement of structures and better opacification of the blood vessels. The use of power injectors also provides a means to reproduce examination parameters and allows different vascular phases to be captured.

EQUIPMENT

Power injector equipment includes an injector assembly that is ceiling mounted next to the scanner or on a movable stand. The injector head typically has two syringes; however, some models may have only a single-syringe delivery system. If the injector head is a double-syringe system, each of the syringe controls is color-coded. The same color-coding system is shown on the injector control module that is next to the CT scan console. The injector must be programmed at the control module, but operational buttons are located on the injector head as well.

The control module for the system is typically placed on or near the operator console of the scanner. Each injector system has controls for flow rate of the injection, pounds per square inch (psi) of pressure used for the injection, amount of contrast medium to be delivered, and time delays. Dual-head systems have dual sets of controls for each syringe. Dual-head systems are used when the radiologist requests a saline flush to follow the contrast injection.

Special pressure syringes and pressure tubing must be used when injecting. The pressure injections must be closely monitored, and care must be taken that no air is in the syringe or tubing. The pressure syringes have oval etchings on the side of the syringe as a safety feature. If the syringe is full of contrast material, the oval etchings appear round when viewed through the syringe owing to light refraction. If no fluid is present, the etchings remain oval in shape (Fig. 25.25).

Correct IV catheter size and placement are vital to the success of the CT examination. Catheters are typically placed in the arm veins in the antecubital fossa; however, veins lower in the forearm can also be used. Small veins should be avoided because of the pressures used

Fig. 25.25 CT pressure syringe partially filled with contrast material. Note oval etching above fluid level and round etching below fluid level.

when injecting. Catheter size depends on the type of CT examination being performed. A routine, non-CTA examination typically uses a 22-gauge Angiocath with an injection rate of 2 mL/s. A CTA study requires a larger bore 18-gauge to 20-gauge Angiocath with an injection rate of 4 to 7 mL/s.

PATIENT CARE AND INJECTION SAFETY

Patient positioning should be considered when placing the IV line. For many CT examinations, the patients must keep their arms resting above the head on a pillow or sponge during the examination. Care should be taken to make the patients as comfortable as possible while keeping their arms as straight as possible. The angiocatheter should not be placed in a site that would be bent when the patient elevates the arms above the head.

Proper placement of the Angiocath should always be confirmed with a hand test injection of saline that mimics the injection rate of the examination. The ease of injection and the injection site should be observed and palpated during the test injection to confirm patency of the vein. Patients should be instructed to notify the CT technologist immediately if they experience any pain or discomfort at the injection site during the procedure.

All connections between the Angiocath, injector tubing, and syringe should be checked and tightened to prevent air from entering the IV line. The pressure syringe should be checked for air bubbles, and the etchings on the side of the syringe should be confirmed as round. The injected head and syringe should be pointed down to ensure that any potential air bubble rises back into the syringe base and away from the IV line.

The patient should be instructed about the timing of the scan, the injection, and sensations of warmth and an odd taste caused by the dilation of the blood vessels. These sensations should be discussed with the patient, and the patient should be reassured that these are normal and fade quickly. The intensity of warmth and taste intensify as the injection amount and rate increase, so these are more intense for a patient having a CTA study.

If the patient complains of discomfort at or near the injection site, the injection should be terminated, and the patient should be checked for a contrast extravasation (contrast material leaking out of the vein). If there is any change in the appearance of the patient's arm (swelling, discoloration), the radiologist should be notified immediately. The CT technologist should be familiar with the department policy for the treatment of extravasation, which typically includes cold or hot compresses and elevation of the arm.

Factors Affecting Image Quality

In CT, the technologist has access to numerous scan parameters that can have a dramatic effect on image quality. The five main factors contributing to image quality are spatial resolution, contrast resolution, temporal resolution, noise, and artifacts.

SPATIAL RESOLUTION

Spatial resolution is determined by the degree of blur or the ability to see the difference between two objects that are close together. The method most commonly used to evaluate spatial resolution is the number of line pairs per centimeter (lp/cm). The scan parameters that affect spatial resolution include scanning section thickness, display FOV, matrix, and reconstruction slice thickness, and algorithm/kernel. The detector aperture width is the most significant geometric factor that contributes to spatial resolution.

CONTRAST RESOLUTION

Contrast resolution is the ability to differentiate between small differences in density within the image. Currently tissues with density differences of less than 0.5% can be distinguished with CT. The scan parameters that affect contrast resolution are slice thickness, reconstruction algorithm, image display (window width), and x-ray beam energy. The size of the patient and the detector sensitivity also have a direct effect on contrast resolution.

TEMPORAL RESOLUTION

Temporal resolution is the ability of the CT system to freeze any motion of a scanned object. It is the shortest amount of time needed to acquire a complete data set. The use of CT in cardiac imaging requires high (shortest time) temporal resolution to decrease heart motion. Factors that improve temporal resolution include multidetector CT (i.e., 64-, 128-, 256-, 320-slice), tube/gantry rotation time, and the development of dual-source CT.

NOISE

The most common cause of *noise* in CT is *quantum noise*. This type of noise arises from the random variation in photon detection. Noise in a CT image primarily affects contrast resolution. As noise increases in an image, contrast resolution decreases. Noise gives an image a grainy quality or a mottled appearance. Among the scan parameters that influence noise are matrix size, slice thickness, x-ray beam energy, and reconstruction algorithm. Scattered radiation and patient size also contribute to the noise of an image. New technology is available to prevent scatter radiation from hitting the detector. Fig. 25.26 shows the ClearRay Anti-Scatter Collimator (Philips Medical Systems), which greatly reduces noise and increases contrast resolution.

ARTIFACTS

Metallic objects, such as dental fillings, pacemakers, and artificial joints, can cause starburst or *streak artifacts*, which can obscure diagnostic information. Dense residual barium from fluoroscopy examinations can cause *artifacts* similar to those caused by metallic objects. Many CT departments do not perform a CT examination in a patient until several days after barium studies to allow the body to eliminate the residual barium from the area of interest. Large differences in tissue densities of adjoining structures can cause artifacts that detract from image quality. Bone-soft tissue interfaces, such as occur with the skull and brain, often cause streak or shadow artifacts on CT images; these artifacts are referred to as *beam hardening* (Fig. 25.27).

New software developments have greatly improved image quality and reduced artifacts. Interactive reconstruction methods include Philips Medical's iDose4 and orthopedic metal artifact reduction (OMAR) (Fig. 25.28).

OTHER FACTORS
Patient factors

Patient factors also contribute to the quality of an image. If a patient cannot or will not hold still, the scan is likely to be nondiagnostic. Body size also can have an effect on image quality. Large patients attenuate more radiation than small patients; this can increase image noise, detracting from overall image quality. An increase in milliampere-seconds (mAs) is usually required to compensate for large body size. This increase results in a higher radiation dose to the patient. Image quality factors under technologist control include slice thickness, *scan time*, *scan diameter*, and patient instructions. Slice thickness is

Fig. 25.26 Philips Medical Systems 2D Anti-Scatter Grid, which can be focused for true three-dimensional cone-beam geometry. Scatter reduction improves low contrast resolution.

(Courtesy Philips Medical Systems.)

Fig. 25.27 Streaking through the posterior fossa represents beam-hardening artifact. Normal appearance of the brain. *1,* Sphenoid sinus; *2,* trigeminal ganglion; *3,* fourth ventricle; *4,* temporal lobe; *5,* pons; *6,* middle cerebellar peduncle; *7,* cerebellar hemisphere.

usually dictated by image *protocol*. As in tomography, the thinner the slice thickness, the better the image-recorded detail. Thin-section CT scans, often referred to as *high-resolution scans*, are used to show structures better (Fig. 25.29). However, thinner slices require more mA, increasing the dose to the patient.

As in conventional radiography, patient instructions are a crucial part of a diagnostic examination. Explaining the procedure fully in terms that the patient can understand increases the level of compliance from almost any patient.

Scan times

Scan times are usually preselected by the computer as part of the scan protocol, but they can be altered by the technologist. When selecting a scan time, the technologist must take into account possible patient motion such as inadvertent body movements, breathing, or peristalsis. A good guideline is to choose a scan time that would minimize patient motion while providing a quality diagnostic image. When it is necessary to scan an uncooperative patient quickly, using the shortest scan time possible may allow the technologist to complete the examination, although the quality of the images obtained is likely to be compromised.

Scan diameter

The amount of the detector utilized for imaging is referred to as the scan FOV (SFOV). When imaging a pediatric patient, the entire detector does not have to be active for such a small patient. The image that appears on the monitor depends on the *display FOV (DFOV)*. The technologist can adjust the DFOV to include the entire cross section of the body part being scanned or to include only a specified region within the part. For most head, chest, and abdomen examinations, the selected scan diameter includes all anatomy of the body part to just outside the skin borders. Certain examinations may require the DFOV to be reduced to include specific anatomy, such as the sella turcica, sinuses, one lung, mediastinal vessels, suprarenal glands, one kidney, or the prostate.

Fig. 25.28 Philips Medical Systems iDos4 and OMAR techniques to reduce noise and artifacts on patient with a hip pinning.

(Courtesy Philips Medical Systems.)

Special Features
DYNAMIC SCANNING

One advantage of CT is that data can be obtained for image reconstruction by the computer at a later time. The scanner can be programmed to scan through an area rapidly. In this situation, raw data are saved, but image reconstruction after each scan is bypassed to shorten scan time.

Dynamic scanning is based on the principle that after contrast agent administration, different structures enhance at different rates. Dynamic scanning can consist of rapid sequential scanning at the same level to observe contrast material filling within a structure, such as is performed when evaluating enhancement within a tumor. Another form is incremental dynamic scanning, which consists of rapid serial scanning at consecutive levels during the bolus injection of a contrast medium, such as is performed when evaluating the patient for aortic aneurysm or perfusion imaging on stroke patients.

SINGLE SLICE SPIRAL OR HELICAL COMPUTED TOMOGRAPHY

Single slice *spiral CT* (SSCT) and *helical CT* are terms used to describe a method of data acquisition in CT. During spiral CT, the gantry is rotating continuously while the table moves through the gantry aperture. The continuous gantry rotation combined with the continuous table movement forms the spiral path from which raw data are obtained one slice per revolution (Fig. 25.30). Slip-ring technology has made continuous rotation of the x-ray tube possible by eliminating the large high-voltage cables between the x-ray tube and the generators.

One of the unique features of spiral CT is that it scans a volume of tissue rather than a group of individual slices. This method makes it extremely useful for the detection of small lesions, because an arbitrary slice can be reconstructed along any position within the volume of raw data. In addition, because a volume of tissue is scanned in a single breath, respiratory motion can be minimized. For a volume scan of the chest, such as shown in Fig. 25.31, the patient is instructed to hold the breath, and a tissue volume of 24 mm is obtained in a 5-second spiral scan.

Two of the resultant images show a small lung nodule without breathing interference of *image misregistration;* a three-dimensional reconstruction of the lung clearly shows the pathologic condition. Spiral CT is especially useful when scanning uncooperative or combative patients; patients who cannot tolerate lying down for long periods; and patients who cannot hold still, such as pediatric patients or trauma patients. The use of spiral CT may

Fig. 25.29 High-resolution 1-mm slice using edge enhancement algorithm, showing nodule in left lung *(arrow)*.

Fig. 25.30 Continuous gantry rotation combined with continuous table rotation, forming a spiral path of data.

Fig. 25.31 (A and B) Spiral images of lung showing lung nodule and associated vasculature. (C) Three-dimensional reconstruction of lung nodule *(arrow)* after spiral scan.

(Courtesy Siemens Medical Systems, Iselin, NJ.)

decrease the amount of contrast medium necessary to visualize structures; this makes the examination safer and more cost-effective.

MULTISLICE SPIRAL OR HELICAL COMPUTED TOMOGRAPHY

Multislice helical CT (MSHCT) or *multidetector CT (MDCT)* systems incorporate a detector array that contains multiple rows of detector (channels) along the z axis compared with the single row of detectors in conventional spiral CT (SSCT). Each channel comprises numerous elements. In a "four-row" scanner, the detector array is connected to four DASs that generate four channels of data (Fig. 25.32). This type of detector array would allow a scan four times faster than the conventional single row spiral/helical scanner. Current technology detector arrays have 4, 8, 16, 32, 64, 128, 256, and 320 rows or channels. The increased width of the detector now requires the x-ray beam to be a cone-beam configuration compared with the fan beam used for SSCT. The 64-, 128-, 256-, and 320-row scanners are referred to as VCT systems because the amount of body section coverage in a single tube rotation. Figs. 25.33 and 25.34 were acquired on the Toshiba 320 row scanner in a single revolution. Fig. 25.33 is a three-dimensional VR pediatric chest image acquired in 0.035 second. Fig. 25.34 shows a 16-cm volume coverage that allows for whole-brain perfusion imaging for evaluation of stroke. Cardiac imaging using VCT is a

Fig. 25.33 Technology employing 320 detector rows makes it possible to scan an infant's chest with fine detail, low radiation dose, and fast acquisition times. This image is a three-dimensional VR acquired in a single rotation completed in 0.035 second.

(Courtesy Toshiba America Medical Systems.)

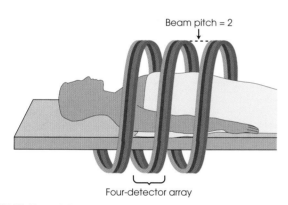

Fig. 25.32 Four-detector array with a beam pitch of 2 covers eight times the tissue volume of a single-slice spiral CT scan.

Fig. 25.34 Whole-brain imaging is possible with 16 cm of volume coverage. This three-dimensional VR whole-brain perfusion study shows evidence of acute stroke.

(Courtesy Toshiba America Medical Systems.)

Fig. 25.35 Images show scan range for various row scanners. (A) 64-row scanner. (B) 128-row scanner. (C) 320-row scanner. The 320-row scanner allows complete imaging of the cranial vessels with one table location.

(Courtesy Toshiba America Medical Systems.)

rapidly growing component of CT imaging. The advantages of MSHCT/MDCT include isotropic imaging and postprocessing, greater anatomic coverage, multiphase studies, faster examination times, and improved spatial resolution. The advancement of VCT, with increasing larger detector arrays, has provided unique clinical opportunities in diagnostic medicine. Fig. 25.35 compares the *z*-axis coverage of 64-, 128-, and 320-row detectors.

COMPUTED TOMOGRAPHY ANGIOGRAPHY

CTA is an application of spiral CT that uses three-dimensional imaging techniques. With CTA, the vascular system can be viewed in three dimensions. The three basic steps required to generate CTA images are as follows:

1. Choice of parameters for IV administration of the *bolus* of contrast medium (i.e., injection rate, injection duration, and delay between bolus initiation and the start of the scan sequence)
2. Choice of spiral parameters to maximize the contrast medium in the target vessel (i.e., *scan duration*, collimation, and *table speed*)
3. Reconstruction of two-dimensional image data into three-dimensional image data

CTA has several advantages over conventional angiography. CTA uses spiral technology; an arbitrary image within the volume of data can be retrospectively reconstructed without exposing the patient to additional IV contrast medium or radiation. During postprocessing of the image data, overlying structures can be eliminated so that only the vascular anatomy is reconstructed. Finally, because CTA is an IV procedure that does not require arterial puncture, only minimal postprocedure observation is necessary.

Currently CTA is replacing angiography as a diagnostic tool for some studies. This is especially true in departments using multirow detectors that allow significantly faster scanning. Fig. 25.36 shows the vessels of the brain, whereas Fig. 25.37 shows the renal vessels in a three-dimensional format. The heart and coronary vessels are shown in Fig. 25.38,

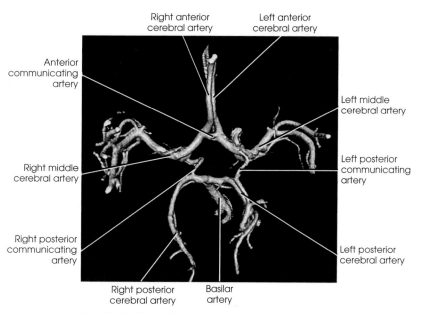

Right anterior
cerebral artery

Left anterior
cerebral artery

Anterior
communicating
artery

Left middle
cerebral artery

Right middle
cerebral artery

Left posterior
communicating
artery

Right posterior
communicating
artery

Left posterior
cerebral artery

Right posterior
cerebral artery

Basilar
artery

Fig. 25.36 Color CT angiography of circle of Willis.

Fig. 25.37 Color CT angiography in three-dimensional format.

(Courtesy Toshiba America Medical Systems.)

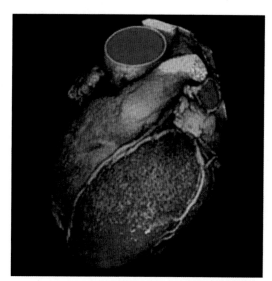

Fig. 25.38 Color three-dimensional cardiac CTA.

and a graft is shown in Fig. 25.39. Fig. 25.40 shows multiple reformations from a cardiac gated dose reduction method performed on a Philips Medical 256-row scanner. Fig. 25.41 is a brain perfusion study showing significant vascular changes on a patient with an acute stroke.

THREE-DIMENSIONAL IMAGING

A rapidly expanding area of CT is three-dimensional imaging. This is a *postprocessing* technique that is applied to raw data to create realistic images of the surface anatomy to be visualized. The introduction of advanced computers and faster software programs has dramatically increased the applications of three-dimensional imaging. The common techniques used in creating three-dimensional images include *maximum intensity projection* (MIP), *shaded surface display* (SSD), and *VR*. All techniques use three initial steps to create the three-dimensional images from the original CT data:

1. *Construction* of a volume of three-dimensional data from the original two-dimensional CT image data. This same process is used in MPR.
2. *Segmentation* to crop or edit the target objects from the reconstructed data. This step eliminates unwanted information from the CT data.
3. *Rendering* or *shading* to provide depth perception to the final image.

Maximum intensity projection

MIP consists of reconstructing the brightest pixels from a stack of two-dimensional or three-dimensional image data into a three-dimensional image. The data are rotated on an arbitrary axis, and an imaginary ray is passed through the data in specific increments. The brightest pixel found along each ray is *mapped* into a grayscale image. MIP is commonly used for CTA.

Shaded surface display

SSD provides a three-dimensional image of the surface of a particular structure. After the original two-dimensional data are reconstructed into three-dimensional data, the different tissue types within the image need to be separated. This process, called *segmentation*, can be performed by drawing a line around the tissue of interest or, more commonly, by setting *threshold values*. A threshold value can be set for a particular CT number; the result is that any pixel that has an equal or greater CT number than the threshold value would

be selected for the three-dimensional image. When the threshold value is set and the data are reconstructed into a three-dimensional image, a shading technique is applied. The shading or rendering technique provides depth perception in the reconstructed image.

Volume rendering

VR techniques incorporate the entire volume of data into a three-dimensional image by summing the contributions of each voxel along a line from the viewer's eye through the data set. This results in a three-dimensional image in which the dynamic range throughout the image is preserved. Rather than being limited to surface data, a VR image can display a wide range of tissues that accurately depict the anatomic relationships between vasculature and viscera. Because VR incorporates and processes the entire data set, much more powerful computers are required to reconstruct three-dimensional VR images at a reasonable speed.

Fig. 25.40 Prospectively gated CT angiograms. Low-dose studies performed with Philips Step and Shoot Cardiac software that has arrhythmia detection that stops scans until ECG stabilizes.

(Courtesy Philips Medical Systems.)

Fig. 25.41 CT brain perfusion study with brain perfusion parameter maps (B) and summary map overlays (A) showing areas of ischemic penumbra *(green)* and infarct *(red)*. Images were acquired using a lower dose protocol on a Philips Brilliance CT scanner.

(Courtesy Philips Medical Systems.)

Fig. 25.39 Color three-dimensional cardiac CTA with graft *(arrows)*.

Referring physicians and surgeons use three-dimensional images to correlate CT images clinically to the actual anatomic contours of their patients (Fig. 25.42). These reconstructions are especially useful in surgical procedures. Three-dimensional reconstructions are often requested as part of patient evaluation after trauma and for presurgical planning. Fig. 25.43 shows examples of the three common three-dimensional rendering techniques.

RADIATION TREATMENT PLANNING

Radiation therapy has been used for nearly as long as radiology has been in existence. The introduction of CT has had a major impact on radiation treatment planning. The use of spiral CT in conjunction with MPR provides a three-dimensional approach to radiation treatment planning. This method helps the dosimetrist plan treatment so that the radiation dose to the target is maximized and the dose to normal tissue is minimized. The three-dimensional simulation software offers the following: volumetric, high-precision localization; calculation of the geometric center of the defined target; patient marking systems; and virtual simulators capable of producing digitally reconstructed radiographs in *real time*. With the new, specially designed software, a single CT simulation procedure can replace a total of three procedures (one conventional CT scan and two conventional simulations) for radiation treatment planning (Fig. 25.44).

If the CT system is being used for radiation treatment planning, the standard curved couch cannot be used. Instead, a flat, firm board should be placed on the couch. Most radiation therapy departments have their own CT units today. A flat patient couch is substituted on the dedicated therapy units. In this way, the actual therapy delivery can be simulated more accurately. Fig. 25.45 shows the external skin markers and structures that would be in the beam's path.

PET/CT SCANNERS

When a CT scanner is coupled with a positron emission tomography (PET) scanner,

Fig. 25.42 (A) MPR of abdominal aorta. (B) Curved MPR of mandible.

Fig. 25.43 Common three-dimensional rendering techniques used in CT.

(Courtesy Elicit, Hackensack, NJ.)

Fig. 25.44 (A) Brain localization in three planes. (B) Three-dimensional prostate therapy localization.

Fig. 25.45 Patient in prone position for radiation treatment planning. Radiopaque markers *(arrows)* show location of treatment field skin marks: tumor *(T)*, heart *(H)*, liver *(L)*, right lung *(RL)*, and left lung *(LL)*.

it is referred to as a PET/CT scanner. The PET/CT scanner comprises two scanners in close proximity to each other, with a single patient couch that travels between the two scanners. In some scanner configurations, there is a small gap between the scanner housings; in other configurations, the scanner appears to be a single unit. Current PET/CT scanners are typically third-generation scanners and incorporate the latest in detector technology. Most modern PET/CT scanners incorporate 8-, 16-, and 64-row detectors. PET/CT is discussed in more detail in Chapter 29; the scanners are typically housed in the nuclear medicine department instead of the CT department. The CT scanner is used for attenuation correction and anatomic correlation for the functional PET scans. Many patients require a more detailed diagnostic CT examination as well, however, which has required nuclear medicine technologists to obtain additional education and certification in CT to be able to perform the diagnostic CT exams. Fig. 25.46 shows sagittal reconstructed CT spine images and the corresponding PET images and PET/CT fusion image.

QUALITY CONTROL

The goal of any quality assurance program in CT is to ensure that the system is producing the best possible image quality with the minimum radiation dose to the patient. A CT system is a complex combination of sensitive and expensive equipment that requires systematic monitoring for performance and image quality. Most CT systems require weekly or biweekly preventive maintenance to ensure proper operation.

Preventive maintenance is usually performed by a service engineer from the manufacturer or a private company. Increasingly, the technologist is being assigned the responsibility of performing and documenting routine quality assurance tests. Many technologists routinely perform daily test scans on a water phantom to measure the consistency of the CT numbers and to record the standard deviation. As data are recorded over time, the CT scanner's current operating condition and its performance over longer time periods can be evaluated. Many units are also capable of *air calibrations*, which do not require the water phantom and can be performed between patients for unit self-calibration.

A CT phantom is typically multisectioned and is constructed from plastic cylinders, with each section filled with test objects designed to measure the performance of specific parameters. Some phantoms are designed to allow numerous parameters to be evaluated with a single scan. The recommended quality assurance tests for evaluating routine performance include contrast scale and mean CT number of water, high-contrast resolution, low-contrast resolution, laser light accuracy, noise and uniformity, slice thickness, and patient dose.

Computed Tomography and Radiation Dose

Calculating the radiation dose received during CT examinations presents a unique set of circumstances. Typically, radiation received during radiologic examinations comes from a fixed source with delivery to the patient in one or two planes (e.g., anteroposterior [AP] and lateral projections). These exposure parameters typically produce a much higher entrance skin dose than the exit skin dose, which creates a large dose gradient across the patient. In contrast, CT exposures (helical/spiral) originate from an essentially continuous source that rotates 360 degrees around the patient. This results in a radially symmetric radiation dose gradient within the patient.

Equipment manufacturers are developing new hardware to reduce patient dose to include off-focal radiation suppression devices, beam shaping filters, z-axis efficiency with increased collimation, and improved DASs. Fig. 25.47 demonstrates

Fig. 25.46 Sagittal reformatted CT scan (A), sagittal PET (B), PET/CT fusion image (C), and coronal PET (D).

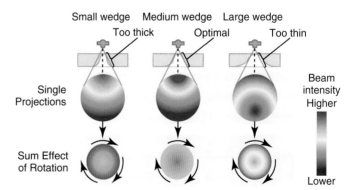

Fig. 25.47 Diagram represents selectable bowtie filters that reduce patient dose and improve image quality. These are referred to as SmartShape wedges on the Philips Brilliance iCT scanner. Note how correct wedge selection affects patient dose. Wedges are typically small (infants 0 to 18 months), medium (cardiac), and large (adult head and body). Wedge selection is built into scan protocols.

(Courtesy Philips Medical Systems.)

the SmartShape wedge from Philips Medical Systems, which is an example of a beam-shaping filter. Note the dose reduction shown on the center image when the appropriate filter is applied. Z-axis efficiency reduces dose effects related to "overscanning," which occurs in helical or spiral scanning systems. CT DASs are utilizing higher efficiency detector material to minimize electronic noise. Also, software development has allowed optimization of image quality based on iterative reconstruction. Using iterative reconstruction allows for a reduction in dose to the patient while maintaining image quality and reducing noise, which improves spatial resolution and low contrast detectability. For the pediatric population, dedicated protocols have been developed and included in the CT purchase.

Measurements of CT dose are typically performed using a circular CT dosimetry phantom that is made of polymethyl methacrylate (PMMA) with implanted thermoluminescent dosimeters (TLDs).

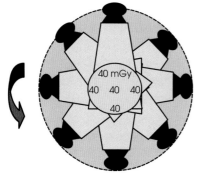

Fig. 25.48 CT dose profile for body.

(Data from McNitt-Gray MF: AAPM/RSNA physics tutorial for residents: topics in CT. Radiation dose in CT. *RadioGraphics* 22:1541, 2002.)

The TLDs are positioned 1 cm below the surface around the periphery of the phantom and at the center (isocenter). The typical phantom sizes are 32 cm for body calculations and 16 cm for head calculations. For a single axial scan location (one full rotation of the tube, no table movement), the typical dose for the body phantom is 20 mGy at the periphery and 10 mGy at the isocenter. The typical dose for the head phantom is higher at 40 mGy at the periphery and 40 mGy at the isocenter. See Fig. 25.48 for the body and Fig. 25.49 for the head. Dose is size dependent (e.g., dose differs depending on head scan or body scan and whether the patient is a child or an adult).

Another component of dose to the patient is distribution of absorbed dose along the length of the patient from one single scan (full rotation at one table location). The radiation dose profile (Fig. 25.50) is not limited just to the slice location; the "tails" of the dose profile contribute to the absorbed dose outside of the primary beam. The size of the contribution to dose from the adjacent sections is directly related to the spacing of the slices and the width and shape of the radiation profile. The first method used to describe dose as a result of multiple scan locations was the *multiple scan average dose* (MSAD). MSAD described average dose resulting from scans over an interval length on the patient. Next was the *computed tomography dose index* (CTDI), which was calculated using a normalized beam width and a standard of 14 contiguous axial slices. This method required a dose profile measured with TLDs or film, neither of which was convenient.

To overcome the measurement limitations, another dose index, the $CTDI_{100}$, was developed. This dose index allowed profile calculations along the full length (100 mm) of a pencil ionization chamber and did not require nominal section widths. To provide a weighted average of the center and peripheral contributions, $CTDI_w$ was created. The final descriptor is $CTDI_{vol}$, which accounts for the helical pitch or axial scan spacing that is used for a specific protocol. The most common reporting method of dose reporting on the present scanners is the *dose-length product* (DLP). This is the $CTDI_{vol}$ multiplied by the length of the scan (cm). It is reported in mGy/cm.

Patient dose must be a part of the permanent record for each examination. Each manufacturer displays dose parameters in various ways. Fig. 25.51 is an example of how Philips Medical Systems displays dose information (note parameters within blue box just above the "go" button). To assist in preventing excessive exposure to patients, the American Association of Physicists in Medicine (AAPM) published a "Notifications Levels Statement" with preestablished *notification values* for individual scans using $CTDI_{vol}$ (mGy). Notification values (NV) are predetermined and set up within the exam protocol; the technologist is notified when any scan series within the complete exam protocol exceeds the preset value. The alert value (AV) notifies the technologist when the cumulative dose index value exceeds the preset value. The dose checking systems will track and report all instances when established diagnostic reference levels (DRLs) have been exceeded.

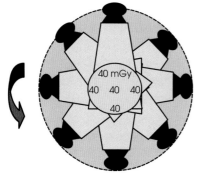

Fig. 25.49 CT dose profile for head.

(Data from McNitt-Gray MF: AAPM/RSNA physics tutorial for residents: topics in CT. Radiation dose in CT. *RadioGraphics* 22:1541, 2002.)

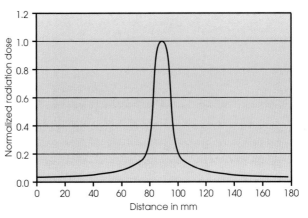

Fig. 25.50 Single-slice CT dose profile.

ESTIMATING EFFECTIVE DOSE

Effective dose takes into account where the radiation dose is being absorbed (e.g., which tissue or organ has absorbed the radiation). The International Commission on Radiological Protection (ICRP) sets the weighting factors for each radiosensitive organ (available at www.ICRP.org). Effective dose is measured in sieverts (Sv) or rems (100 rem = 1 Sv). The effective dose is determined by multiplying the DLP by a region-specific conversion factor. The conversion factors are 0.017 mSv/mGy per cm for chest imaging, 0.019 mSv/mGy per cm for pelvis imaging, and 0.0023 mSv/mGy per cm for head imaging. The conversion factor for head scans is considerably less because fewer radiosensitive organs are irradiated. (The DLP for a given chest examination is 375 mGy; the resulting estimated effective dose is 375 multiplied by 0.017, which equals 6.4 mSv.)

Factors That Affect Dose

The factors that directly influence the radiation dose to the patient are beam energy (kVp), tube current (mA), rotation or exposure time (seconds), section or slice thickness (beam collimation), object thickness and attenuation (size of the patient, pediatric vs. adult), pitch or section spacing (table distance traveled in one 360-degree rotation), dose reduction techniques (mA modulation), patient centering, and distance from the tube to isocenter. Improper patient centering can result in an increase in surface dose. A 3-cm centering mistake can increase the surface dose (breasts) by 18%. A 6-cm mistake can increase surface dose by up to 41%. Patient shielding in the scan area is now possible with bismuth-filled shields, which yield little image artifact but provide 50% to 60% dose reduction. Adult breast shields, various sized pediatric breast shields, thyroid shields, and eye shields are presently available.

Each vendor has optimized the ability to use automatic exposure control in CT, developing a product for automatic tube current modulation (ATCM) and calculating or using patient attenuation measurements in one or more planes. Fig. 25.52 shows a technique of mA modulation that uses an AP and lateral scout image to calculate patient thickness, which results in automatic mA adjustments during the scan (see *red line*). New "selectable" filters (Fig. 25.53) have been developed that allow different filter applications based on body section or patient age or size. These filters can reduce dose by nearly 30% when using 120 kVp and 45% when using 80 kVp. Equipment manufactures include an automated dose-optimized selection of the tube voltage, as in some instances a lower kVp may provide better images with a lower dose.

A

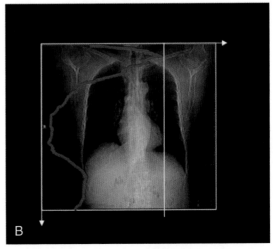

B

Fig. 25.51 Dose amounts must be reported for every series and protocol performed. Each manufacturer displays information differently. Note CTDI and DLP displayed inside the *blue box*.

(Courtesy Philips Medical Systems.)

Fig. 25.52 (A) AP and lateral scout images performed for mA modulation calculations. Note thickness difference A/P versus R/L. (B) Philips DoseRight automated tube current selection (ACS). *Red line* shows z-axis dose modulation. Note technique increase in shoulder and abdomen region and technique decrease in lung region.

(Courtesy Philips Medical Systems.)

Beam collimation (slice thickness) varies in single-detector scanners and multidetector scanners. Beam collimation for single-detector systems has minimal effect on dose; however, this is not the case for multidetector scanners. These scanners have multiple ways to scan and reconstruct images. A multidetector scanner can perform axial scans of 4 × 1.25 mm (5-mm beam width, 1.25-mm slice reconstruction), 4 × 2.5 mm (10-mm beam width, 2.25-mm slice reconstruction), and 4 × 5 mm (20-mm beam width, 5-mm slice reconstruction). When all other parameters are kept constant, there are significant differences in dose. Beam collimation, not reconstruction thickness, results in a difference in some cases of 55% in the head phantom and 65% in the body phantom when comparing single-detector to multidetector scanners. See Table 25.3 for single-detector imaging dose chart, Table 25.4 for multidetector imaging dose chart, and Table 25.5 for multidetector imaging with new dose reduction techniques.

Patient size must be considered carefully when setting up scan parameters. A small adult or pediatric patient absorbs less of the entrance radiation than a larger patient. This results in the exit radiation dose of higher intensity. The American Association of Physicists in Medicine (AAPM) has introduced a parameter known as the size-specific dose estimate (SSDE) that estimates patient dose based on $CTDI_{vol}$ and patient size. See the AAPM Report 204 for further details.

TABLE 25.3

Single-detector doses

Collimation (mm)	$CTDI_w$ head phantom (mGy)	$CTDI_w$ body phantom (mGy)
1	46	20
3	42	19
5	40	18
7	40	18
10	40	18

Fig. 25.53 (A) IntelliBeam adjustable filter that controls beam hardness (quality). Filters are used in conjunction with wedges to reduce patient dose. (B) Graph showing decrease in dose owing to elimination of low-energy photons *(far right diagram)*.

(Courtesy Philips Medical Systems.)

Computed Tomography Dose Reduction and Safety

The following are best practice guidelines to follow to ensure lowest dose and patient safety within CT departments:

- Develop a comprehensive dose reduction strategy (Joint Commission Gap Analysis).
- Establish an exam request review process to eliminate unnecessary radiation—special consideration to multiphase exams.
- Utilize specific exam protocols with consideration given to reason for study, patient history, and as low as reasonably achievable (ALARA) principles.
- Institute specific exam protocol guidelines to ensure consistency across all sites.
- Appoint someone to audit and update exam protocols as needed.

Comparison of Computed Tomography and Magnetic Resonance Imaging

As CT was developing and advancing into a significant diagnostic modality, magnetic resonance imaging (MRI) was also progressing. Similar to CT, MRI was first used to image the brain; whole-body scans were developed shortly afterward. As MRI advanced and the quality of the images improved, it became apparent that MRI images exhibited better low-contrast resolution than CT images. Brain soft tissue detail is not shown as well with CT as with MRI performed at approximately the same level (Fig. 25.54).

The initial introduction of MRI raised concerns that CT scanners would become obsolete. Each modality has been found to have unique capabilities, however. CT and MRI are useful for different clinical applications. As previously mentioned, CT does not show soft tissue as well as MRI; however, CT shows bony structures better than MRI.

Patients often have ferrous metal within their bodies. MRI cannot always be used to scan such patients. CT is one option for these patients. The CT scanner does not affect metal in a patient, but metal can cause artifacts on CT images when the metal lies within the scan plane.

Many patients (especially pediatric and trauma patients) are extremely claustrophobic, combative, or uncooperative. CT is useful for scanning these patients quickly and easily because of the short gantry length, relatively large aperture, and short scan times.

Because equipment costs are less and a greater number of procedures can be accomplished per day, CT often is a less costly examination than MRI. Physicians have found that CT and MRI can be complementary examinations. In many situations, both examinations are ordered to provide as much diagnostic information as possible.

Future Considerations

Since 2010, the diagnostic capabilities of CT have increased significantly, and the dose used is lower than that previously required. The development of iterative reconstruction methods was central to the advancement of CT as a discipline. With the rapid advancements in technology, the CT technologist has an increased responsibility to understand contrast dynamics and the spiral scan parameters of pitch, collimation, scan timing, and table speed. Manufacturers have developed software that can be run from a tablet so the technologist can be in the room providing care to the patient for the greatest amount of time.

Advancements in dose reduction, improvement in spatial resolution, and temporal resolution will continue. Manufacturers are working hard to improve ALARA practices and to meet or exceed the standards published by Image Gently, The Alliance for Radiation Safety in Pediatric Imaging (www.imagegently.org), and Image Wisely: Radiation Safety in Adult Medical Imaging (www.imagewisely.org).

Future Considerations

TABLE 25.4
Multidetector doses

Collimation (mm)	Total beam width (mm)	CTDI$_w$ head phantom (mGy)	CTDI$_w$ body phantom (mGy)
4 × 1.25	5	63	34
2 × 2.5	5	63	34
1 × 5	5	63	34
4 × 2.5	10	47	25
2 × 5	10	47	25
4 × 5	10	47	21

TABLE 25.5
Low-dose protocols (Philips brilliance iCT)

Examination type	Scan mode	kVp	mAs	CTDIvol (mGy)
Adult abdomen and pelvis	Helical	120	160	11.4
Adult chest	Helical	140	20	2
Pediatric head	Helical	120	200	16.3

Fig. 25.54 Axial computed tomography (A) and magnetic resonance imaging (B) scans demonstrating the lateral ventricles: anterior horns and posterior horns, third ventricle, corpus callosum: genu (anterior), splenium (posterior), and head of the caudate nucleus.

(Courtesy MR Voxel Resources.)

Advances in computing power and design have provided workstations that can generate three-dimensional models, rotate the models along any axis, and display the models with varying parameters (Figs. 25.55 and 25.56). Digital subtraction CT, multimodality image superimposition, and translucent shading of soft tissue structures are some newer applications. Virtual colonoscopy (Fig. 25.57), virtual bronchoscopy, virtual cholangiopancreatography, and virtual labyrinthoscopy (inner ear) continue to evolve. As higher-quality images increase the accuracy of diagnosis and treatment, patient care will improve. Because of the superb diagnostic information and cost-effectiveness that CT provides, this imaging modality will continue to be a highly respected diagnostic tool.

Fig. 25.55 Full-body three-dimensional reconstruction from 64-row CT scanner.

Fig. 25.56 Aortic arch stent shown on 500-mm three-dimensional reconstruction.

(Courtesy Philips Medical Systems.)

Fig. 25.57 CT colonography.

(Courtesy Philips Medical Systems.)

Basic Computed Tomography Examination Protocols

Because of the numerous scanner types, parameters, tube rotation speeds, and detector types that are used in CT imaging, it is impossible to list exact examination protocols. Technical factors are directly related to the detector configuration that is used: number of detector rows and fixed array versus adaptive array. Many scans are performed using auto tube current modulation as opposed to fixed mA. This is an overview of basic CT scan protocols using an adaptive array, 16-row scanner. The values listed are close approximations of what can be used for the various examinations.

BASIC HEAD

Anatomical scan range	Scan type	Localizer scans	kVp	mAs	FOV	Scan slice thickness	Recon slice thickness	Gantry tilt	Recon kernel	IV contrast	Oral contrast
Skull base through vertex of head	Axial sequential	AP, LAT	120	250 auto	22cm	5mm	2.5mm	Match skull base	Medium average	No	No

Place patient in supine position with head in head holder. Ensure that patient is not rotated or tilted. Elevate table to bring coronal alignment light to the center of the skull. Landmark per equipment requirements (table movement for scout images). Perform scout images. Prescribe scan locations from skull base to vertex of head. Angle gantry to match skull base (occipital bone) (foramen magnum) and frontal bone (roof of orbit).

CORONAL SINUSES

Anatomical scan range	Scan type	Localizer scans	kVp	mAs	FOV	Scan slice thickness	Recon slice thickness	Gantry tilt	Recon kernel	IV contrast	Oral contrast
Entire sphenoid sinus through entire frontal sinus	Axial sequential	AP, LAT	120	200 auto	16cm	5mm 3mm	2.5mm 1.5mm	90° to max. sinus	Sharp bone	No	No

OPTION 1: Direct coronals—Place patient in prone position with extended chin resting in head holder (see diagram). OPTION 2: Place patient in supine position with head in head holder (basic head positioning). Ensure that patient is not rotated or tilted. Elevate table to bring coronal alignment light to the center of the skull. Landmark per equipment requirements (table movement for scout images). Perform scout images. Prescribe scan locations to include entire sphenoid sinus through entire frontal sinus Angle gantry to 90° orientation to floor of maxillary sinus. Volume scans can be performed with either positioning option with MPRs in opposite planes. Direct coronal positioning provides better information about maxillary meatus.

SOFT TISSUE NECK

Anatomical scan range	Scan type	Localizer scans	kVp	mAs	FOV	Scan slice thickness	Recon slice thickness	Gantry tilt	Recon kernel	IV contrast	Oral contrast
Above floor of frontal fossa to mid aortic arch	Helical	AP, LAT	120	150 auto	20cm	5mm	2.5mm	Usually none	Medium average	Yes 15s delay	No

Place patient supine on table with head resting on radiolucent sponge. Ensure that patient's head and neck are within table scan range. Ensure that patient's head and shoulders are not rotated or tilted. Elevate table to bring coronal alignment light to the center of the neck. Landmark per equipment requirements (table movement for scout images). Tip chin up to bring plane of teeth perpendicular to tabletop. Perform scout images. Prescribe scan locations from above floor of frontal fossa to mid aortic arch. Usually no gantry tilt needed—however, scans should be perpendicular to midcoronal plane. Scans typically performed with IV contrast and a scan delay of 15 seconds.

CERVICAL SPINE

Anatomical scan range	Scan type	Localizer scans	kVp	mAs	FOV	Scan slice thickness	Recon slice thickness	Gantry tilt	Recon kernel	IV contrast	Oral contrast
Occipital condyles to below T2	Helical	AP, LAT	120	250 auto	16cm	3mm	1.5mm	Usually none	Sharp bone	No	No

Place patient supine on table with head resting on radiolucent sponge. Ensure that patient's head and neck are within table scan range. Ensure that patient's head and shoulders are not rotated or tilted. Elevate table to bring coronal alignment light to the center of the neck. Landmark per equipment requirements (table movement for scout images). Perform scout images. Prescribe scan locations from skull base/occipital condyles to below T1. Usually no gantry angle when scanning the entire C-Spine. If individual vertebral bodies are of interest—gantry can be angled to match vertebral bodies/disc spaces. Volume scans performed with MPRs in sagittal and coronal planes.

ROUTINE CHEST

	Anatomical scan range	Scan type	Localizer scans	kVp	mAs	FOV	Scan slice thickness	Recon slice thickness	Gantry tilt	Recon kernel	IV contrast	Oral contrast
	Above lung apices to below adrenal glands	Helical	AP, LAT	120	100 auto	Thorax margin	5mm	2.5mm	None	Medium average	Yes 25s delay	No

Place 22g needle in antecubital space—ensure patency. Place patient in supine position with head on pillow, cushion under patient's knees for comfort. Ensure that patient is not rotated or tilted. Elevate table to bring coronal alignment light to the center of the chest. Landmark per equipment requirements (table movement for scout images). Bring patient's arms above their head and support with sponges/pillows for comfort and to protect IV site. Perform scout images. Prescribe scan locations from above lung apices to below adrenal glands. Define FOV to include lateral margins of chest and use lateral scout to center FOV to include anterior and posterior margins of the chest. Scans typically performed with IV contrast and a scan delay of 25 seconds.

ROUTINE ABDOMEN

	Anatomical scan range	Scan type	Localizer scans	kVp	mAs	FOV	Scan slice thickness	Recon slice thickness	Gantry tilt	Recon kernel	IV contrast	Oral contrast
	Above hemidiaphragms to iliac crest	Helical	AP, LAT	120	200 auto	Body margin	5mm	2.5mm	None	Medium average	Yes 60s delay	Yes 24 hr/ 1 hr

Exams typically performed with oral contrast—give contrast 24 hours and 1 hour before exam or timing as requested by radiologist. Place 22g needle in antecubital space—ensure patency. Place patient in supine position with head on pillow, cushion under patient's knees for comfort. Ensure that patient is not rotated or tilted. Elevate table to bring coronal alignment light to the center of the abdomen. Landmark per equipment requirements (table movement for scout images). Bring patient's arms above their head and support with sponges/pillows for comfort and to protect IV site. Perform scout images. Prescribe scan locations from above hemidiaphragms to iliac crest (scan area must include all of liver). Define FOV to include lateral margins of abdomen and use lateral scout to center FOV to include anterior and posterior margins of the abdomen. Scans typically performed with IV contrast and a scan delay of 60 seconds.

ROUTINE PELVIS

	Anatomical scan range	Scan type	Localizer scans	kVp	mAs	FOV	Scan slice thickness	Recon slice thickness	Gantry tilt	Recon kernel	IV contrast	Oral contrast
	Above Iliac crest to mid symphysis pubis	Helical	AP, LAT	120	200 auto	Body margin	5mm	2.5mm	Usually none	Medium average	Yes 120s delay	Yes 24 hr/ 1 hr

Exams typically performed with oral contrast—give contrast 24 hours and 1 hour before exam or timing as requested by Radiologist. Place 22g needle in antecubital space—ensure patency. Place patient in supine position with head on pillow, cushion under patient's knees for comfort. Ensure that patient is not rotated or tilted. Elevate table to bring coronal alignment light to the center of the pelvis. Landmark per equipment requirements (table movement for scout images). Bring patient's arms above their head and support with sponges/pillows for comfort and to protect IV site. Perform scout images. Prescribe scan locations from above iliac crest to mid symphysis or below symphysis. Define FOV to include lateral margins of pelvis and use lateral scout to center FOV to include anterior and posterior margins of the pelvis. Scans typically performed with IV contrast and a scan delay of 120–180 seconds.

EXTREMITY - KNEE

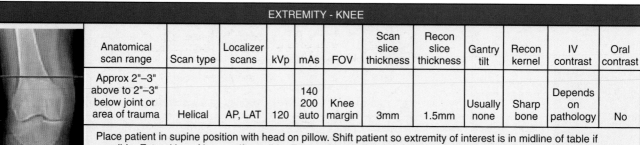

Anatomical scan range	Scan type	Localizer scans	kVp	mAs	FOV	Scan slice thickness	Recon slice thickness	Gantry tilt	Recon kernel	IV contrast	Oral contrast
Approx 2"–3" above to 2"–3" below joint or area of trauma	Helical	AP, LAT	120	140 200 auto	Knee margin	3mm	1.5mm	Usually none	Sharp bone	Depends on pathology	No

Place patient in supine position with head on pillow. Shift patient so extremity of interest is in midline of table if possible. Extend leg of interest if possible. Ensure that patient is not rotated or tilted. Elevate table to bring coronal alignment light to the center of the knee. Landmark per equipment requirements (table movement for scout images). Flex the unaffected knee to bring leg and foot away from scan plane through affected knee if possible. Perform scout images. Prescribe scan locations from approximately 2"–3" above joint to 2"–3" below joint or area of interest. Define FOV to include lateral margins of soft tissues and use lateral scout to center FOV to include anterior and posterior margins of the knee. Volume scans performed followed by MPRs.

PEDIATRIC IMAGING

The following five points should be considered for pediatric imaging: (1) "Child size" the radiation dose, (2) scan only when necessary, (3) scan only indicated areas, (4) multiphase scanning usually not indicated, (5) utilize shielding whenever possible. Most protocols are adjusted based on patient weight as opposed to patient age, with 55kg being the top of the scale for pediatric adjustments. Note: kVp and mAs values listed are typical low/high ranges for imaging based on patient weight.

PEDIATRIC PROTOCOLS

Anatomical region	Pediatric considerations	Scan type	Localizer scans	kVp	mAs	FOV	Scan slice thickness	Recon slice thickness	Gantry tilt	Recon kernel	IV contrast	Oral contrast
Head	Avoid eyes with scan plane	Helical	AP, LAT	80 120	100 200 auto	16-20 cm	5mm 3mm	2.5mm 1.5mm	Match skull base	Medium average	No	No
Soft tissue neck	Typically same coverage as adults	Helical	AP, LAT	80 120	20 80 auto	10-14 cm	5mm 3mm	2.5mm 1.5mm	Usually none	Medium average	Typically yes	No
C-spine	Typically entire C-spine, avoid eyes	Helical	AP, LAT	80 120	40 100 auto	10-14 cm	3mm	1.5mm	Usually none	Sharp bone	No	No
Chest	Restrict to area of interest, typically single phase for peds	Helical	AP, LAT	80 120	20 70 auto	Edge of anatomy	5mm 3mm	2.5mm 1.5mm	Usually none	Medium average	Yes	No
Abdomen	Restrict to area of interest, typically single phase for peds	Helical	AP, LAT	80 120	40 100 auto	Edge of anatomy	5mm 3mm	2.5mm 1.5mm	Usually none	Sharp bone	Yes	Yes
Pelvis	Restrict to area of interest, typically single phase for peds	Helical	AP, LAT	80 120	40 100 auto	Edge of anatomy	5mm 3mm	2.5mm 1.5mm	Usually none	Sharp bone	Yes	Yes
Extremities	Typically same coverage as adults	Helical	AP, LAT	80 120	50 150 auto	Edge of anatomy	3mm	1.5mm	Usually none	Sharp bone	Depends on pathology	No

Definition of Terms

air calibration Scan of air in gantry; based on a known value of −1000 for air, the scanner calibrates itself according to this density value relative to actual density value measured.

algorithm Mathematic formula designed for computers to carry out complex calculations required for image reconstruction; designed for enhancement of soft tissue, bone, and edge resolution. Also referred to as *kernel*.

anisotropic spatial resolution Spatial resolution of a voxel in which all three axes of the volume element are not equal. Slice thickness is not equal to pixel size.

aperture Opening of the gantry through which patient passes during scan.

archiving Storage of CT images on long-term storage device such as cassette tape, magnetic tape, or optical disk.

artifact Distortion or error in image that is unrelated to subject being studied.

attenuation Coefficient CT number assigned to measured remnant radiation intensity after attenuation by tissue density.

axial Describes plane of image as presented by CT scan; same as *transverse*.

bolus Preset amount of radiopaque contrast medium injected rapidly per IV administration to visualize high-flow vascular structures, usually in conjunction with dynamic scan; most often injected using a pressure injector.

channel In multidetector CT, multiple rows of detectors (channels) are arranged along the longitudinal (*z*) axis of the patient. Each detector row (channel) consists of numerous elements.

computed tomography (CT) X-ray tube and detector assembly rotating 360 degrees around a specified area of the body; also called CAT (computed axial tomography) scan.

computed tomography dose index (CTDI) Radiation dose descriptor calculated with normalized beam widths for 14 contiguous sections or slices.

computed tomography dose index$_{100}$ (CTDI$_{100}$) Radiation dose descriptor calculated with the full length of a 100-mm pencil ionization chamber. Measures larger scan distances than CTDI, but only one location is calculated.

computed tomography dose index vol (CTDI$_{vol}$) Radiation dose descriptor that takes into account the parameters that are related to a specific imaging protocol. Considers helical pitch or axial scan spacing in its calculation. More accurate measure of dose per protocol.

computed tomography dose index w (CTDI$_w$) Radiation dose descriptor that provides a weighted average of the center and peripheral contributions to dose within the scan plane. More accurate than CTDI$_{100}$, owing to calculations from more than one location.

CT angiography Use of volumetric CT scanning with spiral technique to acquire image data that are reconstructed into three-dimensional CT angiograms.

CT number Arbitrary number assigned by computer to indicate relative density of a given tissue; CT number varies proportionately with tissue density; high CT numbers indicate dense tissue, and low CT numbers indicate less dense tissue. All CT numbers are based on the density of water, which is assigned a CT number of 0. Also referred to as a *Hounsfield unit*.

contrast resolution Ability to differentiate between small variations in density within the image.

curved planar reformations Post-processing technique applied to stacks of axial image data that can be reconstructed into irregular or oblique planes.

data acquisition system (DAS) Part of detector assembly that converts analog signals to digital signals that can be used by the CT computer.

detector Electronic component used for radiation detection; made of either high-density photo reactive crystals or pressurized stable gases.

detector assembly Electronic component of CT scanner that measures remnant radiation exiting the patient, converting the radiation to an analog signal proportionate to the radiation intensity measured.

direct coronal Describes position used to obtain images in coronal plane; used for head scans to provide images at right angles to axial images; patient is positioned prone for direct coronal images and supine for reverse coronal images.

dose length product (DLP) Commonly reported dose descriptor on CT scanners. Calculated by multiplying the CTDI$_{vol}$ by the length of the scan (cm). DLP = CTDI$_{vol}$ × scan length.

dynamic scanning Process by which raw data are obtained by continuous scanning; images are not reconstructed but are saved for later reconstruction; most often used for visualization of high-flow vascular structures; can be used to scan an uncooperative patient rapidly.

field of view (FOV) Area of anatomy displayed on the monitor; can be adjusted to include entire body section or a specific part of the patient anatomy being scanned.

gantry Part of CT scanner that houses x-ray tube, cooling system, detector assembly, and DAS; often referred to as the "doughnut" by patients.

generation Description of significant levels of technologic development of CT scanners; specifically related to tube/detector movement.

grayscale image Analog image whereby each pixel in the image corresponds to a particular shade of gray.

helical CT Data acquisition method that combines continuous gantry rotation with continuous table movement to form a helical path of scan data; also called *spiral CT*.

high-resolution scans Use of scanning parameters that enhance contrast resolution of an image, such as thin slices, high matrices, high-spatial frequency algorithms, and small-display FOV.

host computer Primary link between system operator and other components of imaging system.

Hounsfield unit (HU) Number used to describe average density of tissue; term is used interchangeably with *CT number*; named in honor of Hounsfield, who is generally given credit for development of the first clinically viable CT scanner.

image misregistration Image distortion caused by combination of table indexing and respiration; table moves in specified increments, but patient movement during respiration may cause anatomy to be scanned more than once or not at all.

index Table movement; also referred to as *table increments*.

isotropic spatial resolution Spatial resolution of a voxel in which all three axes of the volume element are equal. Slice thickness is equal to pixel size.

mapping Assignment of appropriate gray level to each pixel in an image.

matrix Mathematical formula for calculation made up of individual cells for number assignment; CT matrix stores a CT number relative to the tissue density at that location; each cell or "address" stores one CT number for image reconstruction.

maximum intensity projection (MIP) Reconstruction of brightest pixels from stack of image data into a three-dimensional image.

multiplanar reconstruction (MPR) Postprocessing technique applied to stacks of axial image data that can be reconstructed into other orientations or imaging planes.

multiple scan average dose (MSAD) Dose descriptor that calculates average dose resulting from a series of scans over an interval length of scans.

noise Random variation of CT numbers around some mean value within a uniform object; noise produces a grainy appearance in the image.

partial volume averaging Calculated linear attenuation coefficient for a pixel that is a weighted average of all densities in the pixel; the assigned CT number and ultimately the pixel appearance are affected by the average of the different densities measured within that pixel.

pixel (picture element) One individual cell surface within an image matrix used for image display.

postprocessing techniques Specialized reconstruction techniques that are applied to CT images to display the anatomic structures from different perspectives.

primary data CT number assigned to the matrix by the computer; the information required to reconstruct an image.

protocol Instructions for CT examination specifying slice thickness, table increments, contrast administration, scan diameter, and any other requirements specified by the radiologist.

quantum noise Any noise in the image that is a result of random variation in the number of x-ray photons detected.

real time Ability to process or reconstruct incoming data in milliseconds.

reconstruction Process of creating a digital image from raw data.

region of interest (ROI) Measurement of CT numbers within a specified area for evaluation of average tissue density.

rendering Process of changing the shading of a three-dimensional image; commonly used to increase depth perception of an image.

retrieval Reconstruction of images stored on long-term device; can be done for extra film copies or when films are lost.

scan Actual rotation of x-ray tube around the patient; used as a generic reference to one slice or an entire examination.

scan diameter Also referred to as the zoom or focal plane of a CT scan; predetermined by the radiographer to include the anatomic area of interest; determines FOV.

scan duration Amount of time used to scan an entire volume during a single spiral scan.

scan time X-ray exposure time in seconds.

segmentation Method of cropping or editing target objects from image data.

shaded surface display (SSD) Process used to generate three-dimensional images that show the surface of a three-dimensional object.

shading Postprocessing technique used in three-dimensional reconstructions to separate tissues of interest by applying a threshold value to isolate the structure of interest.

slice One scan through a selected body part; also referred to as a *cut*; slice thickness can vary from 0.35 mm to 1 cm, depending on the examination.

slip ring Low-voltage electrical contacts within the gantry designed to allow continuous rotation of an x-ray tube without the use of cables connecting internal and external components.

spatial resolution Ability to identify visibly anatomic structures and small objects of high contrast.

spiral CT Scanning method that combines a continuous gantry rotation with a continuous table movement to form a spiral path of scan data; also called *helical CT*.

streak artifact Artifact created by high-density objects that result in an arc of straight lines projecting across the FOV from a common point.

system noise Inherent property of a CT scanner; the difference between the measured CT number of a given tissue and the known value for that tissue; most often evaluated through the use of water phantom scans.

table increments Specific amount of table travel between scans; can be varied to move at any specified increment; most protocols specify from 1 mm to 20 cm, depending on type of examination; also referred to as *indexing*.

table speed Longitudinal distance traveled by the table during one revolution of the x-ray tube.

temporal resolution Ability of CT system to freeze motions of the scanned object; the shortest amount of time needed to acquire a complete data set.

threshold value CT number used in defining the corresponding anatomy that comprises a three-dimensional object; any pixels within a three-dimensional volume having the threshold value (CT number) or higher would be selected for the three-dimensional model.

useful patient dose Radiation dose received by the patient that is actually and converted into an image.

voxel (volume element) Individual pixel with the associated volume of tissue based on the slice thickness.

window Arbitrary numbers used for image display based on various shades of gray; *window width* controls the overall gray level and affects image contrast; *window level* (center) controls subtle gray images within a certain width range and ultimately affects the brightness and overall density of an image.

Selected bibliography

American Association of Physicists in Medicine (AAPM), AAPM guidelines of ruse of NEMA XR 25 CT dose check standard, 2011, Available at: http://www.aapm.org/pubs/CTProtocols.

Bushong SC: *Radiologic science for technologists: physics, biology, and protection*, ed 10, St Louis, 2017, Mosby.

Griffey RT, Sodickson A: Cumulative radiation exposure and cancer risk estimates in emergency department patients undergoing repeat or multiple CT, *AJR Am J Roentgenol* 192:887, 2009.

Haaga JR, et al: *CT and MRI of the whole body* (vol I and II). ed 5, St Louis, 2009, Mosby.

Image Gently, The Alliance for Radiation Safety in Pediatric Imaging Standards, Available at www.imagegently.org.

Image Wisely, Radiation Safety in Adult Medical Imaging, Available at: imagewisely.org.

Joemai RM, et al: Assessment of patient and occupational dose in established and new applications of MDCT fluoroscopy, *AJR Am J Roentgenol* 192:881, 2009.

Right Dose Information Center, Siemens Healthcare, Available at: www.siemens.com/low-dose.

Seeram E: *Computed tomography: physical principles, clinical applications, and quality control*, ed 3, St Louis, 2009, Saunders.

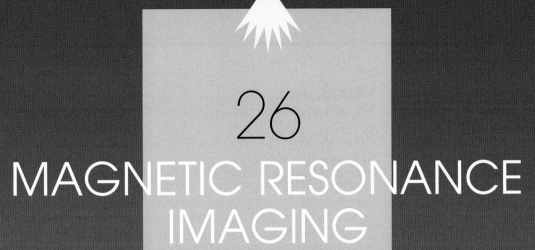

26

MAGNETIC RESONANCE IMAGING

BARTRAM J. PIERCE • CHERYL DUBOSE

Principles of Magnetic Resonance Imaging

Magnetic resonance[a] imaging (MRI) is a noninvasive technique that produces computer-generated cross-sectional images, similar to those of computed tomography (CT) (see Chapter 25), that contain anatomic and physiologic information. Using no ionizing radiation, MRI creates images through the interaction of magnetic fields and radio frequency energy on biologic tissues.

An interesting historical note: MRI was originally called *nuclear magnetic resonance* (NMR) imaging, with the word *nuclear* indicating that the nonradioactive atomic nucleus played an important role in the technique. This term was dropped because of public apprehension about nuclear energy and nuclear weapons—neither of which is associated with MRI in any way.

---

[a]Almost all italicized words on the succeeding pages are defined at the end of this chapter.

Comparison of Magnetic Resonance Imaging and Conventional Radiography

Despite being the mainstay of medical imaging for more than a century, conventional radiography has two significant weaknesses.

On a radiograph, all body structures exposed to the x-ray beam are superimposed into one flat or two-dimensional image. This makes it extremely difficult to separate individual organs or anatomic structures from one another. In many instances, multiple projections must be acquired to visualize these important structures. Cross-sectional imaging techniques, such as MRI, have the ability to create three-dimensional images with little or no superimposition of structures.

Contrast, or the ability to discriminate between two different tissue densities that are very similar, is necessary in imaging soft tissue structures. Because conventional radiography depends on differences in x-ray *attenuation* within the object and the sensitivity of the recording medium (e.g., film or digital detectors), it is difficult for radiographs to detect small differences in contrast. Typically, conventional radiographs can distinguish only tissues with large differences in attenuation of the x-ray beam (air, fat, bone, and metal). Soft tissue structures such as the liver and kidneys cannot be separated by differences in x-ray attenuation alone. For these structures, differences are magnified through the use of contrast agents. MRI is able to distinguish very small differences in contrast among tissues by manipulating biologic tissue with magnetic fields and radio waves.

Historical Development

In the mid-1940s, Felix Bloch, working at Stanford University, and Edward Purcell, working at Harvard University, discovered the principles of NMR. Their work led to the use of nuclear magnetic spectroscopy for the analysis of complex molecular structures and dynamic chemical processes. This technology is still in use today for the nondestructive testing of chemical compounds. In 1952, Bloch and Purcell were jointly awarded the Nobel Prize in physics for their development of new methods in making precise nuclear magnetic measurements.

In 1969, Raymond Damadian proposed the first MRI body scanner. He discovered that the relaxation times (discussed later in this chapter) of tumors differed from the relaxation times of normal tissue. This finding suggested that if images of the body could be obtained by producing maps of relaxation rates it would be possible to differentiate normal from abnormal tissues. In 1973, Paul Lauterbur published the first cross-sectional images of objects obtained with MRI techniques. These first images were crude and only large objects could be distinguished. Sir Peter Mansfield demonstrated how the signals could be rapidly analyzed mathematically, which made it possible to develop useful imaging techniques. Since those discoveries, MRI technology has advanced rapidly. Very small structures are commonly imaged quickly and with increased resolution and contrast. In 2003, the Nobel Prize in Physiology or Medicine was jointly awarded to Lauterbur and Mansfield for their discoveries in MRI.

Physical Principles

SIGNAL PRODUCTION

The structure of an atom is often compared with the structure of the solar system, with the sun representing the central atomic *nucleus* and the planets representing the orbiting electrons. MRI uses properties of the nucleus to generate the signal containing the information that is used to construct the image. Clinical MRI scanners "image" hydrogen because it is the most abundant element in the body and is the strongest nuclear magnet on a per-nucleus basis.

Elements with odd atomic numbers, such as hydrogen, are called *MR-active nuclei* and have magnetic properties causing them to act like tiny bar magnets (Fig. 26.1). Ordinarily, in the absence of a strong magnetic field, these protons point in random directions, as shown in Fig. 26.2, creating no net magnetization. At this point they are not useful for imaging. If the body is placed within a strong uniform magnetic field, the protons will attempt to align themselves in one of two orientations, with the main magnetic field (parallel) or against the main magnetic field (antiparallel). At equilibrium, a slight majority of hydrogen protons will align with, or parallel to, the main magnetic field, also called the *longitudinal plane*, resulting in a slight net magnetization of the imaging volume.

The protons do not line up precisely with the external magnetic field but at an angle, causing them to rotate around the magnetic field in a manner similar to the wobbling of a spinning top. This wobbling motion, depicted in Fig. 26.3, is called *precession* and occurs at a specific *frequency* (rate) for a given atom's nucleus in a magnetic field of a specific strength. These precessing protons can absorb energy only if that energy is presented at the same frequency at which they are wobbling. In MRI, the energy to excite the protons comes from *radio frequency* (RF) energy, typically found in the FM band of the electromagnetic spectrum. The absorption of energy by the precessing protons is referred to as *resonance*. This resonant or precessional frequency, called the Larmor frequency, varies depending on the field strength of the MRI scanner. For example, in a 1-tesla (T) scanner, the Larmor frequency is 42.58 MHz, but in a 3-T scanner the precessional frequency is 127.74 MHz.

When an RF pulse is applied at the Larmor frequency, the protons absorb the energy and begin to resonate, resulting in a reorientation of the net tissue magnetization into a plane perpendicular to the main magnetic field. This is known as the *transverse plane*. The protons in the transverse plane are also precessing at the same resonant frequency. Faraday's law of induction states that a moving magnetic field induces an electrical current in a wire; therefore the precessing protons (a moving magnet) in the tissues create an electrical current, the MRI signal, in the receiving coil or *antenna*.

The MRI signal is picked up by this sensitive antenna or coil, amplified, and processed by a computer to produce a sectional image of the body, which is viewed on a computer monitor. Since the information is in a digital format, it can be postprocessed for additional diagnostic information.

Many other odd-numbered nuclei in the body can be used in MRI. Nuclei from elements such as phosphorus and sodium provide useful or differing diagnostic information than hydrogen nuclei, particularly in efforts to understand the metabolism of normal and abnormal tissues. Metabolic changes may prove to be more sensitive and specific in detecting abnormalities than the more physical and structural changes recognized by hydrogen imaging MRI. Nonhydrogen nuclei may also be used for combined imaging and spectroscopy, in which small volumes of tissue may be analyzed for chemical content.

Fig. 26.1 A proton with magnetic properties can be compared to a tiny bar magnet. *Curved arrow* indicates that a proton spins on its own axis; this motion is different from that of precession.

Fig. 26.2 In the absence of a strong magnetic field, the protons *(arrows)* point in random directions and cannot be used for imaging.

One nucleus   Toy top

Fig. 26.3 Precession. The protons *(arrow)* and the toy top spin on their own axes. Both also rotate *(curved arrows)* around the direction of an external force in a wobbling motion called *precession*. Precessing protons can absorb energy through resonance. B_0 represents the external magnetic field acting on the nucleus. The toy top precesses under the influence of gravity.

SIGNIFICANCE OF THE SIGNAL

As mentioned earlier, conventional radiographic techniques, including CT, produce images based on a single property of tissue: x-ray attenuation or density. MR images are more complex because they contain information about differing properties of tissue—proton density, relaxation rates, and flow phenomena. These properties contribute to the overall strength of the MRI signal. Computer processing converts signal strength to shades of gray on the image. Strong signals are represented by white in the image, and weak signals are represented by black.

One determinant of signal strength is the number of precessing protons in a given volume of tissue. Signal strength that depends on the concentration of protons is termed *proton density*. Most soft tissues, including fat, have a similar number of protons per unit of volume; therefore the use of proton density characteristics alone separates these tissues poorly. Other tissues have few hydrogen nuclei per unit of volume; examples include the cortex of bone and air in the lungs. These tissues have a weak signal as a result of low proton density and can be easily distinguished from other tissues.

MRI signal intensity also depends on the relaxation times of the nuclei. *Relaxation* is the release of energy by the excited protons. Excited nuclei relax through two processes. The process of nuclei releasing their excess energy to the general environment or lattice (the arrangement of atoms in a substance) is called *spin-lattice relaxation*. The rate of this relaxation process is measured in milliseconds and is labeled as T1. *Spin-spin relaxation* is the release of energy by excited nuclei through interaction among themselves. The rate of this process is also measured in milliseconds but is labeled as T2.

Relaxation (T1 and T2) occurs at different rates in different tissues. The environment of a hydrogen nucleus in the spleen differs from that of one in the liver; therefore their relaxation rates differ and the MRI signals created by these nuclei differ. The different relaxation rates in the liver and spleen result in different signal intensities and appearances on the image, enabling the viewer to discriminate between the two organs. Similarly, fat can be separated from muscle, and many types of tissue can be distinguished from others based on the relaxation rates of their nuclei. The most important factor in tissue discrimination is the relaxation time.

The signals produced by MRI techniques contain a combination of proton density, T1, and T2 information. It is possible, however, to obtain images "weighted" toward any one of these three parameters by manipulating nuclei with certain specific *pulse sequences*. In most imaging sequences, a short T1 (fast spin-lattice relaxation rate) produces a high MRI signal on T1-weighted images. Conversely, a long T2 (slow spin-spin relaxation rate) generates a high signal on T2-weighted images.

The final property that influences image appearance is flow. For complex physical reasons, moving substances usually have weak MRI signals. (With some specialized pulse sequences, the reverse may be true; see the discussion of magnetic resonance angiography [MRA] later in the chapter.) With standard pulse sequences, flowing blood in vessels produces a low signal and is easily discriminated from surrounding stationary tissues without the need for the contrast agents required by regular radiographic techniques. Stagnant blood, such as an acute blood clot, typically has a high MRI signal in most imaging schemes as a result of its short T1 and long T2. Specific pulse sequences may facilitate the assessment of vessel patency or the determination of the rate of blood flow through vessels (Fig. 26.4).

Fig. 26.4 T2-weighted image of an abdomen showing the flow void produced by flowing blood. *A,* Aorta; *GB,* gallbladder; *IVC,* inferior vena cava; *K,* kidney; *L,* liver; *S,* spleen.

Equipment

MRI requires a patient area (magnet room), an equipment room, and an operator's console. A separate diagnostic workstation is optional.

CONSOLE

The operator's console is used to control the imaging process (Fig. 26.5). At the console, the operator can interact with the system's computers and electronics to manipulate all necessary examination parameters and perform the appropriate examination. Images are viewed on a computer monitor to ensure that the examination is of appropriate diagnostic quality. Images can be manipulated here, and hard copies of the exam can be produced if necessary. An independent workstation may be used to perform additional imaging manipulation or postprocessing when required.

EQUIPMENT ROOM

The equipment room houses all the electronics and computers necessary to complete the imaging process. The RF cabinet controls transmission of the radio-wave pulse sequences. The gradient cabinet controls the additional time-varying magnetic fields necessary to localize the MRI signal. The array processors and computers receive and process the large amount of *raw data* received from the patient and construct the images the operator sees on the operator's console.

Fig. 26.5 Operator's console. This device controls the imaging process and allows visualization of images.

(Courtesy General Electric Healthcare.)

Equipment

MAGNET ROOM

The magnet is the major component of the MRI system in the scanning room. It must be large enough to surround the patient and any antennas (coils) that are required for radio-wave transmission and reception. Antennas are typically wound in the shape of a positioning device for a particular body part. These are commonly referred to as *coils, or RF antennas.* As the patient lies on the table, coils are placed either on, under, or around the part to be imaged. Once positioned, the patient is advanced into the center of the magnet (isocenter) (Fig. 26.6).

Various magnet types may be used to provide the strong uniform magnetic field required for imaging, as follows:

- *Resistive magnets* are simple but large electromagnets consisting of coils of wire. A magnetic field is produced by passing an electrical current through the wire coils. The greater the current, the higher the field strength. However, the electrical resistance of the wire coils produces heat, which limits the maximum strength of the magnetic field.
- *Superconductive (cryogenic) magnets* are also electromagnets. Their wire loops are cooled to very low temperatures with liquid helium to reduce electrical resistance. This permits higher magnetic field strengths than those produced by resistive magnets.
- *Permanent magnets* are a third source for producing the magnetic field. A permanent magnet has a constant field that does not require additional electricity or cooling. The early permanent magnets were extremely heavy, even compared with the massive superconductive and resistive units. Because of their weight, these magnets were difficult to place for clinical use. The magnetic fields of permanent magnets do not extend as far away from the magnet *(fringe field)* as do the magnetic fields of other types of magnets. Fringe fields are a problem because of their effect on nearby electronic equipment.

Various MRI systems operate at different magnetic field strengths. Magnetic field strength is measured in tesla (T) or *gauss* (G). Most MRI examinations are performed with field strengths ranging from 0.2 to 3 T. Resistive systems generally do not exceed 0.6 T, and permanent magnet systems do not exceed 0.3 T. Higher field strengths require superconductive technology, with popular field strengths of 1.5 T and 3 T.

Prior to the development of actively shielded magnets, installing an MRI system in the hospital was a challenge owing to large magnetic fringe fields. Advances in magnet technology and the use of passive and actively shielded magnets have made the siting of MRI units more commonplace. The fringe fields of both resistive and superconducting magnets can now be "pulled in" or reduced to lessen the interference with nearby electronic and computer equipment. This shielding also reduces the effect of metal objects moving near the magnetic fringe field, such as elevators or automobiles.

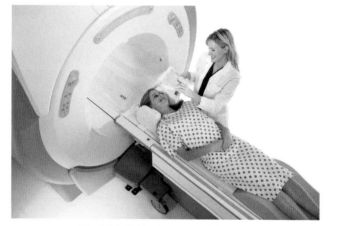

Fig. 26.6 Patient prepared for MRI.

(Courtesy General Electric Healthcare.)

Stray radio waves present another challenge in the placement of MRI units. The radio waves used in MRI may be of the same frequency as the radio waves used for other nearby radio applications. Stray radio waves can be picked up by the MRI antenna coils and interfere with normal image production. MRI facilities require specially constructed rooms, called *Faraday cages,* to shield the receiving antennas from outside radio interference.

Specialty units have become available for limited applications. One example is an extremity MRI scanner (Fig. 26.7). This unit is designed so that the patient can sit comfortably in a chair while having an extremity or musculoskeletal joint imaged. These units are lightweight (approximately 1500 lb) and take up less space than conventional MRI scanners, and they produce good-quality images (Fig. 26.8).

Fig. 26.7 Extremity MRI scanner, 1 T.

(Courtesy ONI Medical Systems, Inc, Wilmington, MA.)

Fig. 26.8 Coronal MRI of the knee obtained with extremity MRI scanner.

(Courtesy ONI Medical Systems, Inc, Wilmington, MA.)

Infection Control

Because of the inherent dangers that exist within the MRI suite (projectiles, torque effects), developing and maintaining a strict infection-control protocol can be a challenge. Although it may be expected that all technologists will practice standard precautions, some may not realize that cleanliness of the magnet room is typically their responsibility. In many institutions, housekeeping is not allowed into the magnet room. It is important for technologists to be aware of the infection-control policies of their institution. Research has shown that various pathogens, including methicillin-resistant *Staphylococcus aureus* (MRSA), will grow within the bore of the magnet. For this reason technologists must be diligent in their practice of infection control.

Safety of Magnetic Resonance Imaging

Because MRI does not use ionizing radiation, it is generally considered safe. However, there are many other potential safety issues that must be mentioned: safety concerns from both direct and indirect effects.

Opinions differ about the safety of the varying magnetic and RF fields to which the patient is directly exposed. Many studies in which experimental animal and cell culture systems were exposed to these fields over long periods have reported no adverse effects, whereas others have reported changes in cell cultures and embryos. RF energy is deposited in the patient during imaging and is dissipated in the body as heat. The resulting changes seem to be less than the levels considered clinically significant, even in areas of the body with poor heat dissipation, such as the lens of the eye. The significance of direct short-term exposure (i.e., exposure of a patient) and long-term exposure (i.e., exposure of an employee who works with MRI) is unclear. No clear association of MRI with adverse effects in humans has been proven, but research is continuing.

Hazards related to the static magnetic field have been well documented. Objects containing ferromagnetic metals (e.g., iron, nickel, cobalt) may be attracted to the imaging magnet with sufficient force to injure patients or personnel who may be interposed between them. Scissors, oxygen tanks, and patient gurneys are among the many items that have been drawn into the magnetic fields at MRI sites. Metallic implants within patients or personnel may become displaced or dislodged and cause injury if they are in delicate locations. Examples include intracranial aneurysm clips, auditory implants, and metallic foreign bodies in the eye. Surgical clips, metal hardware, and artificial joints typically do not pose problems. Electromechanical implants such as non-MRI conditional pacemakers or internal cardiac defibrillators can malfunction when they are exposed to strong magnetic fields or RF energy. Patients who have such implants should not be allowed near the magnet. Fortunately manufacturers continue to develop *MRI safe and conditional* implants, allowing these patients to be scanned safety under specific conditions. Anyone entering the magnet room (patients, visitors, and personnel) should be screened to ensure that they do not carry metallic objects into the magnet room or have objects in their bodies that could be adversely affected by exposure to strong magnetic fields.

Patients can receive local burns from wires, such as electrocardiogram (ECG) leads, and other monitoring devices that may touch their skin during MRI examinations. These injuries have included electrical burns caused by currents induced in the wires or thermal burns caused by heating of the wires. Such burns can be prevented by checking wires for frayed insulation, ensuring that no wire loops are within the magnetic field, and placing additional insulation between the patient and any wires exiting the MRI system. Additional insulation should also be placed between the patient and the bore of the magnet to prevent contact RF burns. Patients should remove all clothing and be gowned in hospital or facility apparel, as many clothing items are now manufactured with metallic threads that can cause contact burns to the patient.

The time-varying magnetic fields (gradients) in an MRI unit act on the machine itself, causing knocking or banging sounds. These noises can be loud enough to produce temporary or permanent hearing damage. Anyone in the magnet room during scanning must use earplugs or some other sound damping device to prevent auditory complications. Claustrophobia can be a significant impediment to MRI in up to 20% of patients (Fig. 26.9). Patient education is perhaps most important in preventing this problem, but medications, appropriate lighting, air movement, and mirrors or prisms that enable a patient to look out of the imager may be helpful. Claustrophobia can also be prevented by having a family member or friend accompany the patient and be present in the room during the scan.

In superconductive magnet systems, rapid venting (quench) of the supercooled liquid gas (helium) from the magnet or its storage containers into the surrounding room space is a rare but potential hazard. As the helium fills the magnet room, it replaces the oxygen, resulting in unsafe levels and posing a risk of unconsciousness or asphyxiation. Oxygen monitoring devices in the magnet or cryogen storage room can signal personnel when the oxygen concentration becomes too low. Personnel may then evacuate the area and activate ventilation systems to exchange the escaped gas for fresh air.

Fig. 26.9 Patient inside a superconducting 1.5-T magnet. Some patients cannot be scanned because of claustrophobia.

(Courtesy General Electric Healthcare.)

Fig. 26.10 Two images (different patients) from a 3-T superconductive MRI scanner, showing excellent resolution of images. (A) This image shows remarkable anatomic detail in a midsagittal image of the head. *A,* Air in sinuses; *B,* brain stem; *C,* cerebrum; *CC,* corpus callosum; *CL,* cerebellum; *V,* ventricle. (B) This coronal image of the pelvis shows anatomic relationships of the prostate *(P),* which is enlarged and elevating the bladder *(B).* Hips *(H)* and acetabula *(A)* are also shown. A loop of the sigmoid *(S)* colon is on top of the bladder. This degree of resolution in coronal or sagittal images would be difficult to obtain by reformatting a series of transverse CT slices.

Examination Protocols

IMAGING PARAMETERS

The availability of many adjustable parameters such as repetition time (TR), echo time (TE), acquisition plane, slice thickness, and imaging matrix makes MRI a complex imaging technique. Knowledge of the patient's clinical condition or disease is also important in choosing the proper technique or exam protocol.

The operator may choose to obtain MR images in any orthogonal (sagittal, coronal, transverse) or oblique plane. These are independently and directly acquired images with equal resolution in any plane (Fig. 26.10). Another MRI technique, especially when numerous thin slices or multiple imaging planes are desired, is three-dimensional imaging. In this technique, MRI data are collected simultaneously from a three-dimensional block of tissue rather than from a series of slices. Special data collection techniques and subsequent computer analysis allow the technologist greater flexibility for postprocessing (Fig. 26.11).

Slice thickness is an important parameter in the production of MR signal and the visualization of pathology. More MRI signal is available from a thicker slice than a thinner slice, so thicker slices may provide images that are less grainy (more signal to noise) but contain less resolution, potentially hiding small pathologic lesions. Slice thickness is adjusted by the technologist based on the type of lesion under investigation.

Fig. 26.11 Single slice from three-dimensional acquisition of the knee on a 3-T MRI unit. Data from an entire volume within the imaging coil are obtained concurrently. The data may be reconstructed into thin slices in any plane, such as the sagittal image shown here. This imaging sequence shows hyaline cartilage *(black arrow)* as a rim of fairly high signal intensity overlying the bone. Meniscal fibrocartilage *(white arrow)* has low signal intensity. High signal intensity from joint fluid in a tear *(curved arrow)* within the anterior horn of the meniscus is visualized.

Imaging matrix (the size of the pixel or voxel) affects not only MR signal but also image resolution and scan time. A finer matrix allows small lesions to be seen but contains less signal to noise and takes longer to acquire. A larger matrix contains more signal but can potentially hide small lesions. It is a balancing act for the technologist to adjust the matrix based on the part being imaged and the patient's condition.

The imaging parameters used in MRI are called *pulse sequences*. A pulse sequence is a combination of gradients and RF pulses chosen to favor a particular tissue (contrast) as quickly as possible (speed) while minimizing artifacts and maximizing the signal-to-noise ratio (SNR). Depending on the choice of pulse sequence and imaging parameters, the resulting images may be more strongly weighted toward proton density, T1, or T2 information. Depending on the relative emphasis given to these factors, normal anatomy (Fig. 26.12) or a pathologic lesion (Fig. 26.13) may be more easily recognized. It is not unusual for a lesion to stand out dramatically when one pulse sequence is used yet be nearly isointense (same MRI signal as surrounding normal tissue) with a different pulse sequence.

Pulse sequences are classed depending on the timing of the gradient and RF pulses. Although the discussion of pulse sequences is outside the scope of this chapter, they can be divided into two categories. *Spin echo* sequences yield true T1-, T2-, or proton density–weighted images and are the standard pulse sequences used for all routine imaging. Classic spin echo sequences tend to have long scan times, so researchers have developed fast or turbo

Fig. 26.12 Axial 3-T images through a normal brain. (A) T1-weighted image shows relatively low differentiation of gray matter (*G*) and white matter (*W*) within the brain. (B) Heavily T2-weighted image shows improved differentiation between gray and white matter. Cerebrospinal fluid within the ventricles (*V*) also changes in appearance with a change in pulse sequence (low signal on T1-weighted image); fat (*F*) normally shows high signal intensity, whereas on the T2-weighted image, the signal intensity of fat is less than that of cerebrospinal fluid.

spin echo, which can dramatically shorten the scan time. Another type of spin echo pulse sequence is inversion recovery. *Inversion recovery* is a sequence that can minimize or null the signal intensity of a particular tissue. Most common are short tau inversion recovery (STIR), which nulls fat signal, and fluid-attenuated inversion recovery (FLAIR), which nulls out signal from cerebrospinal fluid (CSF) in brain imaging. *Gradient echo* sequences are used where the scan time must be short, as in breath-hold abdominal scans. They generate T1- and T2*- weighted images. They are also used in imaging flowing blood (see the discussion of MRA later in this chapter) or pooling blood as a result of hemorrhage or trauma

(susceptibility weighting). Researchers continue to develop new pulse sequences for specific applications.

POSITIONING

Patient positioning for MRI is usually straightforward. Generally, the patient lies supine on a table that is subsequently advanced into the magnetic field. As previously discussed, it is important to make sure that the patient has no contraindications to MRI, such as a cardiac pacemaker or intracranial aneurysm clips. Claustrophobia may be a problem for some patients, as previously noted, because the imaging area is tunnel-shaped in most MRI system configurations (see Fig. 26.9).

Fig. 26.13 Axial MRI showing the use of different pulse sequences and their effect on the visualization of the cerebellopontine angle tumor. (A) T1-weighted image shows that limited contrast exists between the tumor *(T)* and normal brain. (B) The lesion becomes dramatically more obvious using the pulse sequence of the T2-weighted image. (C) The lesion is still visible on a FLAIR pulse sequence but not as well as the T2-weighted image. Choice of pulse sequence is critical. These images also show how the lack of bone artifact makes MRI superior to CT for imaging of posterior fossa lesions.

COILS

Receiving *coils* are used for transmitting the RF pulse and/or receiving the MRI signal (as described earlier in the section on signal production). Some coils can transmit and receive (transmit/receive coils), whereas others may only receive the signal (receive-only coils).

The body part to be examined determines the placement and shape of the surface or receive coil that is used for imaging (Fig. 26.14). Most coils are round or oval, and the body part to be examined is inserted into the coil's open center. Some coils, rather than encircling the body part, are placed directly on the patient over the area of interest. Another form of receive coil is the endocavity coil, which is designed to fit within a body cavity such as the rectum. This enables a receive coil to be placed closer to an internal organ that may be distant from surface coils applied to the exterior body, as when imaging the prostate or uterus. Endocavity coils may also be used to image the wall of the cavity itself (Fig. 26.15).

PATIENT MONITORING

Although most MRI sites are constructed so that the operator can see the patient during imaging, the visibility is often limited, so that the patient is relatively isolated within the MRI room (see Fig. 26.9). At most sites, intercoms are used for verbal communication with the patient, and all units have "panic buttons" with which the patient may summon assistance. These devices may be insufficient, however, to monitor the health status of a sedated, anesthetized, or unresponsive patient. MRI-safe/conditional devices are available to monitor multiple physiologic parameters such as heart rate, respiratory rate, blood pressure, and oxygen concentration in the blood. The technologist should monitor the patient visually and verbally at all times.

Fig. 26.14 Examples of coils used for MRI. *Upper row, left to right,* Foot/ankle coil, breast coil, and knee coil. *Lower row, left to right,* Shoulder coil, functional head coil, and wrist coil.

(Courtesy Invivo Corporation.)

Fig. 26.15 Axial image of prostate obtained with an endorectal coil. The increased resolution allowed by the endorectal coil makes it possible to perform MRS *(PROSE)*. The spectroscopy map shows an elevated citrate level *(arrow)*, consistent with tumor.

(Courtesy GE Healthcare.)

CONTRAST MEDIA

Contrast agents widen the signal differences (contrast to noise) in MR images between various normal and abnormal structures. MRI contrast agents most commonly used in the United States for routine clinical use in the whole body are gadolinium-containing compounds. Gadolinium is a metal with *paramagnetic* qualities. Pharmacologically, an IV-administered gadolinium compound acts similarly to a radiographic iodinated IV agent: it is distributed through the vascular system and its major route of excretion is the urine. A gadolinium compound respects the blood-brain barrier (i.e., it does not leak out from the blood vessels into the brain substance unless the barrier has been damaged by a pathologic process).

New contrast agents used for MRA examinations are known as *blood pool agents* and also contain a gadolinium base. By binding to albumin found in the body, these agents produce shorter T1 relaxation times than regular gadolinium compounds, resulting in a brighter signal on the final image. These agents also prolong retention in the bloodstream, allowing for longer imaging times. Imaging using these agents may allow estimates of tissue perfusion and ischemia. In enhancing heart muscle, they could help to differentiate healthy, ischemic, and infarcted myocardial tissue.

Gadolinium compounds can be used in the evaluation of any body part, including the central nervous system and the musculoskeletal system. The most important clinical action of gadolinium compounds is shortening of the T1 relaxation time. In T1-weighted images, this provides a high-signal, high-contrast focus in areas where gadolinium has accumulated. As seen in Fig. 26.16, gadolinium-containing contrast has leaked through the broken blood-brain barrier into the brain substance. In gadolinium-enhanced T1-weighted images, brain tumors or metastases are better distinguished from their surrounding edema than in routine T2-weighted images. Gadolinium improves the visualization of small tumors or tumors that have a signal intensity similar to that of a normal brain, such as meningiomas. Rapid IV injections of gadolinium are routinely used in dynamic imaging studies of body organs such as the liver and kidneys, similar to techniques using standard radiographic iodinated agents in CT. Contrast-enhanced MRA is routinely performed to image the blood vessels of the neck (carotid) and body.

In general, gadolinium agents are nonspecific; however, organ-specific agents have been developed primarily for imaging the liver. Iron oxide mixtures known as *superparamagnetic* contrast agents have been developed and are available but not widely used. These agents are referred to as T2 contrast agents because they shorten the T2 relaxation times of normal tissue. Research and development of novel contrast agents to improve the specificity of MRI imaging continues.

Despite the fact the gadolinium is a toxic substance, gadolinium-based contrast agents (GBCAs) are well tolerated and typically have fewer side effects than iodine-based contrast agents, and they are not nephrotoxic. Nevertheless, patients with severe kidney disease and reduced renal function are susceptible to developing a life-threatening condition known as nephrogenic systemic fibrosis (NSF).

Gadolinium has also been discovered in the brain and body tissues of patients with normal renal function. Gadolinium-based contrast agents should be used only when clinically necessary.

Fig. 26.16 Use of IV gadolinium contrast medium for lesion enhancement in axial images of the brain. (A) T1-weighted sequence. A single brain lesion (*arrowhead*) is seen as a focal area of low signal intensity in a large area of edema. The borders of the lesion are difficult to delineate. (B) FLAIR image. Areas of high signal (*arrows*) represent tumor and surrounding edema. (C) T1-weighted image obtained using similar parameters after IV administration of gadolinium. Lesion borders and size (*arrow*) are much more conspicuous.

GATING

Respiratory- or cardiac-gated imaging is another technique for improving image quality in areas of the body where breathing or heart motion is a problem. A patient can hold his or her head still for prolonged data acquisition, but heartbeat and breathing cannot be suspended for the several minutes required to do a standard MRI study. Even fast pulse sequences are susceptible to motion *artifact* from the beating heart; this is a problem when images of the chest, heart, or upper abdomen are desired. If special techniques are not used, part of the MRI signal may be obtained when the heart is contracted (systole) and part when the heart is relaxed (diastole). When such information is combined into one image, the heart appears blurred. This problem is analogous to photographing a moving subject with a long shutter speed. Similar problems in MRI occur with the different phases of respiration.

Gating techniques are used to organize the signal so that only the signal received during a specific part of the cardiac or respiratory cycle is used for image production (Fig. 26.17). Gated images may be obtained in one of two ways. In one technique of cardiac gating, the imaging pulse sequence is initiated by the heartbeat (usually monitored by an ECG). The data collection phase of the pulse sequence occurs at the same point in the cardiac cycle. Another method is to obtain data throughout the cardiac cycle but record the point in the cycle at which each data group was obtained. After enough data are collected, they are reorganized so that all data recorded within a certain portion of the cardiac cycle are collated together: data collected during the first eighth of the cycle, second eighth of the cycle, and so on. Each grouping of data can be combined into a single image, producing multiple images at different times in the cycle.

Fig. 26.17 ECG-gated images of the heart. (A) Left ventricular outflow tract (LVOT). (B) Short-axis images. *A,* Aorta; *LV,* left ventricle; *LVW,* left ventricular wall; *P,* papillary muscles; *RV,* right ventricle.

OTHER CONSIDERATIONS

When MRI was first introduced, long imaging times were required to produce diagnostic images. With advances in computer technology and pulse sequence developments, images can now be acquired much more quickly, reducing the time the patient is in the scanner. New pulse sequences have been developed for specialized applications, such as the ability to perform dynamic scans and free-breathing abdominal imaging. These fast sequences can accentuate the bright signal of fluid, allowing for myelographic effects in spine imaging or arthrographic effects in joint imaging (see Fig. 26.11).

Quality assurance is important in a complex technology such as MRI. Calibration of the unit is generally performed by service personnel. Routine scanning of phantoms by the technologist can be useful for detecting any problems that may develop.

Clinical Applications
CENTRAL NERVOUS SYSTEM

MRI is the modality of choice for imaging of the central nervous system. It is routinely used in almost all examinations of the brain with the exception of acute trauma. MRI is superior in the brain because of its inherent ability to differentiate the natural contrast among tissues such as gray and white matter (see Fig. 26.12). This ability allows MRI to be more sensitive than CT in detecting changes in white matter disease, such as multiple sclerosis. The development of specialized pulse sequences such as FLAIR helps visualize lesions in the periventricular area that were previously difficult to detect. MRI is also superior at imaging the posterior fossa (cerebellum and brain stem) because cortical bone does not produce any signal in MRI (see Fig. 26.13). This area is often obscured on CT because of beam-hardening artifact. Almost all brain lesions—such as primary and metastatic tumors, pituitary tumors, acoustic neuromas (tumors of the eighth cranial nerve), and meningiomas—are better seen on MRI. The use of IV gadolinium–based contrast has allowed better differentiation and increased sensitivity in detecting these lesions (Fig. 26.18). Cerebral infarction is identified sooner using diffusion-weighted imaging compared with CT. Diffusion-weighted imaging also gives MRI the ability to determine the age of lesions or differentiate acute from chronic ischemic changes.

Fig. 26.18 Axial MRI of the brain in a patient with an acoustic nerve tumor arising from the complex of the seventh and eighth cranial nerves. (A) Precontrast T1-weighted image shows an inhomogeneous area of abnormality *(white arrows)*, with mass effect expanding the area of the nerve complex. (B) Image obtained at the same level after gadolinium enhancement. Active tumor *(T)* shows high signal intensity.

MRI is also routinely used to image the spinal canal and its contents. The ability of MRI to image directly in the sagittal plane allows for the screening of a large area in a single examination. T2-weighted pulse sequences permit the separation of CSF and the spinal cord, similar to myelography, without the use of a contrast medium (Fig. 26.19). Because of its inherent ability to differentiate slight changes in soft tissue contrast, MRI is exquisitely sensitive to cystic changes associated with tumors within the spinal cord. The visualization of bone marrow is useful in the detection and diagnosis of metastatic disease, pathologic and non-pathologic vertebral fractures, and diskitis (infection). MRI is also commonly used in the imaging of disk disease. Direct visualization of the posterior longitudinal ligament in the sagittal plane and vertebral disks in the oblique plane shows the severity of herniation in disks (Fig. 26.20). The use of IV gadolinium contrast helps differentiate between recurrent disk herniation and postoperative scar tissue, a crucial clinical distinction.

CHEST

Ultrafast pulse sequences and new software algorithms have made it possible to obtain motion-free images of the chest and heart. Cardiac gating (imaging only during a certain part of the cardiac cycle), respiratory gating or triggering, breath-hold scans, and ultrafast imaging sequences have enabled MRI to excel at cardiac imaging. MRI is able to show anatomy and produce functional (ejection fractions, chamber volume) data similar to nuclear medicine and echocardiography. Studies of congenital heart disease, imaging of masses, and heart muscle viability are now routine (Fig. 26.21). MRI may also be used to image the chest wall, thoracic outlet, and brachial plexus region.

Breast MRI, once used only sparingly, has become an essential part of breast imaging. It is routinely used to screen high-risk patients preoperatively to define the extent of disease and screen the contralateral breast for additional disease. Once in treatment, patients undergo breast MRI to monitor adjuvant therapy such as chemotherapy or radiation (Fig. 26.22). In addition, it is the method of choice for imaging the rupture of breast implants.

Fig. 26.19 Sagittal T2-weighted MRI through the thoracic spine. High signal from CSF outlines the normal spinal cord (S), giving a myelogram-like effect without the use of contrast agents.

Fig. 26.20 Sagittal T2-weighted image of the lumbar spine. The spinal canal is filled with high-signal-intensity cerebrospinal fluid (F) except for low-signal-intensity linear nerve roots running within the spinal canal. Normal vertebral disks have a high-signal-intensity nucleus pulposus (N). Desiccated disks (D) show low signal intensity. At L4-5, note the herniated nucleus pulposus (HNP) protruding into the spinal canal and compressing the nerve roots.

Fig. 26.21 Cardiac MRI: four-chamber view from two different patients. (A) T2-weighted image showing normal myocardium in the wall of the left ventricle *(M)* before the administration of contrast medium. (B) Delayed-enhancement image (inversion recovery) showing bright signal in the wall of the left ventricle, representing infarcted or dead myocardium *(D)*.

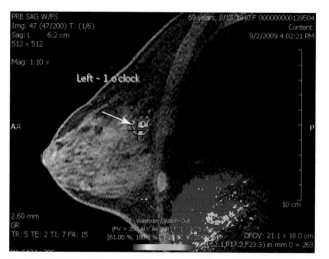

Fig. 26.22 MRI of the breast is postprocessed and showing contrast washin and washout. The patient is a 68-year-old woman with an enhancing mass in the left breast at the 1 o'clock position *(arrow)*.

ABDOMEN

Although abdominal imaging is also affected by respiratory motion, the use of ultrafast scanning techniques with the ability to acquire two- and three-dimensional volumes in a breath-hold has made MRI extremely useful as a problem-solving tool in cases involving the abdomen. Typically not used as a primary diagnostic tool, MRI can serve to follow up questionable results from other modalities such as CT and ultrasound. One exception is liver imaging, in which MRI may be more sensitive in detecting primary and metastatic tumors. The use of liver-specific IV contrast agents has improved sensitivity and specificity in imaging liver lesions. MRI has the ability to predict the histologic diagnosis of certain abnormalities such as hepatic hemangiomas, which have a distinctive appearance. Moreover, the use of in- and out-of-phase images can help to distinguish between benign and malignant adrenal tumors (Figs. 26.23 and 26.24).

PELVIS

Respiratory motion has little effect on the structures of the pelvis. Therefore these structures can be better visualized than structures in the upper abdomen. The ability of MRI to image in the coronal and sagittal planes is helpful in examining the curved surfaces in the pelvis. Bladder tumors are shown well, including tumors at the dome and base of the bladder, which can be difficult to evaluate in the transverse dimension. In the prostate (see Fig. 26.15), MRI is useful in detecting a neoplasm and its spread. In the female pelvis, MRI can be used to image benign and malignant conditions (Fig. 26.25).

MUSCULOSKELETAL SYSTEM

The ability to image in multiple planes with excellent soft tissue contrast and to image bone marrow has rapidly expanded the role of MRI in musculoskeletal imaging.

Fig. 26.23 Multiple images through the liver of a patient with hemangioma *(H)*. (A) Axial T1-weighted image. (B) Axial T2-weighted image. (C) Axial T1-weighted postcontrast image. This image shows the classic fill-in of contrast material from the periphery of the lesion toward the center. MRI also shows the other abdominal organs and their relationship quite well: kidneys *(K)*, pancreas *(P)*, stomach *(S)*, and aorta *(A)*.

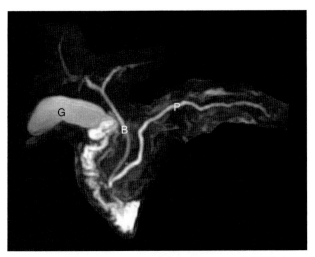

Fig. 26.24 Magnetic resonance cholangiopancreatography (MRCP): heavily T2-weighted images specially designed to image the gallbladder (G), biliary (B), and pancreatic ducts (P).

Fig. 26.25 Multiple images through a female pelvis. (A) Sagittal T2-weighted image. (B) Coronal T1-weighted image after administration of contrast agent. (C) Axial T1-weighted image after administration of contrast agent with fat saturation. All images show the different components of a uterine fibroid (F). The relationship between the uterus (U) and bladder (B) is shown well using multiple imaging planes.

The lack of bone artifact in MRI permits excellent visualization of the bone marrow (Fig. 26.26) and facilitates the more effective diagnosis of pathologic conditions such as stress fractures and avascular necrosis (Fig. 26.27). Local staging of soft tissue and bone tumors is best accomplished with MRI (Fig. 26.28).

MRI has become the imaging modality choice for small and large joints. It has replaced radiographic arthrography in all joints, although MRA is now routinely performed. The ability to assess damage to ligaments, tendons, and menisci as well as to quantify the loss of cartilage is very helpful in treating osteoarthritis of the knee and other joints (see Fig. 26.11).

Fig. 26.26 T1-weighted coronal MRI of the wrist using a surface coil to improve visualization of superficial structures. Marrow within the carpal bones (C), radius (R), and ulna (U) has high signal as a result of its fat content. A *thin black line* of low-signal cortex surrounds the marrow cavity of each bone, and trabecular bone can be seen as low-signal detail interspersed within marrow.

Fig. 26.27 Two T1-weighted images of the left hip from different patients. (A) Normal bone marrow signal (M). (B) Abnormal bone marrow signal consistent with avascular necrosis (AVN).

VESSELS

MRA is the imaging of vascular structures by MR. Two techniques used to obtain images of flowing blood are time-of-flight (TOF) and phase-contrast (PC) imaging. With either of these techniques, MRAs can be obtained in two- or three-dimensional volumes. In TOF imaging, a special pulse sequence is used that suppresses the MRI signal from the anatomic area surrounding the vessels of interest. Consequently, an MRI signal is given only by material that is outside the area of study when the signal-suppressing pulse occurs. Incoming blood vessels appear bright, whereas stationary tissue signal is suppressed (Fig. 26.29). PC imaging takes advantage of the shifts in phase, or orientation, experienced by magnetic nuclei moving through the MRI field. Special pulse sequences enhance these effects in flowing blood, producing a bright signal in vessels when the unchanging signal from stationary tissue is subtracted. PC imaging is used when data about the velocity and direction of blood are needed.

Fig. 26.28 Coronal T1-weighted image of the ankle. Bone marrow shows high signal intensity because of fat. Osteochondral defect seen in the dome of the talus *(T)* shows low signal intensity. *C,* Calcaneus; *F,* fibula; *S,* tibia.

Fig. 26.29 MRA shows intracranial arterial vessels in the AP view. *ACA,* Anterior cerebral arteries; *B,* basilar artery; *IC,* internal carotids; *MCA,* middle cerebral artery. In the center is the circle of Willis.

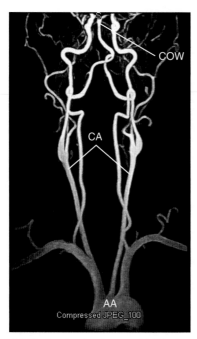

Fig. 26.30 Contrast-enhanced MRA shows carotid arteries *(CA)* from the aortic arch *(AA)* to the circle of Willis *(COW)*.

Fig. 26.31 Contrast-enhanced MRA of the abdominal aorta *(AA)* shows the renal arteries *(RA)*, iliac bifurcation *(IB)*, and iliac arteries *(IA)*.

TOF imaging can be used with the injection of gadolinium-containing IV contrast material. Gadolinium shortens the T1 relaxation time of blood, thus increasing its signal intensity and allowing a decrease in imaging time (breath-hold sequences) and three-dimensional volume imaging in the long axis of the vessel. Imaging of the carotid (Fig. 26.30), thoracic, abdominal, and pelvic arteries (Fig. 26.31) is possible. With the use of a moving table, the aorta can be imaged from the heart to the feet. This is routinely performed to screen for lesions in the peripheral vasculature. Vascular imaging can be used to look for dissections, aneurysms, arteriovenous malformations, plaque, stenosis, and occlusions.

DIFFUSION AND PERFUSION

The sensitivity of MRI to motion can be a handicap or a potential source of information. Motion artifacts interfere with upper abdominal images that are affected by heart and diaphragmatic motion, yet flow-sensitive pulse sequences can image flowing blood in blood vessels.

Specialized techniques have been developed that can image the *diffusion* and *perfusion* of molecules within matter. Molecules of water undergo random motion within tissues, but the cellular membranes (or lack thereof) affect the rate of such diffusion. Tissues have structure, and this structure affects the rates of diffusion and perfusion and their direction; in other words, diffusion and perfusion are not entirely random in a structured tissue. These microscopic motions can be detected by specialized MRI pulse sequences that can image their rate and direction. Diffusion and perfusion motion differ among tissue types. Diffusion patterns of gray matter in the brain differ from the diffusion patterns in more directionally oriented fiber tracts of white matter. This concept is currently used in diffusion tensor imaging.

Diffusion and perfusion imaging is most often used in the brain to visualize ischemic changes such as stroke. Recovery from acute stroke can be predicted by viewing the mismatch between the diffusion and perfusion images. Diffusion and perfusion imaging can produce clinically significant images that may help us to understand white matter degenerative diseases (e.g., multiple sclerosis, ischemia, infarction) (Fig. 26.32), develop possible therapies to return blood flow to underperfused brain tissue, and to characterize brain tumors. Similar applications for the rest of the body have been developed, allowing diffusion and perfusion imaging to be used in imaging of the abdominal and pelvic organs as well as the spine.

Spectroscopy

In routine MRI, the purpose is to produce detailed pictures of the anatomy being imaged. This is accomplished by spatially localizing the MRI signal in a volume of tissue. In magnetic resonance spectroscopy (MRS), the result is a graph, or spectrum, of the chemical composition of the volume of tissue being "imaged." This graph denotes not only the chemical compounds present but also the relationship between the quantity of each compound. In pathologic conditions in which the imaging characteristics are similar or difficult to interpret, MRS can add vital information leading to a more accurate interpretation.

MRS is most commonly used in the brain. It can be helpful in diagnosing metabolic conditions, tumor recurrence versus necrosis, and pathologic processes (Fig. 26.33). The use of MRS is becoming more widespread in breast and prostate imaging to differentiate between normal and abnormal tissue. It has also been used to study normal physiologic changes such as those seen in muscle contraction (Fig. 26.34).

Fig. 26.32 Diffusion-weighted image shows acute ischemic infarct (stroke) (S) in the territory of the right middle cerebral artery. Lack of diffusion in this area turns it bright on this heavily T2-weighted image.

Fig. 26.33 Routine spectroscopy in a patient with a primary brain tumor. Voxel shows normal brain spectra in an area unaffected by the brain tumor.

Fig. 26.34 Spectra from human muscle before *(red line)* and during *(blue line)* exercise. Thin horizontal lines represent separate baselines for each spectrum. Each peak represents a different chemical species, and the area under the peak down to the baseline indicates the amount of substance present. The inorganic phosphate *(Pi)* peak increases with exercise as energy-rich phosphocreatine *(PCr)* is used to provide energy for muscle contraction.

Functional Magnetic Resonance Imaging

Functional MRI (fMRI) records active areas of the brain during certain activities or after the introduction of stimuli, such as visual or auditory stimuli. Typically, fMRI uses the differences in the magnetic properties of oxygenated and deoxygenated blood to visualize active areas of the brain. The use of oxygenated and deoxygenated blood as a contrast agent is known as blood oxygen level–dependent (BOLD) imaging. The human body is composed of approximately 50% oxygenated and 50% deoxygenated blood. Oxygenated blood displays diamagnetic properties; that is, it does not affect molecules in the surrounding area. Deoxygenated blood is a paramagnetic substance, which increases T2* decay and decreases the availability of signal in the area immediately surrounding it (magnetic susceptibility artifact). Because of this increase in magnetic susceptibility artifact, it is possible for MRI to measure the difference between oxygenated and deoxygenated blood. As blood flow increases to areas of activation, the MRI scanner is able to distinguish the subtle differences in signal and register the area of brain activity.

Currently, fMRI is used for many areas of research in an effort to increase our understanding of human brain anatomy and function. Studies involving the visual cortex, memory, Alzheimer disease, schizophrenia, and many others have been performed. fMRI may prove useful in areas of lie detection and mind reading. It holds promise for the future of MRI not only as a diagnostic tool but also as a predictor of future behaviors and disease processes.

Conclusion

Since its development in the 1970s, MRI has evolved into an advanced, widely used tool that is necessary for the diagnosis, staging, and treatment of disease. Today MRI is the imaging modality of choice for studying the central nervous and musculoskeletal systems. The role of MRI in breast, cardiac, and body imaging continues to expand. New techniques in MR spectroscopy and fMRI will enhance its usefulness.

MRI's ability to utilize multiple biological parameters in its image acquisition, the development of new pulse sequences and more sensitive hardware, and the use of newly developed organ-specific contrast agents will keep MRI at the forefront of the imaging world.

Definition of Terms

antenna Device for transmitting or receiving radio waves.

artifact Spurious finding in or distortion of an image.

attenuation Reduction in energy or amount of a beam of radiation when it passes through tissue or other substances.

coil Single or multiple loops of wire (or another electrical conductor such as tubing) designed to produce a magnetic field from current flowing through the wire or to detect a changing magnetic field by voltage induced in the wire.

contrast Degree of difference between two substances in some parameter, with the parameter varying depending on the technique used (e.g., attenuation in radiographic techniques or signal strength in MRI).

cryogenic Relating to extremely low temperature (see *superconductive magnet*).

diffusion Spontaneous random motion of molecules in a medium; a natural and continuous process.

echo planar imaging Fast pulse sequence that can be used to create MR images within a few milliseconds.

fat-suppressed images Images in which the fat tissue in the image is made to be of a lower, darker signal intensity than the surrounding structures.

frequency Number of times that a process repeats itself in a given period (e.g., the frequency of a radio wave is the number of complete waves per second).

fringe field Portion of the magnetic field that extends away from the confines of the magnet; it cannot be used for imaging but can affect nearby equipment or personnel.

gating Organizing data so that the information used to construct the image comes from the same point in the cycle of a repeating motion, such as a heartbeat. The moving object is "frozen" at that phase of its motion, thus reducing image blurring.

gauss (G) Unit of magnetic field strength (see *tesla*).

gradient echo A pulse sequence that uses a gradient instead of a 180-degree RF refocusing pulse to generate T2*-weighted images.

inversion recovery Standard pulse sequence available on most MRI imagers; the name indicates that the direction of longitudinal magnetization is reversed (inverted) before relaxation (recovery) occurs.

longitudinal plane This plane corresponds to the direction of the main magnetic field in superconducting magnets and is the location of protons awaiting excitation.

magnetic resonance (MR) Process by which certain nuclei, when placed in a magnetic field, can absorb and release energy in the form of radio waves. This technique can be used for chemical analysis or for the production of cross-sectional images of body parts. Computer analysis of the radio-wave data is required.

MRI conditional An item that has been demonstrated to pose no known hazards in a specified MRI environment with specified conditions of use.

MRI safe An item that poses no known hazards in any MRI environment.

noise Random contributions to the total signal that arise from stray external radio waves or imperfect electronic apparatus or other interference. Noise cannot be eliminated but it can be minimized; it tends to degrade the image by interfering with accurate measurement of the true MRI signal, similar to the difficulty in maintaining a clear conversation in a noisy room.

nuclear magnetic resonance (NMR) Another name for magnetic resonance; this term is not commonly used.

nucleus The central portion of an atom, composed of protons and neutrons.

paramagnetic Referring to materials that alter the magnetic field of nearby nuclei. Paramagnetic substances are not themselves directly imaged by MRI but instead change the signal intensity of the tissue where they localize, acting as MRI contrast agents. Paramagnetic agents shorten the T1 and T2 of the tissues they affect—actions that tend to have opposing effects on signal intensity.

perfusion Flow of blood through the vessels of an organ or anatomic structure; usually refers to blood flow in the small vessels (e.g., capillary perfusion).

permanent magnet An object that produces a magnetic field without requiring an external supply of electricity.

precession Rotation of an object around the direction of a force acting on that object. This should not be confused with the axis of rotation of the object itself (e.g., a spinning top rotates on its own axis, but it may also precess [wobble] around the direction of the force of gravity that is acting on it).

proton density Measure of proton (i.e., hydrogen, because its nucleus is a single proton) concentration (number of nuclei per given volume); one of the major determinants of MRI signal strength in hydrogen imaging.

pulse See *radio frequency (RF) pulse.*

pulse sequence A coordinated series of gradient activations and RF transmissions designed to excite nuclei in such a way that their energy release has varying contributions from proton density, T1, or T2 processes.

radio frequency (RF) pulse A short burst of radio waves. If the radio waves are of the appropriate frequency, they can give energy to nuclei that are within a magnetic field by the process of resonance. Length of the pulse determines amount of energy given to the nuclei.

raw data Information obtained by radio reception of the MRI signal as stored by a computer. Specific computer manipulation of these data is required to construct an image from them.

relaxation time Measure of the rate at which nuclei, after stimulation, release their absorbed energy.

resistive magnet Simple electromagnet in which electricity passing through coils of wire produces a magnetic field; can be turned on and off.

resonance Process of energy absorption by an object that is tuned to absorb energy of a specific frequency only. All other frequencies would not affect the object (e.g., if one tuning fork is struck in a room full of tuning forks, only the forks tuned to that identical frequency would vibrate [resonate]).

signal In MRI, induction of current into a receiver coil by precessing magnetization.

slice Cross-sectional image; can also refer to the thin section of the body from which data are acquired to produce the image.

spectroscopy Science of analyzing the components of an electromagnetic wave, usually after its interaction with some substance (to obtain information about that substance).

spin echo Standard MRI pulse sequence that can provide T1-weighted, T2-weighted, or proton density–weighted images. The name indicates that a declining MRI signal is refocused to gain strength (similar to an echo) before it is recorded as raw data.

spin-lattice relaxation Release of energy by excited nuclei to their general environment; one of the major determinants of MRI signal strength. T1 is a rate constant measuring spin-lattice relaxation. Also called T1 relaxation.

spin-spin relaxation Release of energy by excited nuclei as a result of interaction among themselves; one of the major determinants of MRI signal strength. T2 is a rate constant measuring spin-spin relaxation. Also called T2 relaxation.

superconductive magnet Electromagnet in which the coils of wire are cooled to an extremely low temperature so that resistance to the conduction of electricity is nearly eliminated (superconductive).

superparamagnetic Material that has a greater effect with a magnetic field; it can dramatically decrease the T2 of tissues, causing a total loss of signal by the absorbing structures.

T1 Spin-lattice relaxation.

T2 Spin-spin relaxation.

tesla (T) Unit of magnetic field strength; 1 T equals 10,000 gauss or 10 kilogauss (other units of magnetic field strength). The earth's magnetic field approximates 0.5 gauss.

transverse plane The plane perpendicular to the longitudinal plane where the MRI signal can be measured.

Selected bibliography

Bloch F: Nuclear induction, *Physiol Rev* 70:460, 1946.

Burghart G, Finn CA: *Handbook of MRI scanning*, St Louis, 2010, Mosby.

Bushong SC, Clarke G: *MRI physical and biological principles*, ed 4, St Louis, 2015, Mosby.

Damadian R: Tumor detection by nuclear magnetic resonance, *Science* 171:1151, 1971.

Expert Panel on MR Safety: *ACR guidance document on MR safe practices: 2013*. Retrieved from https://www.acr.org/Clinical-Resources/Radiology-Safety/MR-Safety. Accessed September 2018.

Kelley LL, Petersen CM: *Sectional anatomy for imaging professionals*, ed 3, St Louis, 2013, Mosby.

Purcell EM, et al: Resonance absorption by nuclear magnetic moments in a solid, *Physiol Rev* 69:37, 1946.

Shellock FG: *Magnetic resonance procedures: health effects and safety*, Boca Raton, FL, 2001, CRC Press.

Shellock FG: *Reference manual for magnetic resonance safety, implants, and devices: 2018*, Playa Del Rey, CA, 2018, Biomedical Research Publishing Group.

Shellock FG, Crues JV: *MRI bioeffects, safety, and patient management*, Playa Del Rey, CA, 2014, Biomedical Research Publishing Group.

Westbrook C, Kaut Roth C, Talbot J: *MRI in practice*, ed 4, Oxford, 2011, Wiley-Blackwell.

27

VASCULAR, CARDIAC, AND INTERVENTIONAL RADIOGRAPHY

LOIS J. LAYNE • LYNETTE PETRIE

Historical Development

In January 1896, just 10 weeks after the announcement of Roentgen's discovery of x-rays, Haschek and Lindenthal announced that they had produced a radiograph showing the blood vessels of an amputated hand using Teichman's mixture, a thick emulsion of chalk, as the contrast agent. This work heralded the beginning of angiography. The advancement of angiography was hindered, however, by the lack of suitable contrast media and low-risk techniques to deliver the media to the desired location. By the 1920s, researchers were using sodium iodide as a contrast medium to produce lower limb studies comparable in quality to studies seen in modern angiography.

The first human cardiac catheterization was reported in 1929 by Forssman, a 25-year-old surgical resident who placed a catheter into his own heart and then walked to the radiology department where a chest radiograph was produced to document his medical achievement. Catheterization of the heart soon became a valuable tool used primarily for diagnostic purposes. Through the 1940s, the basic catheterization study remained relatively uncomplicated and easy for physicians to perform; however, the risk to the patient was significant.

Until the 1950s, contrast media were most commonly injected through a needle that punctured the vessel or through a ureteral catheter that passed into the body through a surgically exposed peripheral vessel. In 1952, shortly after the development of a flexible thin-walled catheter, Seldinger announced a *percutaneous*[a] method of catheter introduction. The Seldinger technique eliminated the surgical risk, which exposed the vessel and tissues. Selective coronary *angiography* was first reported by Sones in 1959, when he inadvertently injected contrast media into the right coronary artery of a patient who was undergoing routine aortography. In 1962, Ricketts and Abrams described the first percutaneous method for selective coronary angiography. This method was further perfected in the late 1960s with the introduction of preformed catheters designed to engage the ostium of the right and left coronary arteries.

It has been said the "Fathers of Interventional Radiology and Cardiology" were Charles Dotter and Andreas Grüntzig, respectively. Dotter performed the first successful dilation of a superficial femoral artery in 1964 using coaxial catheters. In the November 1964 edition of *Circulation*, percutaneous transluminal angioplasty (PTA) was described by Dotter with coauthor Dr. Melvin Judkins. In 1966, Dotter fabricated a reinforced balloon dilating catheter, but it was not used on patients. Dr. Werner Portsman (Berlin, Germany) introduced "*Korsett Balloon Kather*," an 8 Fr outer Teflon catheter with four longitudinal slits in 1973. A latex balloon catheter

---

[a]Almost all italicized words on the succeeding pages are defined at the end of the chapter.

was inflated inside the longitudinal slits. In September 1977, Dr. Andreas Grüntzig successfully used a balloon PTA to treat a left anterior descending coronary artery stenosis. Grüntzig and Hopff introduced the double-lumen, balloon-tipped catheter. One lumen allows the passage of a guidewire and fluids through the catheter. The other lumen communicates with a balloon at the distal end of the catheter. When inflated, the balloon expands to a size much larger than the catheter. Double-lumen, angioplasty balloon catheters are available in sizes ranging from 3 to 9 Fr, with attached balloons varying in length and expanding to diameters of 2 to 20 mm or more. Transluminal angioplasty can be performed in virtually any vessel that can be reached percutaneously with a catheter. In 1978, Molnar and Stockum described the use of balloon angioplasty for dilation of strictures within the biliary system. Balloon angioplasty is also conducted in venous structures, ureters, and the gastrointestinal tract.

The 1980s saw the development of expandable metallic stents. Andrew Cragg, Charles Dotter, Cesare Gianturco, Dierk Maas, Julio Palmaz, and Hans Wallsten were the first stent pioneers. These stents were composed primarily of a stainless steel alloy or thermal memory stents made of nitinol (alloy of nickel and titanium) and were self or balloon expandable. Three stents available for use in 1985 were the Gianturco Z, Palmaz, and Wallstent. Dotter continued advancement of cardiovascular procedures by first using Streptokinase for selective thrombolysis. In the 1980s, Urokinase was used for this widely performed procedure. Continued growth of thrombolysis was due to the advancement of fibrinolytic agents *(recombinant tissue plasminogen activators)*.

Therapeutic vascular occlusion procedures began in 1931 with an open surgical embolization of a carotid cavernous fistula. Dr. Shoji Ishimore used Gelfoam pieces through a polyethylene tube into an exposed carotid artery. Embolization became popular during the 1980s and 1990s with advancement of embolization agents, such as gelatin sponges (Gelfoam), polyvinyl alcohol (Ivalon), liquid and rapidly solidifying polymers including cyanoacrylate glue, coils, and detachable balloons.

Early angiograms consisted of single radiographs or the visualization of vessels by fluoroscopy. Because the advantage of *serial imaging* was recognized, cassette changers, roll film changers, cut film changers, cine and serial spot-filming/digital devices were developed. Until the early 1990s, most angiograms recorded flowing contrast media in a series of images that required *rapid film changers* or cinefluorography devices; however,

presently digital subtraction angiography (DSA) systems are used almost exclusively. The newer imaging equipment has much better image quality and can produce images at a rate of 30 frames per second. In addition, digital imaging is cost-effective because images are stored electronically, reducing the need for expensive film and film storage. Digital images can be archived and retrieved in seconds from within the institution or any network connection. DSA imaging provides the interventionalist with a variety of tools for image manipulation analysis and measurement.

The resolution possible with early digital equipment was a drawback to the use of digital imaging in the cardiovascular laboratory. Larger matrix size, the obvious solution to this problem, allowed for acceptable resolution but also created another problem: how to acquire and store large volumes of digital information. In the late 1970s and early 1980s, the high-speed parallel transfer disk was introduced to solve the acquisition and short-term storage problem. This new disk acquired and stored an entire coronary angiogram and made real-time digital playback during the procedure possible. Permanent storage of the digital images remained a problem,

however. Floppy disk and computer tape storage were inadequate solutions because they required significant time and supplies. Long-term storage of large amounts of digital images has benefited from advances in computer technology, which provide high-speed, large-capacity methods of storage, capable of acquiring large amounts of data (terabytes) with very high resolution. Today, networking, security, redundancy, and image integrity are issues for laboratories equipped with digital technology.

The 1960s and 1970s brought tremendous advances in radiologic and cardiovascular medicine and technology. Radiographic imaging and recording equipment, physiologic monitoring equipment, and cardiovascular pharmaceuticals and supplies became increasingly reliable. The uses of computers in the cardiovascular interventional laboratories have facilitated the development of this rapidly growing subspecialty of the cardiovascular medical and surgical sciences. These advances and trends have enabled angiography to evolve from a simple diagnostic investigation to its current state as a sophisticated diagnostic study and interventional procedure.

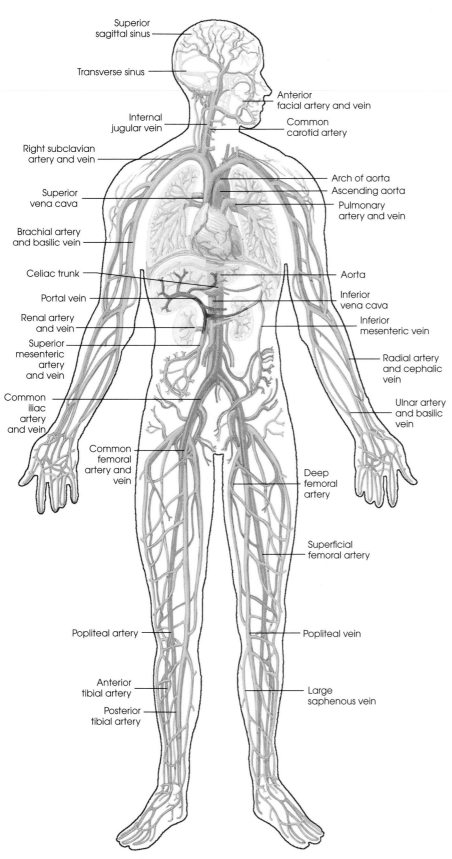

Superior sagittal sinus

Transverse sinus

Internal jugular vein

Right subclavian artery and vein

Superior vena cava

Brachial artery and basilic vein

Celiac trunk

Portal vein

Renal artery and vein

Superior mesenteric artery and vein

Common iliac artery and vein

Common femoral artery and vein

Popliteal artery

Anterior tibial artery

Posterior tibial artery

Anterior facial artery and vein

Common carotid artery

Arch of aorta

Ascending aorta

Pulmonary artery and vein

Aorta

Inferior vena cava

Inferior mesenteric vein

Radial artery and cephalic vein

Ulnar artery and basilic vein

Deep femoral artery

Superficial femoral artery

Popliteal vein

Large saphenous vein

Fig. 27.1 Major arteries and veins: *red,* arterial; *blue,* venous; *purple,* portal.

Circulatory System

The *circulatory system* has two complex systems of intimately associated vessels. Through these vessels, fluid is transported throughout the body in a continuous, unidirectional flow. The major portion of the circulatory system transports blood and is called the *blood-vascular system* (Fig. 27.1). The minor portion, called the *lymphatic system,* collects fluid from the tissue spaces. This fluid is filtered throughout the lymphatic system, which conveys it back to the blood-vascular system. The fluid conveyed by the lymphatic system is called *lymph.* Together, the blood-vascular and lymphatic systems carry oxygen and nutritive material to the tissues. They also collect and transport carbon dioxide (CO_2) and other waste products of metabolism from the tissues to the organs of excretion: the skin, lungs, liver, and kidneys.

Blood-Vascular System

The blood-vascular system consists of the *heart, arteries, capillaries,* and *veins.* The *heart* serves as a pumping mechanism to keep the blood in constant circulation throughout the vast system of blood vessels. *Arteries* convey the blood *away* from the heart. *Veins* convey the blood *back* toward the heart.

Two circuits of blood vessels branch out of the heart (Fig. 27.2). The first circuit is the arterial circuit or the *systemic circulation,* which carries oxygenated blood to the organs and tissues. Every organ has its own vascular circuit that arises from the trunk artery and leads back to the trunk vein for return to the heart. The systemic arteries branch out, treelike, from the aorta to all parts of the body. The arteries are usually named according to their location. The systemic veins usually lie parallel to their respective arteries and are given the same names.

The second circuit is the *pulmonary circulation,* which takes blood to the lungs for CO_2 exchange and for the reoxygenation of the blood, which is carried back to the arterial systemic circulation. The pulmonary trunk arises from the right ventricle of the heart, passes superiorly and posteriorly for a distance of about 2 inches (5 cm), and then divides into two branches, the right and left pulmonary arteries. These vessels enter the root of the respective lung and, following the course of the bronchi, divide and subdivide to form a dense network of capillaries surrounding the alveoli of the lungs. Through the thin walls of the capillaries, the blood discharges CO_2 and absorbs oxygen from the air contained in the alveoli. The oxygenated blood passes onward through the pulmonary veins for return to the heart. In the pulmonary circulation, the deoxygenated blood is transported by the pulmonary arteries, and the oxygenated blood is transported by the pulmonary veins.

Two main trunk vessels arise from the heart. The first is the aorta for the systemic circulation: the arteries progressively diminish in size as they divide and subdivide along their course, finally ending in minute branches called *arterioles.* The arterioles divide to form the capillary vessels, and the branching process is then reversed: the *capillaries* unite to form *venules,* the beginning branches of the veins, which unite and reunite to form larger and larger vessels as they approach the heart. These venous structures empty into the right atrium, then into the right ventricle, and then into the second main trunk that arises from the heart—the pulmonary trunk, or the pulmonary circulation. The process of oxygen exchange is carried out in small venous structures and then in larger and larger pulmonary veins. The pulmonary veins join to form four large veins (two from each lung), which empty into the left atrium, then into the left ventricle, and then into the aorta, which starts the circulation again throughout the body.

The pathway of venous drainage from the abdominal viscera to the liver is called the *portal system.* In contrast to the systemic and pulmonary circuits, which begin and end at the heart, the portal system begins in the capillaries of the abdominal viscera and ends in the capillaries and sinusoids of the liver. The blood is filtered and then exits the liver via the hepatic venous system, which empties into the *inferior vena cava (IVC)* just proximal to the right atrium.

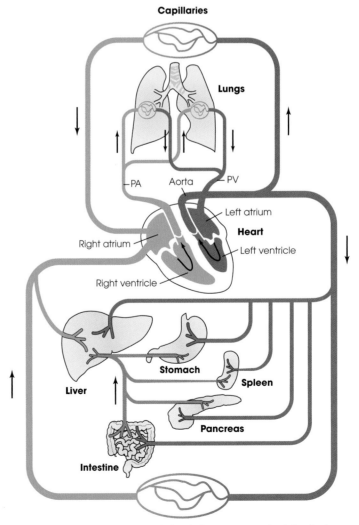

Fig. 27.2 Pulmonary, systemic, and portal circulation: oxygenated *(red)*, deoxygenated *(blue)*, and nutrient-rich *(purple)* blood.

The systemic veins are arranged in a superficial set and in a deep set with which the superficial veins communicate; both sets converge at a common trunk vein. The systemic veins end in two large vessels opening into the heart: the *superior vena cava* (SVC) leads from the portion of the body above the diaphragm, and the inferior vena cava (IVC) leads from below the level of the diaphragm.

The capillaries connect the arterioles and venules to form networks that pervade most organs and all other tissues supplied with blood. The capillary vessels have exceedingly thin walls through which the essential functions of the blood-vascular system take place: the blood constituents are filtered out, and the waste products of cell activity are absorbed. The exchange takes place through the medium of tissue fluid, which is derived from the blood plasma and is drained off by the lymphatic system for return to the blood-vascular system. The tissue fluid undergoes modification in the lymphatic system. As soon as this tissue fluid enters the lymphatic capillaries, it is called *lymph*.

The *heart* is the central organ of the blood-vascular system and functions solely as a pump to keep the blood in circulation. It is shaped like a cone and measures approximately $4\frac{3}{4}$ inches (12 cm) in length, $3\frac{1}{2}$ inches (9 cm) in width, and $2\frac{1}{2}$ inches (6 cm) in depth. The heart is situated obliquely in the central mediastinum, primarily to the left of the midsagittal plane. The base of the heart is directed superiorly, posteriorly, and to the right. The apex of the heart rests on the diaphragm against the anterior chest wall and is directed anteriorly, inferiorly, and to the left.

The muscular wall of the heart is called the *myocardium*. Because of the force required to drive blood through the extensive systemic vessels, the myocardium is about three times as thick on the left side (the arterial side) as on the right (the venous side). The membrane that lines the interior of the heart is called the *endocardium*. The heart is enclosed in the double-walled *pericardial sac*. The exterior wall of this sac is fibrous. The thin, closely adherent membrane that covers the heart is referred to as the *epicardium* or, because it also serves as the serous inner wall of the pericardial sac, the *visceral pericardium*. The narrow, fluid-containing space between the two walls of the sac is called the *pericardial cavity*.

The heart is divided by septa into right and left halves, with each half subdivided by a constriction into two cavities, or chambers. The two upper chambers are called *atria*, and each atrium consists of a principal cavity and a lesser cavity called the *auricle*. The two lower chambers of the heart are called *ventricles*. The opening between the right atrium and right ventricle is controlled by the right atrioventricular (tricuspid) valve, and the opening between the left atrium and left ventricle is controlled by the left atrioventricular (mitral or bicuspid) valve.

The atria and ventricles separately contract (systole) in pumping blood and relax or dilate (diastole) in receiving blood. The atria precede the ventricles in contraction; while the atria are in systole, the ventricles are in diastole. One phase of contraction (referred to as the heartbeat) and one phase of dilation are called the *cardiac cycle*. In the average adult, one cardiac cycle lasts 0.8 second. The heart rate, or number of pulsations per minute, varies, however, with size, age, and gender. Heart rate is faster in small persons, young individuals, and females. The heart rate is also increased with exercise, food, and emotional disturbances.

The atria function as receiving chambers. The superior and inferior venae cava empty into the right atrium (Fig. 27.3); the two right and left pulmonary veins empty into the left atrium. The ventricles function as distributing chambers. The right side of the heart handles the venous, or deoxygenated, blood, and the left side handles the arterial, or oxygenated, blood. The left ventricle pumps oxygenated blood through the aortic valve into the aorta and the systemic circulation. The three major portions of the aorta are the ascending aorta, the aortic arch, and the descending aorta. The right ventricle pumps deoxygenated blood through the pulmonary valve into the pulmonary trunk and the pulmonary circulation.

Blood is supplied to the myocardium by the right and left coronary arteries. These vessels arise in the aortic sinus immediately superior to the aortic valve (Fig. 27.4). Most of the cardiac veins drain into the coronary sinus on the posterior aspect of the heart, and this sinus drains into the right atrium (Fig. 27.5).

The ascending aorta arises from the superior portion of the left ventricle and passes superiorly and to the right for a short distance. It then arches posteriorly and to the left and descends along the left side of the vertebral column to the level of L4, where it divides into the right and left common iliac arteries. The common iliac arteries pass to the level of the lumbosacral junction, and divide into the internal iliac, or hypogastric, artery and the external iliac artery. The internal iliac artery passes into the pelvis. The external iliac artery passes to a point about midway between the anterior superior iliac spine and pubic symphysis and then enters the upper thigh to become the common femoral artery.

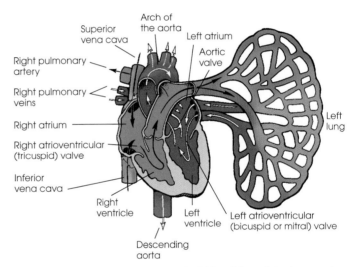

Fig. 27.3 Heart and great vessels: deoxygenated blood flow *(black arrows)*; oxygenated blood flow *(white arrows)*.

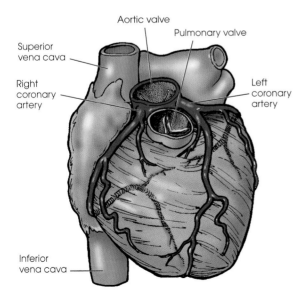

Fig. 27.4 Anterior view of coronary arteries.

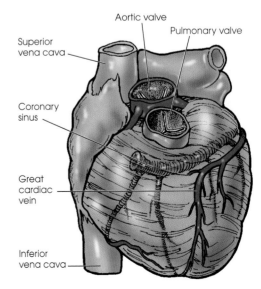

Fig. 27.5 Anterior view of coronary veins.

The velocity of blood circulation varies with the rate and intensity of the heartbeat. Velocity also varies in the different portions of the circulatory system based on distance from the heart. The speed of blood flow is highest in the large arteries arising at or near the heart because these vessels receive the full force of each wave of blood pumped out of the heart. The arterial walls expand with the pressure from each wave. The walls then rhythmically recoil, gradually diminishing the pressure of the advancing wave from point to point, until the flow of blood is normally reduced to a steady, nonpulsating stream through the capillaries and veins. The beat, or contraction and expansion of an artery, may be felt with the fingers at several points and is called the *pulse.*

Complete circulation of the blood through the systemic and pulmonary circuits, from a given point and back again, requires about 23 seconds and an average of 27 heartbeats. In certain contrast examinations of the cardiovascular system, tests are conducted to determine the circulation time from the point of contrast media injection to the site of interest.

Lymphatic System

The lymphatic system consists of an elaborate arrangement of closed vessels that collect fluid from the tissue spaces and transport it to the blood-vascular system. Almost all lymphatic vessels are arranged in two sets: (1) a superficial set that lies immediately under the skin and accompanies the superficial veins and (2) a deep set that accompanies the deep blood vessels and with which the superficial lymphatics communicate (Fig. 27.6). The lymphatic system lacks a pumping mechanism such as the heart of the blood-vascular system. The lymphatic vessels are richly supplied with valves to prevent backflow, and the movement of the lymph through the system is believed to be maintained primarily by extrinsic pressure from the surrounding organs and muscles.

The lymphatic system begins in complex networks of thin-walled, absorbent capillaries situated in the various organs and tissues. The capillaries unite to form larger vessels, which form networks and unite to become still larger vessels as they approach the terminal collecting trunks. The terminal trunks communicate with the blood-vascular system.

The lymphatic vessels are small in caliber and have delicate, transparent walls. Along their course the collecting vessels pass through one or more nodular structures called *lymph nodes.* The nodes occur singly but are usually arranged in chains or groups of 2 to 20. The nodes are situated so that they form strategically placed centers toward which the conducting vessels converge. The nodes vary from the size of a pinhead to the size of an almond or larger. They may be spherical, oval, or kidney shaped. Each node has a hilum through which the arteries enter and veins and efferent lymph vessels emerge; the afferent lymph vessels do not enter at the hilum. In addition to the lymphatic capillaries, blood vessels, and supporting structures, each lymph node contains masses, or follicles, of lymphocytes that are arranged around its circumference and from which cords of cells extend through the medullary portion of the node.

Numerous conducting channels, here called *afferent lymph vessels*, enter the node opposite the hilum and break into wide capillaries that surround the lymph follicles and form a canal known as the *peripheral* or *marginal lymph sinus.* The network of capillaries continues into the medullary portion of the node, widens to form medullary sinuses, and then collects into several *efferent lymph vessels* that leave the node at the hilum. The conducting vessels may pass through several nodes along their course, each time undergoing the process of widening into sinuses. Lymphocytes—a variety of white blood cells formed in the lymph nodes—are added to the lymph while it is in the nodes. It is thought that most of the lymph is absorbed by the venous system

from these nodes, and only a small portion of the lymph is passed on through the conducting vessels.

The absorption and interchange of tissue fluids and cells occur through the thin walls of the capillaries. The lymph passes from the beginning capillaries through the conducting vessels, which eventually empty their contents into terminal lymph trunks for conveyance to the blood-vascular system. The main terminal trunk of the lymphatic system is called the *thoracic duct.* The lower, dilated portion of the duct is known as the *cisterna chyli.* The thoracic duct receives lymphatic drainage from all parts of the body below the diaphragm and from the left half of the body above the diaphragm. The thoracic duct extends from the level of L2 to the base of the neck, where it ends by opening into the venous system at the junction of the left subclavian and internal jugular veins.

Three terminal collecting trunks—the right jugular, the subclavian, and the bronchomediastinal trunks—receive the lymphatic drainage from the right half of the body above the diaphragm. These vessels open into the right subclavian vein separately or occasionally after uniting to form a common trunk called the *right lymphatic duct.*

Lymphography is seldom performed in current practice because of the superior imaging capabilities of newer modalities such as magnetic resonance imaging (MRI), computed tomography (CT), and positron emission tomography (PET) (Fig. 27.7). At present, it is primarily used to assess the clinical extent of lymphomas or to stage radiation treatment. Lymphography may also be indicated in patients who have clinical evidence of obstruction or other impairment of the lymphatic system. A more detailed description of lymphography is provided in previous editions of this text.

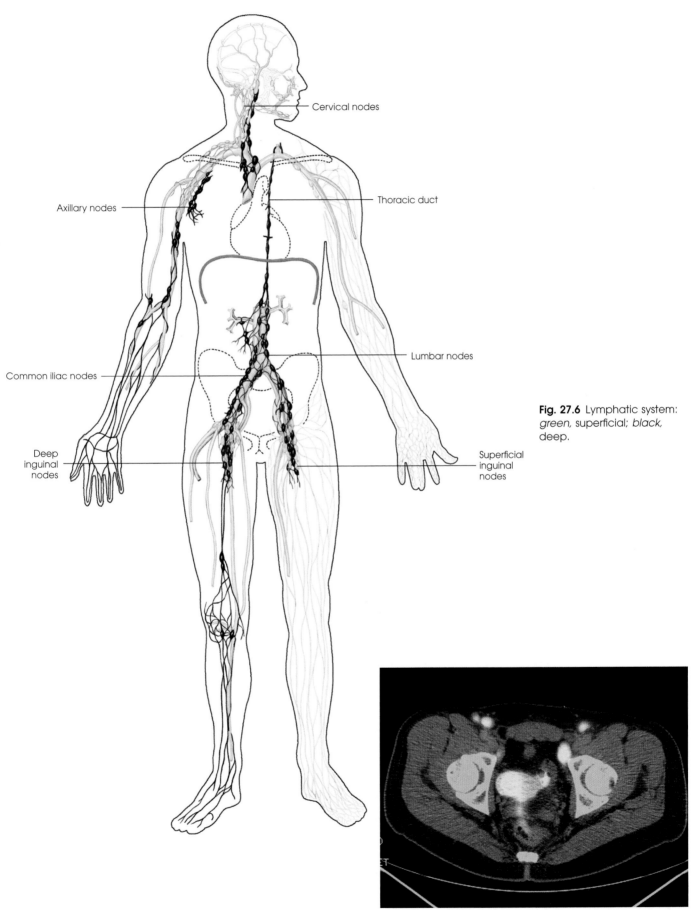

Cervical nodes

Thoracic duct

Axillary nodes

Lumbar nodes

Common iliac nodes

Fig. 27.6 Lymphatic system: *green,* superficial; *black,* deep.

Deep inguinal nodes

Superficial inguinal nodes

Fig. 27.7 Axial PET/CT of lymph nodes with lymphoma.

Definitions and Indications

Blood vessels are not normally visible on conventional radiography because no natural contrast exists between them and other soft tissues of the body. These vessels must be filled with a radiopaque contrast media to delineate them for radiography. *Angiography* is a general term that describes the radiologic examination of vascular structures within the body after the introduction of an iodinated contrast media or gas.

The visceral and peripheral angiography procedures identified in this chapter can be categorized generally as either *arteriography* or *venography*. Examinations are more precisely named for the specific blood vessel opacified and the method of injection.

Angiography is primarily used to identify the anatomy or pathologic process of blood vessels. Chronic cramping leg pain after physical exertion, a condition known as *claudication*, may prompt a physician to order an arteriogram of the lower limbs to determine whether atherosclerosis is diminishing the blood supply to the leg muscles. A *stenosis* or *occlusion* is commonly caused by *atherosclerosis* and is an indication for an arteriogram. Cerebral angiography is performed to detect and verify the existence and exact position of an intracranial vascular lesion such as an *aneurysm*. Although most angiographic examinations are performed to investigate anatomic variances, some evaluate the motion of the part. Other vascular examinations evaluate suspected tumors by opacifying the organ of concern; after a diagnosis is made, these lesions may be amendable to some type of intervention. Interventional radiology assists in the diagnosis of lesions and then is used to treat these lesions through an endovascular approach.

Contrast Media

Opaque contrast media containing organic iodine solutions are used in angiographic studies. At the kilovolt peak (kVp) used in angiography, iodine is slightly more radiopaque (atom for atom) than lead. This allows for excellent radiopacity. The iodine in the contrast media is incorporated into water-soluble molecules formed as tri-iodinated benzene rings, meaning there are three iodine atoms on each particle in solution (a 3:1 ratio).

Although usually tolerated, the injection of iodinated contrast media may cause undesirable consequences. The contrast medium is subsequently filtered out of the bloodstream by the kidneys. It causes physiologic cardiovascular side effects, including peripheral vasodilation, hypotension, and renal toxicity. It may also produce nausea and an uncomfortable burning sensation. Most significantly, the injection of iodinated contrast media may invoke allergic reactions. These reactions may be minor (e.g., hives, slight difficulty in breathing) and require minimal treatment, or they may be severe and require immediate medical intervention. Severe reactions are characterized by a state of shock in which the patient exhibits shallow breathing and a high pulse rate and may lose consciousness. The administration of contrast media is one of the significant risks in angiography.

There are two major classes of tri-iodinated contrast: ionic and nonionic. Ionic contrast agents have high solubility, low viscosity and high osmolar properties. Nonionic contrast agents have high viscosity and low osmolar properties. Nonionic contrast media cause fewer physiologic cardiovascular side effects, less intense sensations, and fewer allergic reactions.

Another form of contrast medium is a dimer, in which the two benzene rings are bonded together as the anion. Ionic contrast media with a dimer result in six iodine atoms for every two particles in solution, which yields the same 3:1 ratio as nonionic contrast media. The ionic dimer has advantages over the ionic monomeric molecule, primarily by reducing osmolality, but it lacks some of the properties of the nonionic molecule. Nonionic contrast media can also be found as a dimer, which yields a ratio of 6:1 because it does not dissociate into two particles, producing an osmolality similar to blood.

All forms of iodinated contrast media are available in various iodine concentrations. The agents of higher concentration are more opaque. Typically, 30% iodine concentrations (300 mg/mL) are used for cerebral and limb arteriography, whereas 35% concentrations (350 mg/mL) are used for visceral angiography. Peripheral venography may be performed with 30% or lower concentrations. Ionic agents of higher concentration and nonionic agents are more viscous and produce greater resistance in the catheter during injection.

Patients with a predisposition to allergic reaction may be pretreated with a regimen of antihistamines and steroids to help prevent anaphylactic reactions to contrast media. Patients who have a history of severe reaction to iodinated contrast media or with compromised renal function may undergo procedures in which CO_2 is used as a contrast agent. CO_2 is less radiopaque than blood and appears as a negative or void in angiographic imaging. CO_2 is approved for use only below the diaphragm because the possibility of emboli is too great near the brain. CO_2 imaging is possible only in the DSA environment because it requires a narrow contrast window and the ability to stack or combine multiple images to provide a single image free of bubbles or fragmented vascular opacification. Specific kVp values should be employed to display the CO_2 optimally in contrast to the rest of the body. Faster filming rates are also required, usually 10 frames per second, because the CO_2 dissipates quickly within the blood.

Injection Techniques

Angiography primarily involves placing the catheter within a vessel and injecting a contrast media so that the vessel and its major branches are opacified. In a selective injection, the catheter tip is positioned into the orifice of a specific artery so that only that specific vessel is opacified. This technique has the advantage of more densely opacifying the vessel and limiting the superimposition of other vessels.

A contrast medium may be injected by hand with a syringe, but ideally it should be injected with an automatic injector. The major advantage of automatic injectors is that a specific quantity of contrast media can be injected during a predetermined period. Another advantage to automatic injectors is the ability to operate these remotely from a shielded control room. This reduces radiation exposure to physician and staff while still allowing visualization of images and patient. Automatic injectors have controls to set the injection rate, injection volume, and maximum pressure. Another useful feature is a control to set a time interval during which the injector gradually achieves the set injection rate, which is the linear rise. This may prevent a catheter from being dislodged by whiplash.

Because the opacifying contrast media are often carried away from the area of interest by blood flow, the injection and demonstration of opacified vessels usually occur simultaneously. The injector is often electronically connected to the rapid serial radiographic imaging equipment to coordinate the timing between the injector and the onset of imaging.

Digital Subtraction Angiographic Procedures

Under fluoroscopic guidance the intravascular catheter is positioned within the target vessel and a suitable imaging position and field of view are selected. At this point, an image that does not have a large dynamic range should be established; no part of the image should be significantly brighter than the rest of the image. This image can be accomplished by proper positioning, but it often requires the use of compensating filters. Most newer imaging systems have built-in compensating filters. If compensating filters are not properly placed, image quality is reduced significantly. Automatic controls in the system adjust the exposure factors so that the brightest part of the image is at that level. An unusually bright spot satisfies the automatic controls and causes the rest of the image to lie at significantly reduced levels, where the camera performance is worse. Proper positioning and technique are essential for high-quality imaging.

As the imaging sequence begins, an image that will be used as a subtraction mask (without contrast media) is acquired,

digitized, and stored in the digital memory. This mask image and those that follow are produced when the x-ray tube is energized and x-rays are produced, usually 1 to 30 exposures per second at 65 to 95 kVp and between 5 and 1000 mAs. The dose for each image acquisition may be reduced or the same as that used for a conventional radiograph. Images can be acquired at variable rates, from 1 image every 2 to 3 seconds up to 30 images per second.

The *acquisition rate* or filming rate can also be varied during a filming sequence, or run. Most commonly, images are acquired at a faster rate during the passage of contrast media through the arteries and then at a reduced rate in the venous phase, during which the blood flow is much slower. This procedure minimizes the radiation exposure to the patient but provides a sufficient number of images to show the clinical information. Each of these digitized images is electronically *subtracted* from the mask, and the subtraction image is amplified (contrast enhanced) and displayed in real time so that the subtraction images appear essentially instantaneously during the imaging

procedure. The images are simultaneously stored on a *digital imaging system.*

Some DSA equipment allows the table or the image receptor, such as a flat panel detector system, to be moved during acquisition. The movement is permitted to "follow" the flow of contrast media as it passes through the arteries. Sometimes called the "bolus chase" or "DSA stepping" method, this technique is particularly useful for evaluating the arteries in the pelvis and lower limb. Previously, several separate imaging sequences would be performed with the image receptor positioned in a different location for each sequence, but this method required an injection of contrast media for each sequence. The bolus chase method requires only one injection of contrast media and the imaging sequence follows (or "chases") the contrast media as it flows down the limb. The imaging sequence may be preceded or followed by a duplicate sequence without contrast media injection to enable subtraction. Occasionally, this method may need to be repeated because the contrast media in one leg may flow faster than in the other.

Misregistration, a major problem in DSA, occurs when the mask and the images displaying the vessels filled with contrast media do not exactly coincide. Misregistration is sometimes caused by voluntary movements of the patient, but it is also caused by involuntary movements such as bowel peristalsis or heart contractions. Preparing the patient by describing the sensations associated with injection of contrast media and the importance of holding still can help eliminate voluntary movements. It is also important to have the patient suspend respiration during the filming sequence.

During the imaging procedure, the subtraction images appear on the display monitor (Fig. 27.8). Often a preliminary diagnosis can be made at this point or as the images are reviewed immediately after each exposure sequence. A formal reading session occurs after the patient study has been completed; the final diagnosis is made at that time.

Some *postprocessing* is performed after each exposure sequence to improve visualization of the anatomy of interest or to correct misregistration. More involved postprocessing, including quantitative analysis, is performed after the patient study has been completed. The processed images are available on the computer monitor for review by the radiologist. In most institutions DSA images are stored in a *picture archive and communication system (PACS)*. These digital images can be transmitted via a computer network throughout the hospital or to remote locations for consultation with an expert or referring physician. As an alternative to digital storage, hard-copy images may be produced using a *laser printer*, with several images appearing on each radiograph.

Rapid serial imaging used in angiography requires x-ray tubes to have high heat load ratings. They also require multiple focal-spot sizes. Large focal-spot sizes of 0.8 to 1.2 mm are most capable of withstanding a high heat load and are used for abdominal and thoracic angiography. Small focal-spot sizes of 0.4 to 0.6 mm provide more detailed imaging and are therefore used for cerebral and peripheral angiography. Magnification studies require focal spot sizes of 0.1 to 0.3 mm. X-ray tubes may have to be specialized to satisfy these extreme demands. Rapid serial imaging also necessitates radiographic generators with high-power output. Because short exposure times are needed to compensate for all patient motion, the generators must be capable of producing high-milliampere output. Imaging systems may be used either singly or in combination at right angles to obtain simultaneous frontal and lateral images of the vascular system under investigation with one injection of contrast media. This arrangement of units is called a biplane imaging system (Fig. 27.9).

Fig. 27.8 DSA image of common carotid artery showing stenosis *(arrow)* of internal carotid artery.

Fig. 27.9 Modern biplane digital angiography suite.

(Courtesy GE Medical.)

MAGNIFICATION

Magnification occurs intentionally and unintentionally in angiographic imaging sequences. Different magnification levels can be utilized by employing different focusing filters inside the image receptor. Varying the distance of the image receptor can increase this type of magnification. Intentional use of magnification can result in a significant increase in resolution of fine-vessel recorded detail. Fractional focal-spot tubes of 0.3 mm or less are necessary for direct radiographic magnification techniques. The selection of a fractional focal spot necessitates the use of low milliamperage. Short exposure time (1 to 200 ms) is necessary because of the size and load capacity of the smaller focal spot.

The formula for manual magnification is as follows:

$$M = \frac{SID}{SOD} \quad or \quad \frac{SID}{SID - OID}$$

The SID is the *source-to-image-receptor distance*, the SOD is the *source-to-object distance*, and the OID is the *object-to-image-receptor distance*. For a 2:1 magnification study using SID of 40 inches (101 cm), the focal spot and the image receptor are positioned 20 inches (50 cm) from the area of interest. A 3:1 magnification study using a 40-inch (101-cm) SID is accomplished by placing the focal spot 13 inches (33 cm) from the area of interest and the image receptor 27 inches (68 cm) from the area of interest.

Unintentional magnification occurs when the area of interest cannot be placed in direct contact with the image receptor. The magnification that occurs as a result of these circumstances is frequently 20% to 25%. A 25% magnification occurs when a vessel within the body is 8 inches (20 cm) from the image receptor—OID of 8 inches (20 cm)—and SID is 40 inches (101 cm).

Angiographic images do not represent vessels at their actual size, and this must be taken into account when direct measurements are made from angiographic images. Increasing SID while maintaining OID can reduce unintentional magnification. Increasing SID may not be an option, however, if the increase in technical factors would exceed tube output capacity or exposure time maximum. When any measurement is necessary, the DSA postprocessing quantitative analysis programs require the radiologist to calibrate the system by measuring an object in the imaging field of known value. Some systems calibrate by using the known position of the table, the image receptor, and x-ray tube and the tube angulation.

THREE-DIMENSIONAL INTRAARTERIAL ANGIOGRAPHY

To acquire a three-dimensional model of a vascular structure, a C-arm is rotated around the region of interest (ROI) at speeds up to 60 degrees per second. The C-arm makes a preliminary sweep while mask images are acquired. Images are acquired at 7.5 to 30 frames per second. The C-arm returns to its initial position, and a second sweep is initiated. Just before the second sweep, a contrast medium is injected to opacify the vascular anatomy. The second sweep matches mask images from the first sweep, producing a rotational subtracted DSA sequence. The DSA sequence is sent to a three-dimensional rendering computer where a three-dimensional model is constructed. This model provides an image that can be manipulated and analyzed. It has proved to be a valuable tool for interventional approaches and for evaluation before surgery. Various methods of vessel analysis are available with three-dimensional models. Aneurysm volume calculation, interior wall analysis, bone fusion, and device display all are possible (Figs. 27.10 and 27.11).

A comprehensive angiography suite contains a considerable amount of equipment other than radiologic imaging devices (Fig. 27.12). Monitoring systems record patient electrocardiogram (ECG) data, blood pressure readings, and pulse oximetry. Emergency equipment includes resuscitation equipment (e.g., a defibrillator for the heart), anesthesia apparatus, and ultrasound machine.

Fig. 27.10 Three-dimensional angiography provides for reconstruction of the vessels and the skeletal anatomy.

Fig. 27.11 Three-dimensional reconstruction of left internal carotid artery. Note the anterior communicating artery aneurysm *(arrow)*.

Fig. 27.12 Modern single-plane digital angiography suite.

(Courtesy GE Medical.)

VASCULAR ACCESS

Vascular access needles are necessary when performing percutaneous procedures. Needle size is based on the external diameter of the needle and is assigned a gauge size. To allow for appropriate guidewire matching, the internal diameter of the needle must be known. Vascular access needles come in different types, sizes, and lengths. The most commonly used access needle for adult cardiovascular procedures is an 18-gauge needle that is 2.75 inches (7 cm) long. This particular needle is compatible with a 0.035-inch guidewire, which is the most frequently used guidewire in cardiovascular procedures. Appropriate needle size is predicated on the type or size of guidewire needed, the size of the patient, and the targeted entry vessel. To decrease the chances of vascular complications, the smallest gauge needle that meets the above-mentioned criteria is used for vascular access. Access needles for pediatric patients come in smaller gauge sizes with shorter lengths (Fig. 27.13).

GUIDEWIRES

Guidewires are used in angiography and other special procedures as a platform over which the catheter is to be advanced. To decrease the possibilities of complications, the guidewire should be advanced into the vasculature ahead of the catheter. After the guidewire is positioned in the area of interest, the position of the guidewire is fixed, and the catheter is advanced until it meets the tip of the guidewire. Similar to needles, guidewires come in various sizes, shapes, and lengths, and care must be taken to match the proper guidewire to the selected access needle and catheter.

Most guidewires are constructed of stainless steel, with a core or mandrel encased circumferentially within a tightly wound spiral outer core of spring wire. The mandrel gives the guidewire its stiffness and body. The length of the mandrel within the wire determines the flexibility of the wire. The shorter the mandrel, the more flexible the wire, and the more likely it is to traverse tortuous anatomy. A safety ribbon is built into the tip of the guidewire to prevent wire dislodgment in case the wire fractures. Many stainless steel guidewires are coated with polytef (Teflon) to provide lubricity and to decrease the friction between the catheter and wire. Similarly, the Teflon coating is thought to help decrease the thrombogenicity of the guidewire.

Plastic alloy guidewires consist of a hydrophilic plastic polymer coating These wires provide a smooth outer coating, with a pliable tip, and exhibit a high degree of torque or maneuverability (Fig. 27.14).

Fig. 27.13 Various needles used during catheterization.

Fig. 27.14 A guidewire allows the user a high degree of torque and maneuverability. Various lengths and shaped tips are available.

MICROPUNCTURE ACCESS SETS

Micropuncture access sets allow vascular access using a smaller gauge needle, typically 21-gauge that accepts a 0.018-inch guidewire. Once the 0.018 guidewire is in the vessel a coaxial short access catheter with a removable inner dilator is advanced over the 0.018 guidewire. The wire and inner dilator are removed, leaving the access catheter in the vessel. The access catheter has a lumen that will accept a 0.038 guidewire (Fig. 27.15).

INTRODUCER SHEATHS

Introducer sheaths are frequently used in angiographic procedures when multiple catheters are used. When the sheath has been placed, controlled access of the vasculature is ensured while reducing vessel trauma by limiting numerous catheter passages through the vessel wall.

Introducer sheaths are short catheters consisting of a slotted, rubberized back-bleed valve and a sidearm extension port. The back-bleed valve prevents the loss of blood volume during catheter exchanges or guidewire manipulations. The sidearm extension port may be used to infuse medications, monitor blood pressure, or inject contrast media to visualize the vessel or adjacent vessels.

Similar to vascular catheters, introducer sheaths come in various sizes and lengths. Typically, most introducer sheaths range in length from 4 to 35 inches (10 to 90 cm). Catheters are measured by their outside diameters and expressed in units of French size (Fr), and introducer sheaths are named according to the French size catheter they can accommodate. To accomplish this, the outer diameters of introducer sheaths are 1.5 to 2 Fr sizes larger than the catheter they can accept. A 5-Fr introducer has an outer diameter of nearly 7 Fr and accepts a 5-Fr catheter (Fig. 27.16).

Fig. 27.15 Micro puncture access set. From left: 21-gauge needle; 0.018 guidewire; 5-Fr coaxial short access catheter with 3-Fr removable inner dilator; 5-Fr access catheter with 3-Fr inner dilator remove (accepts 0.038 guidewire; #-French inner dilator).

(From Kaufman JA: Fundamentals of angiography. In Kaufman JA, Lee MJ, editors: *Vascular and interventional radiology: the requisites,* ed 2, Philadelphia, 2014, Elsevier.)

Fig. 27.16 Various types of introducer sheaths used during catheterization.

CATHETERIZATION

Catheterization for filling vessels with contrast media is preferred to needle injection of the media. The advantages of catheterization are as follows:

1. The risk of *extravasation* is reduced.
2. Most body parts can be reached for selective injection.
3. The patient can be positioned as needed.
4. The catheter can be safely left in the body while radiographs are being examined.

The femoral, axillary, brachial, and radial arteries are the most commonly punctured vessels. The common femoral artery is the most widely used access site because it is associated with the fewest risks, although the radial artery is quickly becoming the preferred access site, especially during cardiac catheterization.

The most widely used catheterization method is the Seldinger technique.[1] Seldinger described the method as puncture of both walls of the vessel (the anterior and posterior walls). The steps of the technique are described in Fig. 27.17. The modified Seldinger technique allows for puncture of the anterior wall only and has become the preferred method. The procedure is performed under sterile conditions. The catheterization site is suitably cleaned and surgically draped. The patient is given local anesthesia at the catheterization site. With this percutaneous technique, the arteriotomy or venotomy is no larger than the catheter itself, so hemorrhage is minimized. Patients can usually resume normal activity within 24 hours after the examination. Most outpatient angiographic studies can be performed in the morning, allowing the patient to be discharged later that same day. The risk of infection is less than in surgical procedures because the vessel and tissues are not exposed.

After a catheter is introduced into the blood-vascular system, it is maneuvered by pushing, pulling, and turning the part of the catheter outside the patient so that the part of the catheter inside the patient travels to the desired location. A guidewire is often positioned inside the catheter to help manipulate and guide the catheter. When the wire is removed from the catheter, the catheter is aspirated to ensure blood return and then infused, or flushed, with sterile solution, most commonly heparinized saline, to help prevent clot formation. Assisting the physician in the catheterization process is often the responsibility of the technologist.

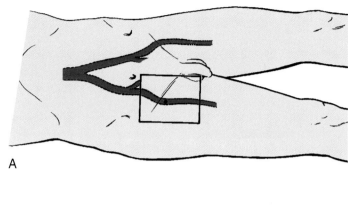

Fig. 27.17 Seldinger technique. (A) The ideal puncture occurs in the femoral artery just below the inguinal ligament. (B) Beveled compound needle containing an inner cannula pierces through the artery. (C) Needle is withdrawn slowly until there is blood flow. (Modified Seldinger would puncture only here, on the anterior wall.) (D) The needle's inner cannula is removed, and a flexible guidewire is inserted. (E) Needle is removed; pressure fixes the wire and reduces hemorrhage. (F) Catheter is slipped over the wire and into the artery. (G) Guidewire is removed, leaving the catheter in the artery.

Digital Subtraction Angiographic Procedures

When the examination is complete, the catheter and sheath are removed. Pressure is applied to the site until complete hemostasis is achieved, but blood flow through the vessel is maintained. The patient is placed on complete bed rest and observed for the development of bleeding or *hematoma*. Vascular closure devices, which close the vessel percutaneously, reduce vascular compression time and allow the patient to ambulate sooner. These devices work either by placing a collagen plug, a thrombin-collagen slurry, or a sealant gel between the artery and the skin, or by closing the arteriotomy with suture or a small surgical clip. These devices are designed for closing arteriotomies in the femoral artery after using sheath sizes between 4 and 8 Fr (Fig. 27.18).

When peripheral artery sites are unavailable, a catheter may sometimes be introduced into the aorta using the translumbar aortic approach. For this technique, the patient is positioned prone, and a special catheter introducer system is inserted percutaneously through the posterolateral aspect of the back and directed superiorly so that the catheter enters the aorta around the T11–12 level.

Fig. 27.18 Vascular closure devices. (A) Angio-Seal; (B) Perclose; (C) StarClose; (D) Mynx.

(A, Courtesy St. Jude Medical, Inc., St. Paul, MN; B and C, courtesy Abbott Vascular, Redwood City, CA; D, courtesy AccessClosure, Inc., Santa Clara, CA.)

Catheters are produced in various forms, each with a particular advantage in shape, maneuverability or torque, and maximum injection rate (Fig. 27.19). Angiographic catheters are made of pliable plastic that allows them to straighten for insertion over the guidewire. They normally resume their original shape after the guidewire is withdrawn. Some catheters have multiple side holes to facilitate high injection rates but are used only in large vascular structures for flush injections. A pigtail catheter is a special multiple-side hole catheter that allows higher volumes of contrast media to be injected with less whiplash effect, causing less damage to the vessel being injected. Catheters with a predetermined design or shape are maneuvered into the origins of vessels for selective injections. These selective catheters usually have only an end hole, allowing contrast media to be injected in one direction only.

Common angiographic catheters range in size from 4 Fr (0.05 inch) to 7 Fr (0.09 inch), although smaller or larger sizes may be used. Most angiographic catheters have inner lumens that allow them to be inserted over guidewires ranging from 0.032 to 0.038 inches in diameter. Micro-catheters and micro-guidewires are often used for distal catheterization. These micro-catheter systems are threaded through a diagnostic catheter, coaxially (Fig. 27.20).

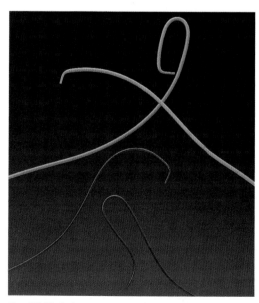

Fig. 27.19 Selected catheter shapes used for angiography.

(Courtesy Cook, Inc., Bloomington, IN.)

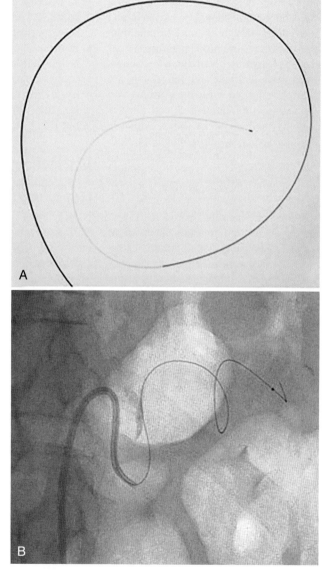

Fig. 27.20 (A) Typical microcatheter that tapers from 3-Fr to 2.3-Fr with radiopaque marker at tip. (B) Microcatheter is advanced over a 0.016-inch guidewire into distal splenic artery through a larger diagnostic selective catheter.

(From Kaufman JA: Fundamentals of angiography. In Kaufman JA, Lee MJ, editors: *Vascular and interventional radiology: the requisites,* ed 2, Philadelphia, 2014, Elsevier.)

Patient Care

Before the initiation of an angiographic procedure, it is appropriate to explain the process and the potential complications to the patient. Written consent is obtained after an explanation. Potential complications include a vasovagal reaction; stroke; heart attack; death; infection; bleeding at the puncture site; nerve, blood vessel, or tissue damage; and an allergic reaction to the contrast media. Bleeding at the puncture site is usually easily controlled with pressure to the site. Blood vessel and tissue damage may require a surgical procedure. A vasovagal reaction is characterized by sweating and nausea caused by a decrease in blood pressure. The patient's legs should be elevated, and intravenous (IV) fluids may be administered to help restore blood pressure. Minor allergic reactions to iodinated contrast media, such as hives and congestion, are usually controlled with medications and may not require treatment. Severe allergic reactions may result in shock, which is characterized by shallow breathing, high pulse rate, and possibly loss of consciousness. Angiography is performed only if the benefits of the examination outweigh the risks.

Patients are usually restricted to clear liquid intake and routine medications before undergoing angiography. Adequate hydration from liquid intake may minimize kidney damage caused by iodinated contrast media. Solid food intake is restricted to reduce the risk of aspiration related to nausea. Contraindications to angiography are determined by physicians and include previous severe allergic reaction to iodinated contrast media, severely impaired renal function, impaired blood clotting factors, and inability to undergo a surgical procedure or general anesthesia.

Because the risks of general anesthesia are greater than the risks associated with most angiographic procedures, conscious sedation may be used for the procedure. Thoughtful communication from the technologist and physician calms and reassures the patient. The technologist or physician should warn the patient about the sensations caused by the contrast media and the noise produced by the imaging equipment. This information also reduces the patient's anxiety and helps ensure a good radiographic series with no patient motion.

Preparation of Examining Room

The angiography suite and every item in it should be scrupulously clean. The room should be fully prepared, with every item needed or likely to be needed on hand before the patient is admitted. Cleanliness and advance preparation are of vital importance in procedures that must be carried out under aseptic conditions. The technologist should observe the following guidelines in preparing the room:
- Ensure patient information is entered correctly on acquisition equipment.
- Check the angiographic equipment and all working parts of the equipment, and adjust the controls for the procedure being performed.
- Ensure all patient safety equipment is available, including emergency equipment.
- Ensure all appropriate sterile supplies for the procedure are available as needed.

Radiation Protection

As in all radiographic examinations, radiation protection during angiography is extremely important for patients and staff. Angiography procedures, especially interventional procedures, can include extended periods of fluoroscopy and multiple filming sequences. The technologist is expected to know how to effectively use the imaging equipment to produce quality images while limiting the radiation dose.

There are many radiation safety features inherent in angiography equipment, such as shielding, collimators, low-dose parameters for imaging, low pulse rates for fluoroscopy, and last image hold on monitors designed to limit the radiation dose. Patient gonadal shielding should be available and used when it does not interfere with the procedure. Keeping the IR as close to the patient as possible reduces radiation scatter, and keeping the tube as far from the patient as possible reduces skin dose. All staff must wear lead protective clothing during fluoroscopy studies and maintain as much distance as they can from the tube during exposures. Lead equivalent shielding should be utilized as much as possible to reduce the radiation dose to staff; when possible, staff should leave the examination room when filming sequences are performed. Angiography suites are designed to allow observation of the patient at all times and provide adequate protection to the physician and staff. These goals are usually accomplished with leaded glass observation windows between the examination room and control room.

Angiography Team

The angiography team primarily consists of the physician (usually an interventional radiologist), the radiologic technologist, and a nurse. Other specialists, such as an anesthetist or respiratory technologist, may be necessary, depending on patient condition. The radiologic technologist assists in performing procedures that require sterile technique. Other duties may include operating monitoring devices, emergency equipment, and radiographic equipment. Instruction in patient care techniques and sterile procedure is included in the basic preparation of the technologist.

Angiography in the Future

Although noninvasive imaging techniques such as ultrasound, magnetic resonance angiography (MRA), and CT angiography (CTA) are used as primary means in diagnosing vascular diseases, there is still some diagnostic information that can only be obtained through conventional angiographic imaging. Selective injections of contrast media using selective catheterization more accurately localize and define vascular diseases. Diagnostic angiography is still routinely performed prior to performing endovascular interventional procedures.

Conventional angiographic methods are also the foundation for endovascular interventional procedures such as vascular access and guide wire and catheter manipulations. The field of angiography and endovascular intervention continues to develop and grow, with advances in catheter and guide wire technologies allowing smaller devices to be used with fewer complications.

Aortography

Visualization of the aorta is achieved by placing a multihole catheter into the aorta at the desired level, using the modified Seldinger technique. *Aortography* is usually performed with the patient in the supine position for simultaneous frontal and lateral imaging, with the central ray perpendicular to the imaging system. For introduction of a translumbar aortic catheter, the patient must be in the prone position.

THORACIC AORTOGRAPHY

Thoracic aortography may be performed to rule out an aortic aneurysm or to evaluate congenital or postsurgical conditions. The examination is also used in patients with *aortic dissection.*

The technologist does the following:

• For lateral projections, move the patient's arms superiorly so that they do not appear in the image.

• For best results, increase lateral SID, so that magnification is reduced.

• A 45-degree right posterior oblique (RPO) or left anterior oblique (LAO) projection often produces an adequate study of the aorta.

• For all projections, direct the perpendicular central ray to the center of the chest at the level of T7. The entire thoracic aorta should be visualized, including the proximal brachiocephalic, carotid, and subclavian vessels.

• Contrast media injection rates range from 15 to 25 mL/s for a total volume of 30 to 50 mL.

• Make the exposure at the end of suspended inspiration (Fig. 27.21).

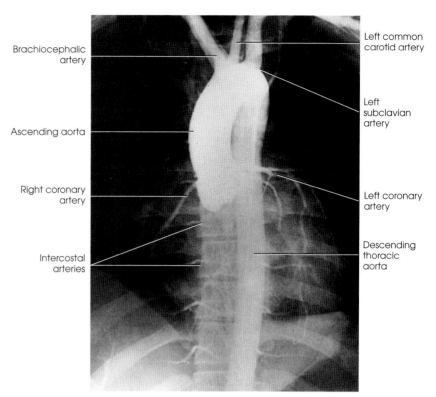

Fig. 27.21 AP thoracic aorta that also shows right and left coronary arteries.

Brachiocephalic artery

Ascending aorta

Right coronary artery

Intercostal arteries

Left common carotid artery

Left subclavian artery

Left coronary artery

Descending thoracic aorta

Aortography

Hepatic
artery

Splenic
artery

Right renal
artery

Left renal
artery

Abdominal
aorta

Right common
iliac artery

Fig. 27.22 AP abdominal aorta.

Celiac axis

Superior
mesenteric
artery

Abdominal
aorta

Fig. 27.23 Lateral abdominal aorta.

ABDOMINAL AORTOGRAPHY

Abdominal aortography may be performed to evaluate abdominal aortic aneurysm (AAA), occlusion, or atherosclerotic disease.

- For the lateral projection, move the patient's arms superiorly so that they are out of the image field.
- Usually, collimate the field in the anterior aspect of the lateral projection.
- Direct the perpendicular central ray at the level of L2 so that the aorta is visualized from the diaphragm to the aortic bifurcation. The AP projection shows best the renal artery origins, the aortic bifurcation, and the course and general condition of all abdominal visceral branches. The lateral projection best shows the origins of the celiac and superior mesenteric arteries because these vessels arise from the anterior abdominal aorta.
- Contrast media injection rates range from 15 to 20 mL/s for a total volume of 25 to 40 mL.
- Make the exposure at the end of suspended expiration (Figs. 27.22 and 27.23).

PULMONARY ARTERIOGRAPHY

Under fluoroscopic control, a catheter is passed from a peripheral vein through the vena cava and right side of the heart and into the pulmonary arteries. This technique is usually employed for a selective injection, and the examination is primarily performed for the evaluation of pulmonary embolic disease (Fig. 27.24). Pulmonary angiography has widely been replaced with pulmonary CT angiography because it provides superior imaging.

- Position the patient in the supine position.
- Image in both AP and oblique views.
- May need multiple views to cover apex and base of lung.
- Contrast media injection rates range from 10 to 20 mL/s for a total volume of 20 to 40 mL.
- Make exposures at end of suspending inspiration.

VISCERAL ARTERIOGRAPHY

Abdominal visceral arteriographic studies (Fig. 27.25) are usually performed to visualize tumor vascularity or to rule out atherosclerotic disease, thrombosis, occlusion, and bleeding. An appropriately shaped catheter is introduced, usually from a transfemoral artery puncture, and advanced into the orifice of the desired artery.

- Position the patient in the supine position.
- Direct the central ray perpendicular to the image receptor.
- If necessary, use oblique projections to improve visualization or avoid superimposition of vessels.
- For all abdominal visceral studies, obtain angiograms during suspended expiration.

Selective abdominal visceral arteriograms are described in the following sections.

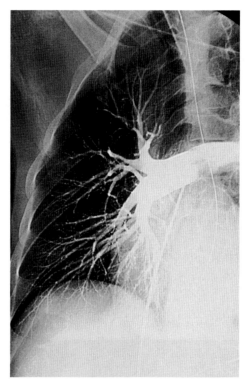

Fig. 27.24 Right pulmonary artery.

Fig. 27.25 Abdominal aortogram showing visceral arteries.

Fig. 27.26 Superselective celiac artery injection.

Celiac arteriogram

The celiac artery normally arises from the aorta at the level of T12 and carries blood to the stomach and proximal duodenum, liver, spleen, and pancreas.

- For the angiographic examination, center the patient to the image receptor.
- Direct the central ray to L1 (Fig. 27.26).
- Contrast media injection rates range from 5 to 10 mL/s for a total volume of 20 to 35 mL.
- To visualize the portal venous system, it is necessary to extend the filming sequence.

Hepatic arteriogram

The common hepatic artery branches from the right side of the celiac artery and supplies circulation to the liver, stomach and proximal duodenum, and pancreas.

- Position the patient so that the upper and right margins of the liver are at the respective margins of the image receptor (Fig. 27.27).
- Contrast media injection rates range from 5 to 10 mL/s for a total volume of 10 to 30 mL.

Fig. 27.27 Superselective hepatic artery injection.

Splenic arteriogram

The splenic artery branches from the left side of the celiac artery and supplies blood to the spleen and pancreas.

- Position the patient to place the left and upper margins of the spleen at the respective margins of the image receptor (Fig. 27.28).
- Injection of the splenic artery can show the portal venous system on the late venous images.
- To show the portal vein, center the patient to the image receptor.

Superior mesenteric arteriogram

The superior mesenteric artery (SMA) supplies blood to the small intestine and the ascending and transverse colon. It arises at about the level of L1 and descends to L5–S1.

- To visualize the SMA, center the patient to the midline of the image receptor.
- Direct the central ray to the level of L3 (Fig. 27.29).
- It may be necessary to inject a number of times with overlapping fields of view to visualize the entire area supplied by the SMA.
- Contrast media injection rates range from 5 to 10 mL/s for a total volume of 10 to 35 mL.
- When attempting to visualize bleeding sites, extend the exposure duration to 60 seconds or as requested by the radiologist.

Fig. 27.28 Superselective splenic artery injection.

Fig. 27.29 Selective SMA injection.

Inferior mesenteric arteriogram

The inferior mesenteric artery (IMA) supplies blood to the splenic flexure, descending colon, and rectosigmoid area. It arises from the left side of the aorta at about the level of L3 and descends into the pelvis.

- To visualize the IMA best, use a 15-degree right anterior oblique (RAO) or left posterior oblique (LPO) position that places the descending colon and rectum at the left and inferior margins of the image (Fig. 27.30).
- It may be necessary to inject a number of times with overlapping fields of view to visualize the entire area supplied by the IMA.
- Contrast media injection rates range from 3 to 5 mL/s for a total volume of 9 to 15 mL.

Renal arteriogram

The renal arteries arise from the right and left side of the aorta between L1 and L2 and supply blood to the respective kidney. A renal flush aortogram may be accomplished by injecting 10 to 20 mL/s for a total volume of 20 to 40 mL of contrast media through a multiple–side-hole catheter positioned in the aorta at the level of the renal arteries. A representative selective injection is 5 mL/s for a 10-mL total volume.

- For a right renal arteriogram, position the patient so that the central ray enters at the level of L2 midway between the center of the spine and the patient's right side.

- For a selective left renal arteriogram, position the patient so that the central ray enters at the level of L1 midway between the center of the spine and the patient's left side (Fig. 27.31).

Other abdominal arteriograms

Other arteries branching from the aorta may be selectively studied to show anatomy and possible pathology. The positioning for these procedures depends on the area to be studied and the surrounding structures (these may include spinal, lumbar, adrenal, and phrenic).

Fig. 27.30 Selective IMA injection.

Fig. 27.31 Selective left renal artery injection in early arterial phase.

Peripheral Angiography
UPPER LIMB ARTERIOGRAMS

Upper limb arteriography is most often performed to evaluate traumatic injury, atherosclerotic disease, or other vascular lesions. Arteriograms are usually obtained using the modified Seldinger technique to introduce a catheter, most often at a femoral artery site for selective injection into the subclavian or axillary artery. The contrast media may also be injected at a more distal site through a catheter. The area to be radiographed may be a hand or another selected part of the arm or the entire upper extremity and thorax.

The recommended projection is a true AP projection with the arm extended and the hand supinated. Hand arteriograms may be obtained in the supine or prone arm position (Figs. 27.32 and 27.33). The injection varies from 3 to 4 mL/s through a catheter positioned distally to 10 mL/s through a proximally positioned catheter. Images are obtained by using a bolus chase technique or by performing serial runs over each segment of the extremity.

UPPER LIMB VENOGRAMS

Upper limb venography is most often performed to look for thrombosis or occlusions. The contrast medium is injected through a needle, IV line, or catheter into a superficial vein at the elbow or wrist. Radiographs should cover the vasculature from the wrist or elbow to the superior vena cava (Fig. 27.34).

Fig. 27.32 Right hand arteriogram (2:1 magnification) showing severe arterial occlusive disease *(arrows)* affecting digits after cold temperature injury.

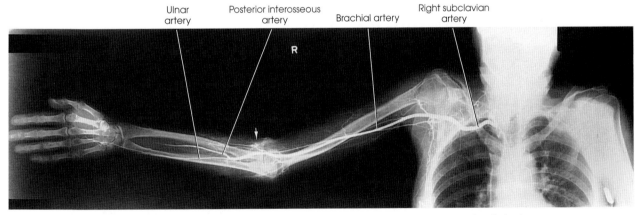

Fig. 27.33 Right subclavian artery injection showing iatrogenic occlusion of radial artery *(arrow).*

Fig. 27.34 Normal right upper limb venogram.

LOWER LIMB ARTERIOGRAMS

Aortofemoral arteriography is usually performed to determine whether atherosclerotic disease is the cause of *claudication*. A catheter is usually introduced into a femoral artery using the modified Seldinger technique. The catheter tip is positioned superior to the aortic bifurcation so that bilateral arteriograms are obtained simultaneously. When only one leg is to be examined, the catheter tip is placed below the bifurcation, or the contrast media is injected through a catheter or sheath placed in the femoral artery on the side of interest.

- For a bilateral examination, place the patient in the supine position for single-plane AP projections and center the patient to the midline of the image receptor to include the area from the renal arteries to the ankles (Fig. 27.35).
- Internally rotate the legs 30 degrees.

- Subtracted or unsubtracted bolus chase selections can be used to follow the contrast media down the legs, or alternately, a number of stationary DSA filming sequences can be performed to cover the area of interest.
- Make exposures of the opacified lower abdominal aorta and aortic bifurcation with the patient in suspended expiration. Examinations of a specific area of the leg such as the popliteal fossa or foot are occasionally performed.
- The preferred injection site is usually the femoral artery.
- AP, lateral, or both projections may be obtained with the patient centered to the designated area.
- Contrast media injection rates range from 5 to 10 mLs/s for a total of 40 to 60 mL for bolus chase, or from 5 to 10 mLs/s for a total of 10 to 30 mL for stationary DSA sequences.

LOWER LIMB VENOGRAMS

Lower limb venography is usually performed to visualize thrombosis of the deep veins of the leg. Ultrasound of the legs is the first-line diagnostic tool to diagnose deep vein thrombosis. CT or MR venography can also be performed for noninvasive diagnostic imaging. In cases where interventional procedures are expected to be performed, lower limb venography can also be obtained with contrast media injected through a sheath or catheter placed directly into the popliteal vein with the patient prone (Fig. 27.36).

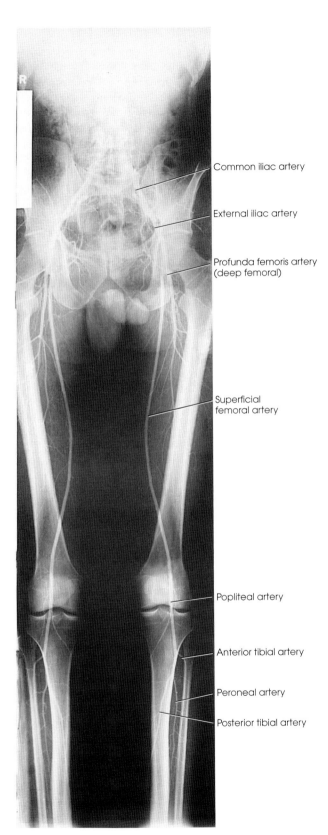

Common iliac artery

External iliac artery

Profunda femoris artery
(deep femoral)

Superficial
femoral artery

Popliteal artery

Anterior tibial artery

Peroneal artery

Posterior tibial artery

Fig. 27.35 Normal abdominal
aortogram and bilateral femoral
arteriogram in late arterial phase.

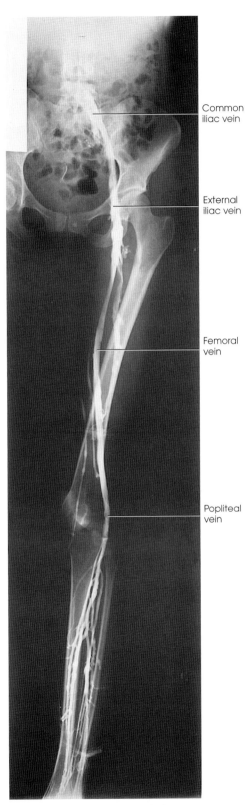

Common
iliac vein

External
iliac vein

Femoral
vein

Popliteal
vein

Fig. 27.36 Normal left lower limb venogram.

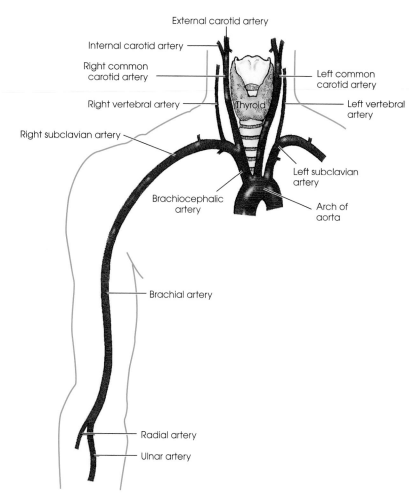

Fig. 27.37 Major arteries of upper chest, neck, and arm.

Cerebral Anatomy

Cerebral angiography is the radiologic and angiographic examination of the blood vessels of the brain. The procedure was introduced by Egas Moniz[2] in 1927. It is performed to investigate intracranial vascular lesions such as aneurysms, arteriovenous malformations (AVMs), tumors, and atherosclerotic or stenotic lesions.

The brain is supplied by four trunk vessels or great vessels (Fig. 27.37): the right and left common carotid arteries, which supply the anterior circulation; and the right and left vertebral arteries, which supply the posterior circulation. These paired arteries branch from the arch of the aorta and ascend through the neck.

The first branch of the aortic arch is the *innominate artery* or the *brachiocephalic artery*. It bifurcates into the right common carotid and the right subclavian artery. The second branch of the aortic arch is the left common carotid, followed by the left subclavian artery. Each of the vessels originates directly from the aortic arch. Both vertebral arteries most commonly take their origins from the subclavian arteries. Although this branching pattern is common in most patients, there can be some *anomalous* origins of these great vessels. Each common carotid artery passes superiorly and laterally alongside the trachea and larynx to the level of C4 and then divides into internal and external carotid arteries. The external carotid artery contributes blood supply to the extracranial and extra-axial circulation. There can be some collateral circulation into the internal carotid circulation in some situations. The internal carotid artery (ICA) enters the cranium through the carotid foramen of the temporal bone and bifurcates into the anterior and middle cerebral arteries (Fig. 27.38). These vessels branch and rebranch to supply the anterior circulation of the respective hemisphere of the brain.

Fig. 27.38 Right common carotid artery injection showing right internal carotid artery *(arrows)* and anterior cerebral blood circulation, including reflux across anterior communicating artery *(small arrow)*.

The vertebral arteries ascend through the cervical transverse foramina and pass medially to enter the cranium through the foramen magnum. The vertebral arteries unite to form the basilar artery, which, after a short superior course along the posterior surface of the dorsum sellae, bifurcates into the right and left posterior cerebral arteries. The blood supply to the posterior fossa (cerebellum) originates from the vertebral and basilar arteries (Fig. 27.39).

The anterior and posterior cerebral arteries are connected by communicating arteries at the level of the midbrain to form the *circle of Willis*. The anterior communicating artery forms an anastomosis between the anterior cerebral arteries, which communicate between the right and left hemispheres. The right and left posterior communicating arteries each form an anastomosis between the ICA and the posterior cerebral artery connecting the anterior and posterior circulation. A chart detailing intracerebral circulation is provided in Figs. 27.40 and 27.41.

Fig. 27.39 Left vertebral artery injection showing posterior cerebral blood circulation, including reflux into posterior communicating artery *(arrows)*.

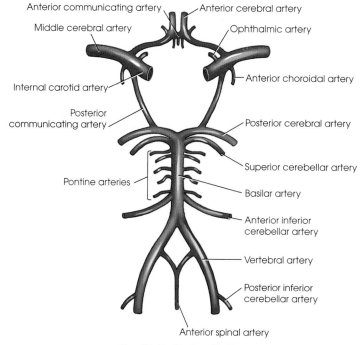

Anterior communicating artery

Anterior cerebral artery

Middle cerebral artery

Ophthalmic artery

Internal carotid artery

Anterior choroidal artery

Posterior communicating artery

Posterior cerebral artery

Superior cerebellar artery

Pontine arteries

Basilar artery

Anterior inferior cerebellar artery

Vertebral artery

Posterior inferior cerebellar artery

Anterior spinal artery

Fig. 27.40 Circle of Willis.

Technique

Cerebral angiography should be performed only in facilities equipped to produce studies of high technical quality with minimal risk to the patient. The ability to obtain rapid-sequence biplane images with automatic injection represents the minimum standard. This equipment is available in all major medical centers and in most large hospitals (see Fig. 27.9).

Cerebral angiography is most commonly performed from a transfemoral approach; however, a brachial or axillary artery approach can be employed. Selective catheterization techniques also allow the internal and external carotid circulation to be studied separately, which is useful in delineating the blood supply of some forms of cerebral tumors and vascular malformations.

The final position of the catheter depends on the information sought from the angiographic study. When atherosclerotic disease of the extracranial carotid, subclavian, and vertebral arteries is being evaluated, injection of the aortic arch with imaging of the extracranial portion of these vessels is an appropriate way to begin.

LATERAL PROJECTION ANTEROPOSTERIOR PROJECTION

Carotid artery

Internal carotid arteriogram

Vertebral artery

Vertebral arteriogram

Superior sagittal sinus

Transverse sinus

Superior sagittal sinus

Transverse sinus

Internal carotid venogram

Fig. 27.41 Diagram of intracranial circulation: arterial and venous phase.

(From Bean BC: A chart of the intracerebral circulation, ed 2. *Med Radiogr Photogr* 34:25, 1958; courtesy Dr. Berton C. Bean and Eastman Kodak Co.)

Technique

Fig. 27.42 Right internal carotid injection, lateral projection, shows arterial phase of circulation. Note posterior communicating artery *(arrow)*.

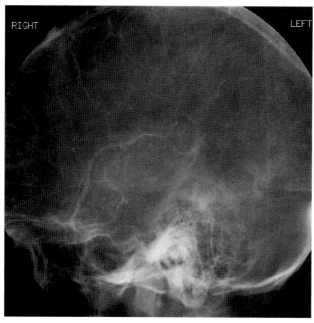

Fig. 27.43 Right internal carotid injection, lateral projection, shows capillary phase of carotid circulation.

CIRCULATION TIME AND IMAGING PROGRAM

Egas Moniz[3] stated that the transit time of the cerebral circulation is only 3 seconds for the blood to circulate from the ICA to the jugular vein, with the circulation time being slightly prolonged by the injected contrast solution. Greitz,[4] who measured the cerebral circulation time as "the time between the points of maximum concentration (of contrast media) in the carotid siphon and in the parietal veins," found a normal mean value of 4.13 seconds. This time is a highly important factor in cerebral angiography.

Certain pathologic conditions significantly alter the cerebral circulation time. AVMs shorten the transit time; arterial vasospasm may cause a considerable delay.

A standard radiographic program should include a radiograph taken before the arrival of contrast media to serve as a subtraction mask and rapid-sequence images at 2 to 4 images per second in the AP and lateral projections during the early, or arterial, phase (first $1\frac{1}{2}$ to $2\frac{1}{2}$ seconds) of the arteriogram (Fig. 27.42). After the arterial phase, imaging may be slowed to one image per second for the capillary, or parenchymal, phase (Fig. 27.43) and maintained at one image per second or every other second for the venous phase (Fig. 27.44) of the angiogram. The entire program should cover 7 to 10 seconds, depending on the preference of the angiographer. The imaging program must be tailored to show the suspected pathologic condition.

Injection rates and volumes through the catheter are coupled with the imaging program, usually by automatic means. Injections at rates of 5 to 9 mL/s for 1 to 2 seconds are most often employed in the cerebral vessels, with variations dependent on vessel size and the patient's circulatory status.

EQUIPMENT

Rapid-sequence biplane imaging with DSA electronically coupled with an automatic injector is employed almost universally in cerebral angiography. Collimating to the area of the head and neck is essential for improving image quality in a nonmagnified study. The standard tube collimator may be used for this purpose.

POSITION OF HEAD

The centering and angulation of the central ray required to show the anterior circulation differ from those required to show the posterior circulation. The same head position is used for the basic AP and lateral projections of both regions.

- For the initial right-angle studies, center the head to the AP and lateral image receptors.
- Adjust the patient's head to place its midsagittal plane exactly perpendicular to the headrest and consequently exactly parallel with the laterally placed image receptor.
- Place the infraorbitomeatal line (IOML) perpendicular to the horizontal plane when positioning is done manually.
- Angle the central ray for caudally inclined AP and AP oblique projections from the vertically placed IOML, or adjust the central ray so that it is parallel to the floor of the anterior fossa, as indicated by a line extending from the supraorbital margin to a point $\frac{3}{4}$ inch (1.9 cm) superior to the external acoustic meatus (EAM).

Frontal projections are described in this section as AP projections, but equivalent PA projections also exist. Angiographic imaging systems place the image receptor above the tabletop and the x-ray tube below. Because patients usually lie supine for cerebral angiography, the central ray, coming from below, enters the posterior cranium and exits the anterior cranium on its course to the image receptor. The position of the central ray results in PA projections equivalent to the AP projections described. Fluoroscopy is often used to determine the final position of the head and the angulation of the central ray required to achieve the desired image.

The literature on cerebral angiography contains numerous position variations concerning the degree of central ray angulation, the base from which the central ray should be angled or the line that it should parallel, and the degree of part rotation for oblique studies. This chapter discusses the most frequently employed images and reasonably standard specifications for obtaining them.

The number of radiographs required for satisfactory delineation of a lesion depends on the nature and location of the lesion. Oblique projections or variations in central ray angulation are used to separate the vessels that overlap in the basic positions and to evaluate any existing abnormality.

Fig. 27.44 Right internal carotid injection, lateral projection, shows venous phase of circulation.

Aortic Arch Angiogram (for Cranial Vessels)

An aortic arch angiogram is most commonly obtained to visualize atherosclerotic or occlusive disease of the extracranial or common carotid, vertebral, and subclavian arteries. A multiple–side-hole catheter is positioned in the ascending thoracic aorta so that the subsequent injection fills all of the vessels simultaneously.

SIMULTANEOUS BIPLANE OBLIQUE PROJECTIONS

For best results, simultaneous biplane oblique projections are produced so that superimposition of vessels is minimized (Fig. 27.45).

- Place the image receptor in a 35-degree RPO (LAO) position. This position opens the aortic arch and clearly demonstrates the origins of the brachiocephalic, left common carotid, and left subclavian arteries.

- Raise the patient's chin to superimpose the inferior margin of the mandible onto the occiput so that as much of the neck as possible is exposed in the frontal image.

- Move the patient's shoulders inferiorly so that they are removed as much as possible from the lateral image.

- Position the lateral image receptor in a 35–45-degree LPO (RAO) projection to better demonstrate the bifurcation of the brachiocephalic and the origin of the left vertebral artery.

- The image receptor is positioned to include the inferior boarder of the aortic arch at the bottom of the imaging field.

Fig. 27.45 Digital subtracted images of thoracic aortogram showing the origins of the great vessels. *IN,* Innominate; *LVA,* left vertebral artery; *LSA,* left subclavian artery; *RCC,* right common carotid; *RVA,* right vertebral artery; *RSA,* right subclavian artery.

Anterior Circulation
LATERAL PROJECTION

- Center the patient's head to the vertically placed image receptor.
- Extend the patient's head enough to place the IOML perpendicular to the horizontal.
- Adjust the patient's head to place the midsagittal plane vertical and parallel with the plane of the image receptor.
- Adapt immobilization to the type of equipment being employed.
- Perform lateral projections of the anterior, or carotid, circulation with the central ray directed horizontally to a point slightly cranial to the auricle and midway between the forehead and the occiput. This centering allows for patient variation (Figs. 27.46–27.48).

NOTE: See Fig. 27.41 for assistance in identifying the cerebral vessels in the image.

Fig. 27.46 Cerebral angiogram: lateral projection as part of a biplane setup.

Fig. 27.47 Lateral projection.

Fig. 27.48 Left internal carotid artery injection. Cerebral angiogram: lateral projection showing anterior circulation. Note posterior communicating artery (arrow).

Fig. 27.49 Carotid angiogram: PA axial (supraorbital) projection.

Fig. 27.50 AP axial (supraorbital).

AP AXIAL PROJECTION (SUPRAORBITAL)

Adjust the patient's head so that the midsagittal plane is centered over and perpendicular to the midline of the image receptor and so that it is extended enough to place the IOML vertically.

- Immobilize the patient's head.
- Keep in mind that achieving the goal in this angiogram requires superimposition of the supraorbital margins on the superior margin of the petrous ridges so that the vessels are projected above the floor of the anterior cranial fossa.
- To obtain this result in most patients, direct the central ray 20 degrees caudally for the AP axial projection or 20 degrees cephalad for the PA axial projection along a line passing $\frac{3}{4}$ inch (1.9 cm) superior to and parallel with a line extending from the supraorbital margin to a point $\frac{3}{4}$ inch (1.9 cm) superior to the EAM; the latter line coincides with the floor of the anterior fossa (Figs. 27.49–27.51).

Fig. 27.51 Left common carotid artery injection showing AP axial (supraorbital) projection. Arterial phase of circulation.

AP AXIAL OBLIQUE PROJECTION (TRANSORBITAL)

The oblique transorbital projection shows the internal carotid bifurcation and the anterior communicating and middle cerebral arteries within the orbital shadow.

- From the position for the basic AP transorbital projection, rotate the patient's head approximately 30 degrees away from the injected side, or angle the central ray 30 degrees toward the injected side.
- Angle the central ray 20 degrees cephalad and center it to the mid-orbit of the uppermost side (Figs. 27.52 and 27.53).

Posterior Circulation
LATERAL PROJECTION

- Center the patient's head to the vertically placed image receptor.
- Extend the patient's head enough to place the IOML perpendicular to the horizontal plane, and adjust the head to place the midsagittal plane vertically and parallel with the plane of the image receptor.

- Rigidly immobilize the patient's head.
- Perform lateral projections of the posterior, or vertebral, circulation with the central ray directed horizontally to the mastoid process at a point about $\frac{3}{8}$ inch (1 cm) superior to and $\frac{3}{4}$ inch (1.9 cm) posterior to the EAM.
- Restrict the exposure field to the middle and posterior fossae for lateral studies of the posterior circulation (Figs. 27.54 and 27.55). Inclusion of the entire skull

Fig. 27.52 AP axial oblique (transorbital) projection.

Fig. 27.53 Right internal carotid artery injection showing AP axial oblique (transorbital) projection.

Fig. 27.54 Lateral projection for posterior circulation.

Fig. 27.55 Right vertebral artery injection showing lateral projection of vertebrobasilar system.

Fig. 27.56 AP axial projection for posterior circulation.

Fig. 27.57 Right vertebral artery injection showing AP axial projection of vertebrobasilar system.

is neither necessary nor, from the standpoint of optimal technique, desirable.

AP AXIAL PROJECTION

- Adjust the patient's head so that the midsagittal plane is centered over and perpendicular to the midline of the grid, and extend the head enough so that the IOML is vertical.
- Immobilize the patient's head.
- Direct the central ray to the region approximately $1\frac{1}{2}$ inches (3.8 cm) superior to the glabella at an angle of 30 to 35 degrees caudad. The central ray exits at the level of the EAM. For this projection, the supraorbital margins are positioned approximately $\frac{3}{4}$ inch (1.9 cm) below the superior margins of the petrous ridges (Figs. 27.56 and 27.57).

Venous blood in veins flows proximally toward the heart. Injection into a central venous structure may not opacify the peripheral veins that *anastomose* to it. The position of peripheral veins can be indirectly documented, however, by the filling defect from unopacified blood in the opacified central vein.

- Place the patient in the supine position for either a single-plane AP or PA projection or biplane projections.
- Move the patient's arms out of the field of view.
- Obtain lateral projections at increased SID, if possible, to reduce magnification.
- Remember that collimation to the long axis of the vena cava improves image quality but may prevent visualization of peripheral or *collateral veins*.

Superior Venacavogram

Venography of the superior vena cava is performed primarily to rule out the existence of thrombus or the occlusion of the superior vena cava. The contrast media may be injected through a needle or an angiographic catheter introduced into a vein in an antecubital fossa, although superior opacification results from injection through a catheter positioned in the axillary or subclavian vein. Radiographs should include the opacified subclavian vein, brachiocephalic vein, superior vena cava, and right atrium (Fig. 27.58).

Inferior Venacavogram

Venography of the IVC is performed primarily to identify the location of the renal veins for placement of an IVC filter. The contrast media are injected through a multiple–side-hole catheter inserted through the femoral vein and positioned in the common iliac vein or the inferior aspect of the IVC (Fig. 27.59).

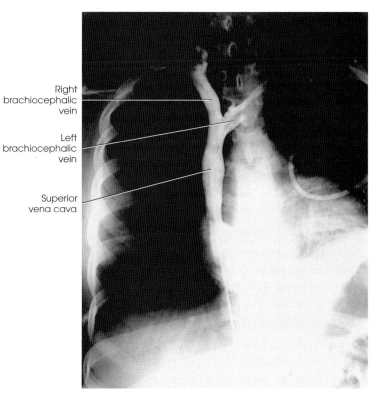

Right brachiocephalic vein

Left brachiocephalic vein

Superior vena cava

Fig. 27.58 AP superior vena cava.

Inferior vena cava

Right common iliac vein

Fig. 27.59 AP inferior vena cava.

Visceral Venography

The visceral veins are often visualized by extending the imaging program of the corresponding visceral artery injection. The veins that drain the small bowel are normally visualized by extending the imaging program of a superior mesenteric arteriogram. Portal venography (Fig. 27.60) can be performed by injecting the portal vein directly from a percutaneous approach, but it is usually accomplished by late-phase imaging of a splenic artery injection or SMA injection.

HEPATIC VENOGRAM

Hepatic venography is usually performed to rule out stenosis or thrombosis of the hepatic veins. These veins are also catheterized to obtain pressure measurements from the interior of the liver. The hepatic veins carry blood from the liver to the IVC. (The portal vein carries nutrient-rich blood from the viscera to the liver.) The hepatic veins are most easily catheterized from a jugular vein or an upper limb vein approach, but a femoral vein approach may also be used.

- Place the patient in the supine position for AP or PA projections that include the liver tissue and the extreme upper IVC (Fig. 27.61).
- Make exposures at the end of suspended expiration.

RENAL VENOGRAM

Renal venography is usually performed to rule out thrombosis of the renal vein. The renal vein is also catheterized for blood sampling, usually to measure the production of renin, an enzyme produced by the kidney when it lacks adequate blood supply. The renal vein is most easily catheterized from a femoral vein approach.

- Place the patient in the supine position for a single-plane AP or PA projection.
- Center the selected kidney to the image receptor, and collimate the field to include the kidney and area of the IVC (Fig. 27.62).
- Make exposures at the end of suspended expiration.

Fig. 27.60 Portal venogram. *c*, Coronary varices; *i*, inferior mesenteric vein; *m*, main portal vein; *s*, superior mesenteric vein; *sp*, splenic vein.

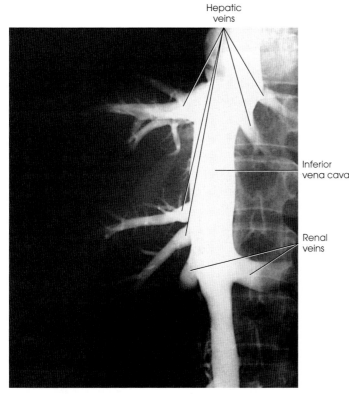

Hepatic veins

Inferior vena cava

Renal veins

Fig. 27.61 Hepatic vein visualization from reflux from inferior vena cava injection. (Note reflux into bilateral renal veins.)

Left renal veins

Fig. 27.62 Selective left renal venogram. AP projection.

Interventional radiology has a therapeutic rather than diagnostic purpose in that it intervenes in, or interferes with, the course of a disease process or other medical condition. Since the conception of this form of radiology in the early 1960s, its realm has become so vast and sophisticated that publishers of periodicals struggle to keep abreast of this rapidly advancing specialty.

Interventional radiology allows the radiologist to assume an important role in the management and treatment of disease in many patients. Interventional radiologic procedures reduce hospital stays in many patients and help some patients avoid surgery, with consequent reductions in medical costs.

Every interventional radiologic procedure must include two integral processes. The first is the interventional or medical side of the procedure, in which a highly skilled radiologist uses wires, catheters, and special medical devices (e.g., occluding coils, stents) to improve the patient's status or condition. The second process involves the use of fluoroscopy and radiography to guide and document the progress of the steps taken during the first process. A radiologic technologist must receive special education in the angiographic and interventional suite. This skilled technologist has an important role in assisting the radiologist in the interventional procedures.

The more frequently performed interventional procedures are described in this section. Resources containing more detailed information are cited in the selected bibliography at the end of the chapter.

Percutaneous Transluminal Angioplasty and Stenting

PTA is a therapeutic radiologic procedure designed to dilate or reopen stenotic or occluded areas within a vessel using a catheter introduced by the Seldinger technique. In 1964, Dotter and Judkins[5] first described PTA using a coaxial catheter method. First, a guidewire is passed through the narrowed area of a vessel. A smaller catheter then is passed over the guidewire through the stenosis to begin the dilation process. Finally, a larger catheter is passed over the smaller catheter to cause further dilation. This method is referred to as the "Dotter method." Although this method can achieve dilation of stenosis, it has the significant disadvantage of creating an arteriotomy as large as the dilating catheters, and it is seldom used as a first-line therapy.

In 1974, Grüntzig and Hopff[6] introduced the double-lumen, balloon-tipped catheter. One lumen allows the passage of a guidewire and fluids through the catheter. The other lumen communicates with a balloon at the distal end of the catheter. When inflated, the balloon expands to a size much larger than the catheter. Double-lumen angioplasty balloon catheters are available in sizes ranging from 3 to 9 Fr, with attached balloons varying in length and expanding to diameters of 2 to 20 mm or more (Fig. 27.63).

Fig. 27.64 illustrates the process of *balloon angioplasty*. The stenosis is initially identified on a previously obtained angiogram. The balloon diameter used for a procedure is often the measured diameter of the normal artery adjacent to the stenosis. The angioplasty procedure is often performed at the same time and through the same catheterization site as the initial diagnostic examination.

Fig. 27.63 Balloon angioplasty catheters with varied diameters and lengths.

(2014 C. R. Bard, Inc. Used with permission. Bard is a registered trademark of C. R. Bard, Inc.)

Fig. 27.64 Balloon angioplasty of atherosclerotic stenosis. (A) Guidewire advanced through stenosis. (B) Balloon across stenosis. (C) Balloon inflated. (D) Postangioplasty stenotic area.

After the guidewire is positioned across the stenosis, the angiographic catheter is removed over the wire. The angioplasty balloon catheter is introduced and directed through the stenosis over the guidewire. The balloon is usually inflated with a diluted contrast media mixture for 15 to 45 seconds, depending on the degree of stenosis and the vessel being treated.

The balloon is deflated and repositioned or withdrawn from the lesion. Contrast media can be injected through the angioplasty catheter for a repeat angiogram to determine whether or not the procedure was successful. The success of the angioplasty procedure may also be determined by comparing transcatheter blood pressure measurements from a location distal and a location proximal to the lesion site. Nearly equal pressures indicate a reopened stenosis.

Transluminal angioplasty can be performed in virtually any vessel that can be reached percutaneously with a catheter (Figs. 27.65 and 27.66). In 1978, Molnar and Stockum[7] described the use of balloon angioplasty for dilation of strictures within

Fig. 27.65 Digital subtracted images of the abdominal aortogram and bilateral iliac arteries. (A) High-grade stenosis of right common iliac artery *(arrow)*. (B) Abdominal aortogram and bilateral iliac arteries, postangioplasty, showing widely patent iliac system.

Fig. 27.66 Abdominal aortogram before and after angioplasty of the left renal artery. (A) High-grade stenosis of left renal artery *(arrow)*. (B) Postangioplasty and stent placement within left renal artery *(arrow)*.

the biliary system. Balloon angioplasty is also conducted in venous structures, ureters, and the gastrointestinal tract.

Balloon angioplasty has been used successfully to manage various diseases that cause arterial narrowing. The most common form of arterial stenosis treated by transluminal angioplasty is caused by atherosclerosis. Dotter and Judkins[5] speculated that this atheromatous material was soft and inelastic and could be compressed against the artery wall. Later research showed, however, that the plaque does not compress. If plaque surrounds the inner diameter of the artery, the plaque cracks at its thinnest portion as the arterial lumen is expanded. Continued expansion cracks the inner layer of the arterial wall, the *intima*, then stretches and tears the middle layer, the *media*, and finally stretches the outer layer, the *adventitia*. The arterial lumen is increased by permanently enlarging the artery's outer diameter. Restenosis, when it occurs, is usually caused by deposits of new plaque, rather than arterial wall collapse.

A final possibility for percutaneous treatment of vessel stenoses is the placement of vascular stents. A vascular *stent* is composed of a metal material, stainless steel or nitinol, and can be covered or uncovered with a surgical graft material that is introduced through a catheter system and positioned across a stenosis to keep the narrowed area spread apart. These devices remain in the vessel permanently (Figs. 27.67 and 27.68).

The success of PTA and/or stent placement in the management of atherosclerosis has made it a significant alternative to surgical procedures in the treatment of this disease. PTA is not indicated in all cases, however. Long segments of occlusion may be best treated by surgery. PTA has a lower risk than surgery but is not totally risk-free. Generally, patients must be able to tolerate the surgical procedure that may be required to repair vessel damage that can be caused by PTA. Unsuccessful transluminal angioplasty and stent procedures rarely prevent or complicate necessary subsequent surgery. In selected cases, the procedure is effective and almost painless and can be repeated as often as necessary with no apparent increase in risk to the patient. The recovery time is often no longer than the time required to stabilize the arteriotomy site, usually a matter of hours, and general anesthesia is normally not required. The hospital stay and the cost to the patient are reduced.

Abdominal Aortic Aneurysm Endografts

An interventional therapy started in the late 1990s treats abdominal aortic aeurysms (AAAs) with a transcatheter approach and stenting. AAAs historically have been treated with an open repair of the aneurysm by a vascular surgeon. This approach has risks associated with abdominal surgery and a long hospital stay for recovery of the incision. The stent graft or endograft is a metal stent covered in synthetic graft material that comes in pieces or one intact device depending on the manufacturer (Fig. 27.69). A cutdown approach to bilateral femoral arteries is done, and sheaths and delivery catheters are advanced to deliver the device. A large amount of planning is done before a

Fig. 27.67 Intravascular stents. (A) Gianturco-Rosch biliary Z-stent. (B) Memotherm. (C) Palmaz; unexpanded and expanded. (D) Symphony. (E) Wallstent.

Fig. 27.68 Stent and balloon for angioplasty shown collapsed and inflated.

Fig. 27.69 Stent graft or endograft used to repair aneurysm in the aorta and iliac region.

patient can undergo this approach to treating AAA. Patients preferably should have an AAA that is infrarenal or occurring below the renal arteries. The endograft would occlude any arteries originating from the portion of the aorta being treated. Some newer devices are designed to treat aneurysms that extend to involve the renal artery and even mesenteric artery origins. These fenestrated endografts are usually custom made for each individual patient (Fig. 27.70).

Preliminary abdominal and iliac arteriograms may be obtained using a calibrated catheter that the radiologist or vascular surgeon can use for measuring (Fig. 27.71). CT is the preferred imaging

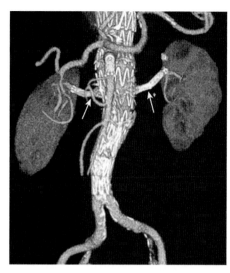

Fig. 27.70 Fenestrated, or branched, endograft. Volume rendering of a computed tomographic angiography showing a fenestrated endograph (Zenith, Cook, Bloomington, IL). There are extensions into both renal arteries *(arrows)*, the superior mesenteric artery, and celiac artery.

(From Kaufman JA: Abdominal aorta and pelvic arteries. In Kaufman JA, Lee MJ, editors: *Vascular and interventional radiology: the requisites,* ed 2, Philadelphia, 2014, Elsevier. Courtesy Roy Greenberg, MD, Cleveland, OH.)

Fig. 27.71 (A) Abdominal aortogram. (B) Placement of endograft. (C) Follow-up aortogram showing repair.

modality and is used as the primary source for measurements. This procedure is done either in the catheterization laboratory or in the operating room depending on the hospital. If done in the operating room, a portable C-arm is needed with DSA capability. Some hospitals are building hybrid surgical suites that have a C-arm built in to the room like a standard angiography suite.

Although most PTA procedures are conducted in the angiography suite, angioplasty involving the arteries of the heart, *percutaneous transluminal coronary angioplasty (PTCA)*, is generally performed in the cardiac catheterization laboratory because of the possibility of potentially serious cardiac complications. PTCA is discussed later in this chapter.

Transcatheter Embolization

Transcatheter embolization was first described by Brooks[8,9] in 1930. He described vessel occlusion for closure of arteriovenous fistula. Transcatheter embolization involves the therapeutic introduction of various substances to occlude or drastically reduce blood flow within a vessel (Box 27.1). The three main purposes for embolization are (1) to stop active bleeding sites, (2) to control blood flow to diseased or malformed vessels (e.g., tumors or AVMs), and (3) to stop or reduce blood flow to a particular area of the body before surgery.

The patient's condition and the situation must be considered when choosing an embolic agent. The interventionalist usually identifies the appropriate agent to be used. Embolic agents must be administered with care to ensure that they flow to the predetermined vessel or target without embolizing nontarget vessels. Embolization can be a permanent treatment; the effects on the lesion are irreversible. Many embolic agents are available (Box 27.2), and the choice of agent depends on whether the occlusion is to be temporary or permanent (Table 27.1).

Temporary agents such as Gelfoam[b] or Avitene may be used as a means to reduce the pressure head of blood to a specific site. These temporary agents reduce flow into a bleeding site so that hemostasis may be achieved. Temporary agents can also be used to prevent inadvertent embolization of normal vessels.

---

[b]Gelfoam is the trademark for a sterile, absorbable, water-insoluble, gelatin-base sponge.

BOX 27.1

Lesions amendable to embolization

Aneurysm
Pseudoaneurysm
Hemorrhage
Neoplasms
  Malignant
  Benign
Arteriovenous malformations
Arteriovenous fistula
Infertility (varicocele)
Impotence owing to venous leakage
Redistribution of blood flow

BOX 27.2

Embolic agents

Particulate agents
Polyvinyl alcohol
Embosphere
Avitene
Gelfoam

Metal coils
Gianturco coils
Metal coils
Detachable coils
  Platinum
  Coated

Vascular occluder plug
Liquid agents (occluding, sclerosing)
  Ethanol
  Thrombin
  Hypertonic glucose
  Sodium tetradecyl sulfate
  Ethibloc
  EVAL
  Onyx
Detachable balloons
  Latex—Debrun
  Silicone—Hieshima
Liquid adhesives
  N-butyl 2-cyanoacrylate
Autologous material

TABLE 27.1

Particulate agent sizes

Agent	Size
Gelfoam powder	40–60 μ
Gelfoam sponges	Pledgets-torpedoes
Avitene	100–150 μ
Polyvinyl alcohol	100–1,200 μ
Embosphere	100–1,200 μ

Vasoconstricting drugs can be used to reduce blood flow temporarily. Vasoconstrictors such as vasopressin (Pitressin) drastically constrict vessels, resulting in hemostasis.

When permanent occlusion is desired, as in trauma to the pelvis that causes hemorrhage or when vascular tumors are supplied by large vessels, stainless steel coils may be used. This coil (Fig. 27.72), which functions to produce thrombogenesis, is simply a looped segment of guidewire with Dacron fibers attached to it. The coil is initially straight and is easily introduced into a catheter that has been placed into the desired vessel. This coil is then deployed by being pushed out of the catheter tip with a guidewire. The coil assumes its looping shape immediately as it enters the bloodstream. It is important that the catheter tip be specifically placed in the vessel so that the coil springs precisely into the desired area. Numerous coils can be placed as needed to occlude the vessel. Detachable coils are mounted on a wire and are deployed either manually or with an electrical current to allow for more precise placement. If the placement is not correct the coil can be removed without being deployed. Newer generations of coils promise more effective embolization by using various coatings on the outside of the coil. One such coil uses a coating that initiates a foreign body/scarring response. Another type of coil is coated with an expansile gel that

Fig. 27.72 Embolization coils. (A) Coils are packaged preloaded in tubes. Shown is a Gianturco stainless steel coil with polyester fibers. (B) The coil is delivered through a catheter *(arrow).* The coil can be pushed with a guidewire, or injected.

(A, Courtesy Cook Group, Bloomington, IN. From Kaufman JA: Vascular interventions. In Kaufman JA, Lee MJ, editors: *Vascular and interventional radiology: the requisites,* ed 2, Philadelphia, 2014, Elsevier.)

Transcatheter Embolization

swells in the presence of blood, occluding the vessel (Fig. 27.73). Another newer permanent occlusion device is a vascular plug, which is deployed by manually unscrewing the device from the delivery wire when in the desired position within the vessel. The vascular plug is used for large vessel occlusion.

Fig. 27.74 shows a hypervascular uterine fibroid that was causing significant symptoms. Embolization of this uterine fibroid was successfully accomplished with total occlusion of the lesion. Embolization combined with arterial catheter directed infusion of chemotherapy drugs is known as *chemoembolization*. This is most commonly performed for treatment of primary and metastatic hepatic lesions. In recent years embolic spheres or *microspheres* have been designed to absorb therapeutic agents, such as chemotherapy drugs, to ensure a more controlled and sustained release of the drug.[10] *Radioembolization* is also used to treat hepatic lesions. This procedure uses radioactive microspheres to both cut off blood supply to the tumor and to destroy tumor tissue by emitting powerful, but short, penetrating, beta radiation.

Transcatheter embolization has also been used in the cerebral vasculature of the brain. Vascular lesions within the cerebral vasculature, such as aneurysms, AVMs, and tumors, can be managed using multiple embolic agents, PVA, or tissue adhesive. Microcatheters (2 or 3 Fr) are passed through a larger catheter, a coaxial system that is positioned in the cerebral vessels. The smaller catheter is manipulated into the appropriate cerebral vessel, and lesions such as an aneurysm and the embolic material are delivered through it until the appropriate embolization is achieved (Fig. 27.75).

Fig. 27.73 Coil coated with a hydrogel that swells when in contact with blood. (A) Coil as packaged. (B) Coil after hydration. The process requires approximately 20 minutes in the blood to complete.

(Courtesy MicroVention Inc., Tustin, CA. From Kaufman JA: Vascular interventions. In Kaufman JA, Lee MJ, editors: *Vascular and interventional radiology: the requisites*, ed 2, Philadelphia, 2014, Elsevier.)

Fig. 27.74 Hypervascular uterine fibroid. (A) Bilateral uterine artery injections using coaxial microcatheters, showing hypervascular uterine fibroid. (B) Bilateral iliac artery injections, postembolization, showing total occlusion of both uterine arteries *(arrows)*.

Fig. 27.75 Left vertebral artery injection. (A) Basilar tip aneurysm *(arrow)*. (B) Left vertebral artery injection postembolization with the use of Guglielmi detachable coils (GDCs).

Vena Cava Filter Placement

Vena cava filters are designed to trap venous emboli from migrating to the pulmonary arteries causing a pulmonary embolus (PE). Most commonly filters are placed in the IVC, although filters can also be placed in the superior vena cava (SVC) when necessary. A pulmonary embolus is a blood clot that forms as a thrombus and usually develops in the deep veins of the leg. When such a thrombus becomes dislodged and migrates, it is called an *embolus*. An embolus originating in the leg may migrate through the IVC and right side of the heart and finally lodge in the pulmonary arteries. A filter can be percutaneously placed in the IVC to trap such an embolus.

Lower limb vein thrombosis is not an indication for IVC filter placement. Normally, blood-thinning medications are administered to treat deep vein thrombosis.

When anticoagulant therapy is contraindicated because of bleeding or the risk for hemorrhage, filter placement may be indicated. Filter placement itself has associated risks, including thrombosis of the vein through which the filter is introduced and thrombosis of the vena cava. These risks normally are not life threatening, however. IVC filter placement is not a treatment for deep vein thrombosis of the leg but a therapy intended to reduce the chance of pulmonary embolism.

The idea of interrupting the pathway of an embolus is not a new one. Surgical interruption of the common femoral vein was first described in 1784, and surgical interruption of the IVC was described in 1868. These procedures and the partial surgical interruption procedures that evolved from them had a high rate of complications, not only owing to the surgical process but also owing to inadequate venous drainage from the lower limbs. Catheterization technology led to the development of detachable balloons for occluding the IVC, but that procedure also resulted in complications because of inadequate venous flow from the lower limbs.

The first true filter designed to trap emboli while maintaining vena cava patency was introduced in 1967 by Mobin-Uddin. It consisted of six metal struts joined at one end to form a conical shape that was covered by a perforated plastic canopy. The plastic canopy proved to be too occlusive, which is the reason that the Mobin-Uddin filter is no longer in use. Because of this filter's striking resemblance to an open umbrella, vena cava filters of all types for many years were referred to as "umbrella filters."

IVC filters are available in various shapes. All of these filters are initially compacted inside an introducer catheter delivery system and assume their functional shape as they are released (Fig. 27.76). The introducers are passed through sheaths ranging in size from 6 to 15 Fr.

Fig. 27.76 Examples of permanent inferior vena cava (IVC) filters. (A) Greenfield (Boston Scientific); (B) Simon Nitinol (Bard); (C) Bird's Nest (Cook); (D) Vena Tech (B. Braun Medical); (E) Vena Tech LP (B. Braun Medical); (F) TrapEase (Cordis Corporation). Optional IVC filters.

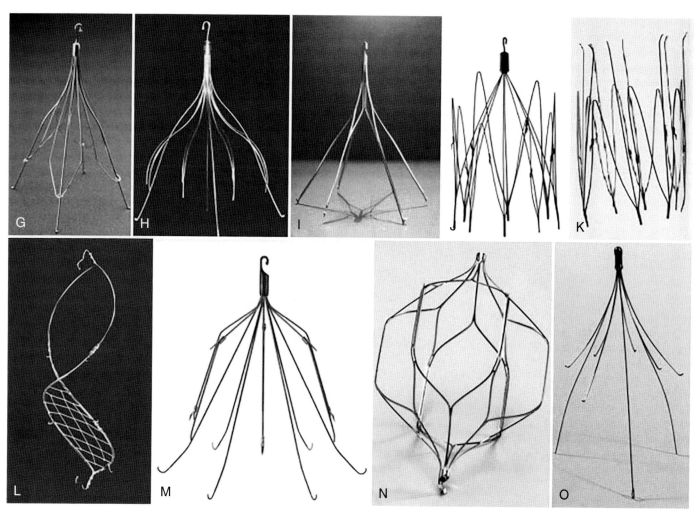

Fig. 27.76, cont'd (G) Gunther Tulip (Cook); (H) Celect (Cook); (I) Option (Argon Medical); (J) Convertible filter in closed position (B. Braun Medical); (K) Convertible filter with cap removed (B. Braun Medical); (L) Crux filter (Crux BioMedical); (M) Meridian (Bard); (N) OPTEASE (Cordis); (O) ALN (ALN Implants).

(From Kaufman JA: Inferior vena cava and tributaries. In Kaufman JA, Lee MJ, editors: *Vascular and interventional radiology: the requisites,* ed 2, Philadelphia, 2014, Elsevier.)

Most filters are designed as a conical shape to trap clots in the central lumen. They are designed to be placed in vena cava ranging up to 20 to 30 mm in diameter. Fig. 27.76 shows the currently available IVC filters. Several newer filters are designed to be retrievable within a specified time frame. These are known as optional filters as physicians have the option to remove the filter,

or leave the filter in permanently, depending on the risks and benefits to the patient. These retrievable filters have hooks, either at the top or bottom, that allow them to be grasped by a catheter snare device and be removed percutaneously (Fig. 27.77).

Regardless of whether the filter is permanent or temporary, the purpose is to prevent new onset of pulmonary embolus

by trapping venous emboli. These filters do not treat preexisting clots.

The filters are percutaneously inserted through a femoral, jugular, or antecubital vein, usually for placement in the IVC just inferior to the renal veins. Placement inferior to the renal veins is important to prevent renal vein thrombosis, which can occur if the vena cava is occluded

Fig. 27.77 The process of filter retrieval. (A) Initial cavogram confirming patency of the filter and inferior vena cava (IVC) (Gunther Tulip, Cook Medical). (B) The filter has been snared *(arrow)* and the sheath *(arrowhead)* advanced over the filter to constrain it. The sheath is advanced over the feet of the filter for safe removal. (C) Completion cavogram after filter removal showing a normal IVC.

(From Kaufman JA: Inferior vena cava and tributaries. In Kaufman JA, Lee MJ, editors: *Vascular and interventional radiology: the requisites*, ed 2, Philadelphia, 2014, Elsevier.)

superior to the level of the renal veins by a large thrombus in a filter. An inferior vena cavagram is performed using the modified Seldinger technique. The inferior vena cavagram defines the anatomy, including the level of the renal veins, determines the diameter of the vena cava, and rules out the presence of a thrombus (Fig. 27.78). Filter insertion from the jugular or antecubital approach may be indicated if a thrombus is present in the iliac veins and/or in the IVC.

The diameter of the vena cava may influence the choice of filter because each filter has a maximum diameter. The filter insertion site is dilated to accommodate the filter introducer. The filter remains sheathed until it reaches the desired level and is released from its introducer by the radiologist. The introducing system is then removed, and external compression is applied to the venotomy site until hemostasis is achieved. A postplacement image is obtained to document the location of the filter (Fig. 27.79).

Fig. 27.78 Inferior vena cavogram. Note reflux into renal veins *(white arrows)* and hepatic veins *(black arrows)*.

Fig. 27.79 Postplacement image showing Greenfield filter in place *(arrow)*.

Transjugular Intrahepatic Portosystemic Shunt

The *portal circulation* consists of blood from the digestive organs, which drains into the liver. The portal system consists of the splenic vein, the superior mesenteric vein, and the inferior mesenteric vein. The blood passes through the liver tissue and is returned to the IVC via the hepatic veins. Disease processes can increase the resistance of blood flow through the liver, elevating the blood pressure of the portal circulation—a condition known as *portal hypertension*. It may cause the blood to flow through collateral veins. Venous *varices* are the result and can be life threatening if they bleed. The creation of a portosystemic shunt can decrease portal hypertension and the associated variceal bleeding by allowing the portal venous circulation to bypass its normal course through the liver. The percutaneous intervention for creating an artificial low-pressure pathway between the portal and hepatic veins is called a *transjugular intrahepatic portosystemic shunt (TIPS)*.

Prior to a TIPS procedure ultrasonography is used to confirm patency of the portal venous system. Hepatic venography and portography are performed during a TIPS procedure to delineate anatomy. Transcatheter blood pressure measurements are often used to confirm the existence of a pressure gradient between the portal and hepatic veins.

The most common approach for a TIPS procedure is from a right internal jugular venous puncture site to the middle or right hepatic vein. A hepatic venogram may be obtained using contrast material or CO_2 or both. A special long needle is passed into the hepatic vein and advanced through the liver tissue into the portal vein. The needle is exchanged for an angioplasty balloon catheter, and the tract through the liver tissue is dilated. An angiographic catheter may be passed through the tract and advanced into the splenic vein for a splenoportal venogram. An intravascular stent is positioned across the tract to maintain its patency (Figs. 27.80 and 27.81). The tract and stent may be enlarged further with an angioplasty balloon catheter until the desired reduction in pressure gradient between the portal and hepatic veins is achieved. If large gastric or splenic varices persist after the shunt creation, embolization of these varices using coils, sclerosants, or glue may be performed. Once the shunt is created, portal pressures are reduced, and flow through the varices diverted, the sheath is removed from the internal jugular vein, and external pressure is applied until hemostasis at the venotomy occurs.

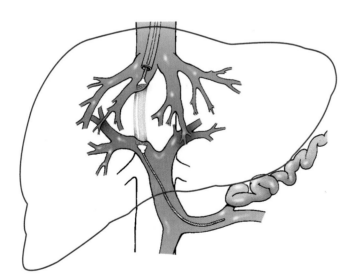

Fig. 27.80 Intravascular stent placement in a TIPS procedure.

Fig. 27.81 TIPS procedure. (A) Stent placement. (B) Stent with contrast. (C) Initial contrast agent injection.

Pharmacological Thrombolysis and Mechanical Thrombectomy

When an angiogram shows thrombus (blood clot) within a vessel, interventional catheters and devices can be used to remove the thrombus and restore blood flow in both arterial and venous systems. These methods are effective in restoring arterial blood flow quickly in acute emergent situations such as large vessel ischemic stroke, limb-threatening ischemia, and in acute myocardial infarction (MI), discussed later in this chapter. Pharmacological thrombolysis uses blood clot–dissolving medications that are infused through an angiographic catheter positioned against the thrombus. Special infusion catheters with side holes are manipulated directly into the clot. Periodic repeat *angiograms* evaluate the progress of *lysis* (dissolution). The catheter may have to be advanced under fluoroscopic control to keep it against or in the clot as lysis progresses. Mechanical thrombectomy uses catheters and/or devices to physically remove the clot. Mechanisms for physical thrombus removal include aspiration, maceration, and fragmentation. Fig. 27.82 demonstrates mechanical thrombectomy in the cerebral arteries using specialized aspiration catheters and a stent retriever device to restore blood flow to brain tissue.

Fig. 27.82 Stroke intervention with a thrombus retrieval device (the Solitaire retrievable stent, Medtronic, Minneapolis, MN). (A) Carotid arteriogram showing abrupt occlusion in right internal carotid artery *(arrow)*. (B) Arteriogram after first pass with stent retriever showing right anterior cerebral is now open *(arrowhead)*. (C) Completion arteriogram showing reperfusion in the right anterior and middle cerebral arteries. (D) The thrombus *(arrow)* removed, trapped in the stent retriever *(arrowhead)*.

(From Kaufman JA, Nesbit GM: Carotid and vertebral arteries. In Kaufman JA, Lee MJ, editors: *Vascular and interventional radiology: the requisites*, ed 2, Philadelphia, 2014, Elsevier.)

Other Procedures

The insertion of vascular access catheters, such as central lines, hemodialysis catheters, tunneled catheters for long-term use, and implantable vascular access devices, such as port-a-caths used for chemotherapy infusion, are often performed in interventional radiology.

Interventional devices can be used to remove foreign bodies, such as catheter fragments or broken guidewires, percutaneously from the vasculature. Various snares can be used for this purpose. A snare catheter introduced using the Seldinger technique is manipulated under fluoroscopic control to grasp the foreign body. The snare and foreign body are then withdrawn as a unit.

In addition to vascular interventional procedures, there are many nonvascular interventional procedures that are performed in interventional radiology. Technologists are expected to have comprehensive knowledge of anatomy and pathophysiology of the gastrointestinal, biliary, urinary systems, and to demonstrate understanding of interventional procedures such as needle biopsy, percutaneous drainage, and stent placement.

Radiology: Present and Future

In recent years the role of catheter-directed angiography as a diagnostic tool has diminished as noninvasive diagnostic imaging techniques have evolved. The emphasis has shifted toward providing minimally invasive catheter-directed interventional procedures. New catheters, guidewires, and medical devices, along with safer, less invasive procedures, are constantly being introduced into this field. These procedures are highly technical, and a team approach is crucial.[11] Although these procedures are most often performed in interventional radiology by radiologists, other medical specialists, such as vascular surgeons, interventional cardiologists, and neurointerventionists may utilize the equipment and staff in interventional radiology to perform these procedures themselves. The cardiovascular and interventional technologist plays an active role on this multidisciplinary interventional team (Fig. 27.83).

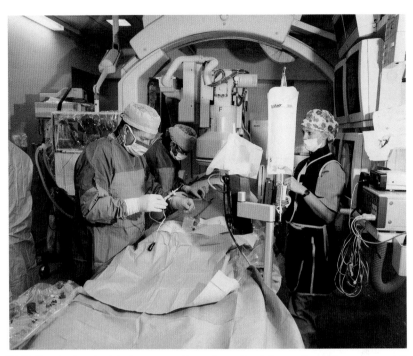

Fig. 27.83 The technologist plays an active role on the interventional team by assisting the interventionalist *(left)* or by circulating within the angiography suite *(right)*.

Cardiac catheterization is a comprehensive term used to describe a minor surgical procedure involving the introduction of specialized catheters into the heart and surrounding vasculature for the purpose of diagnostic evaluation and intervention associated with various cardiovascular-related disorders in children and adults. Cardiac catheterization is classified as either a diagnostic or an interventional procedure. The primary purpose of diagnostic procedures is to collect data necessary to evaluate the patient's condition. Cardiac interventional procedures involve the application of therapeutic measures through catheter-based systems or other mechanical means to treat disorders of the vascular and conduction systems within the heart.

GENERAL INDICATIONS

Cardiac catheterization is performed to identify the anatomic and physiologic condition of the heart. The data gathered during catheterization provide the physician with information to develop management strategies for patients who have cardiovascular disorders. *Coronary angiography* is currently the most defini-tive procedure for visualizing the coronary anatomy. The anatomic information gained from this procedure may include the presence and extent of obstructive coronary artery disease, thrombus formation, coronary artery collateral flow, coronary anomalies, aneurysms, and spasm. Coronary artery size can also be determined.

Coronary artery disease is the most common disorder necessitating catheterization of the adult heart. This disease is caused primarily by the accumulation of fatty intracoronary *atheromatous* plaque, which leads to *stenosis* and *occlusion* of the coronary arteries. Coronary artery disease is symptomatically characterized by chest pain (angina pectoris) or a heart attack (MI). Treatment of coronary artery disease includes medical, surgical, and catheter-directed interventions.

Diagnostic cardiac catheterization of an adult patient with coronary artery disease is conducted to assess the appropriateness and feasibility of various therapeutic options. Cardiac catheterization is performed before open-heart surgery to provide *hemodynamic* and *angiographic* data to document the presence and severity of disease. In selected circumstances, postoperative catheterization is performed to assess the results of surgery. An interventional procedure (e.g., PTCA, intracoronary stent, or atherectomy) may be indicated for the relief of arteriosclerotic coronary artery stenosis.

Diagnostic studies of the adult heart also aid in evaluating a patient who has confusing or obscure symptoms (e.g., chest pain of undetermined cause). These studies are also used to assess diseases of the heart not requiring surgical intervention, such as certain cardiomyopathies.

In children, diagnostic heart catheterization is employed to evaluate congenital and valvular disease, disorders of the cardiac conduction system, and selected cardiomyopathies. Interventional techniques are also performed in children, primarily to alleviate symptoms associated with certain congenital heart defects.

The indications for cardiac catheterization as established by a special task force to the American College of Cardiology and the American Heart Association (ACC/AHA) are summarized in Table 27.2. Commonly performed procedures based on diagnosis are also presented. The ACC/AHA[11] has classified the indications

TABLE 27.2

Indications for cardiac catheterization

Indications	Procedures
1. Suspected or known coronary artery disease	
a. New-onset angina	LV, COR
b. Unstable angina	LV, COR
c. Evaluation before a major surgical procedure	LV, COR
d. Silent ischemia	LV, COR, ERGO
e. Positive ETT	LV, COR, ERGO
f. Atypical chest pain or coronary artery spasm	LV, COR, ERGO
2. Myocardial infarction	
a. Unstable angina postinfarction	LV, COR
b. Failed thrombolysis	LV, COR, RH
c. Shock	LV, COR, RH
d. Mechanical complications (ventricular septal defect)	LV, COR, RH (rupture of wall or papillary muscle)
3. Sudden cardiovascular death	LV, COR, R + L
4. Valvular heart disease	LV, COR, R + L, AO
5. Congenital heart disease (before anticipated corrective surgery)	LV, COR, R + L, AO
6. Aortic dissection	AO, COR
7. Pericardial constriction or tamponade	LV, COR, R + L
8. Cardiomyopathy	LV, COR, R + L, BX
9. Initial and follow-up assessment for heart transplant	LV, COR, R + L, BX

AO, Aortography; *BX,* endomyocardial biopsy; *COR,* coronary angiography; *ERGO,* ergonovine provocation of coronary spasm; *ETT,* exercise tolerance test; *LV,* left ventriculography; *R + L,* right and left heart hemodynamics; *RH,* right heart oxygen saturations and hemodynamics (e.g., placement of Swan-Ganz catheter).
From Kern MJ: *The cardiac catheterization handbook,* ed 4, St Louis, 2003, Mosby.

and appropriateness for coronary angiography by placing the previously discussed disease categories into three classifications, as follows:

Class 1: Conditions for which there is general agreement that coronary angiography is justified

Class 2: Conditions for which coronary angiography is frequently performed, but for which a divergence of opinion exists with respect to its justification in terms of value and appropriateness

Class 3: Conditions for which coronary angiography ordinarily is not justified

Other procedures that may be performed concurrently with coronary angiography are listed in Table 27.3. Some of these procedures are discussed later in the text.

TABLE 27.3
Procedures that may accompany coronary angiography

Procedures	Comment
1. Central venous access (femoral, internal jugular, subclavian)	Used as IV access for emergency medications or fluids, temporary pacemaker (pacemaker not mandatory for coronary angiography)
2. Hemodynamic assessment	
a. Left heart pressures (aorta, left ventricle)	Routine for all studies
b. Right and left heart combined pressures	Not routine for coronary artery disease; mandatory for valvular heart disease; routine for CHF, right ventricular dysfunction, pericardial diseases, cardiomyopathy, intracardiac shunts, congenital abnormalities
3. Left ventricular angiography	Routine for all studies; may be excluded with high-risk patients, left main coronary or aortic stenosis, severe CHF
4. Internal mammary selective angiography	Not routine unless used as coronary bypass conduit
5. Pharmacologic studies	
a. Ergonovine	Routine for coronary vasospasm
b. IC/IV/sublingual nitroglycerin	Optionally routine for all studies
6. Aortography	Routine for aortic insufficiency, aortic dissection, aortic aneurysm, with or without aortic stenosis; routine to locate bypass grafts not visualized by selective angiography
7. Digital subtraction angiography	Not routine for coronary angiography; excellent for peripheral vascular disease
8. Cardiac pacing and electrophysiologic studies	Arrhythmia evaluation
9. Interventional and special techniques	Intracoronary flow-pressure for lesion assessment
	Coronary angioplasty (PTCA)
	Myocardial biopsy
	Transseptal or direct left ventricular puncture
	Balloon catheter valvuloplasty
	Conduction tract catheter ablation
10. Arterial closure devices	Available for patients with conditions prone to puncture site bleeding

CHF, Congestive heart failure.
From Kern MJ: *The cardiac catheterization handbook*, ed 4, St Louis, 2003, Mosby.

CONTRAINDICATIONS, COMPLICATIONS, AND ASSOCIATED RISKS

Cardiac catheterization has associated inherent risk factors. Many physicians agree that the only absolute contraindications to this procedure are the refusal of the procedure by a mentally competent person and the lack of adequate equipment or catheterization facilities.

There are few contraindications for cardiac catheterization when the appropriateness of the procedure is based on the benefit-risk ratio. Relative contraindications according to the guidelines of the ACC/AHA[11] include the following:

- Active gastrointestinal bleeding
- Acute or chronic renal failure
- Recent stroke
- Fever from infection or the presence of an active infection
- Severe electrolyte imbalance
- Severe anemia
- Short life expectancy because of other illness
- Digitalis intoxication
- Patient refusal of therapeutic treatment such as PTCA or bypass surgery
- Severe uncontrolled hypertension
- Coagulopathy and bleeding disorders

- Acute pulmonary edema
- Uncontrolled ventricular arrhythmias
- Aortic valve endocarditis
- Previous anaphylactic reaction to contrast media

Some of these conditions may be temporary, or they may be treated and reversed before cardiac catheterization is attempted. Cardiac catheterization may proceed if any of the above-listed conditions exist in a patient who is deemed to be unstable from a suspected cardiac cause.

As with any invasive procedure, complications can be expected during cardiac catheterization. The Society for Cardiac Angiography and Interventions (SCA&I) reviewed the catheterizations in more than 300,000 patients from three different time periods and found the major complication rate for the entire group was less than 2%. The risks associated with cardiac catheterization have decreased since the early days of the procedure. As the severity of the patient's disease increases, however, so do the risks associated with the procedure.

The risks of cardiac catheterization vary according to the type of procedure and the status of the patient undergoing the procedure. Significantly influencing the outcome of the procedure is the stability of the patient's condition before the procedure. Patients presenting with left main coronary stenosis have a greater than twofold higher risk of complications from coronary angiography than patients who have no left main coronary stenosis. The SCA&I database identified the main predictors of major complications after cardiac catheterization and determined that the following increased the risk of complications:[12]

- Moribund patient (patient with poor response to life-threatening condition)
- Cardiogenic shock
- Acute MI (within 24 hours)
- Renal insufficiency
- Cardiomyopathy

Risk variables of less significance include the anatomy to be studied, type of catheter and approach used, history of drug allergy, presence of basic cardiovascular disease or noncardiac disease such as asthma or diabetes, hemodynamic status, and age or other patient characteristics. The expected benefits of cardiac catheterization must be weighed against the associated risks when determining whether to perform the procedure.

SUPPLIES AND EQUIPMENT

Cardiovascular equipment consists of supplies and equipment needed to perform the procedure. In addition to the equipment mentioned previously for angiographic procedures, there are variations in catheter design to accommodate the coronary arteries. The guidewires used also have several variations in length, stiffness, and coatings depending on the tortuosity of the aorta and iliac arteries leading to the heart. Because of the complexity and types of procedures performed in a cardiac catheterization laboratory, only a few of the main component items are discussed.

Catheters

The catheters used for left heart cardiac catheterization are similar to the angiographic catheters previously described except cardiac catheters are specifically shaped for the cardiac vasculature (Fig. 27.84). Left heart catheterization involves accessing the arterial system to locate the coronary arteries and left side of the heart. Right heart catheterizations involve accessing the venous system to locate the right side of the heart and the pulmonary arteries. Specialized catheters are used for right heart catheterization procedures. In contrast to angiographic catheters, the main purpose of which is to serve as a conduit for contrast media, right heart catheters are typically flow-directed catheters that use an inflated balloon on the tip of the catheter to ease passage through the various chambers of the heart. Various types of flow-directed catheters are capable of performing more tasks than the standard angiographic catheter. Depending on the type of procedure to be performed, the cardiologist determines which catheter(s) to use.

The catheter (or catheters) placed in a patient's vasculature can function as a fluid-filled column for hemodynamic data or as a conduit for contrast media, thrombolytic agents, and mechanical devices. Blood samples can be drawn directly from selected cardiac chambers for the purpose of oximetry or other laboratory analysis. To perform these and other tasks, three or four valves (*stopcocks*) are combined to form a *manifold*, which is attached to the proximal end of the catheter (Fig. 27.85). Using a manifold allows such functions as drawing blood samples, administering medications, and recording blood pressures without disconnecting from the catheter.

Contrast media

Injection of contrast media is essential for angiographic visualization of the cardiac anatomy. Several iodinated radiographic contrast media are approved for intravascular, intracardiac, and intracoronary use in adults and children. Transient (temporary) ECG changes during and immediately after the injection of contrast media are common.

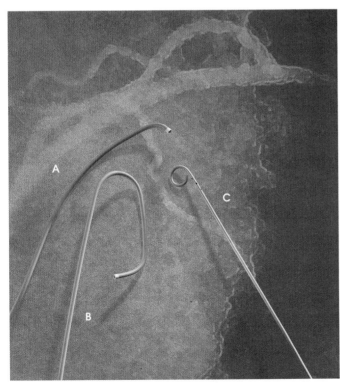

Fig. 27.84 Catheters used during cardiac catheterization. (A) Judkins right. (B) Judkins left. (C) Pigtail.

(Courtesy Cordis Corp., Miami, FL.)

Fig. 27.85 Disposable three-valve Compensator Morse manifold, with a Selector catheter (A), rotating adapter (B), pressure transducer (C), and angiographic control syringe (D).

(Courtesy SCHNEIDER/NAMIC, Glens Falls, NY.)

Pressure injector

The pressure injector for the administration of radiographic contrast media (Fig. 27.86) is also used during cardiac catheterization. During cardiac catheterization, the pressure injector is used to inject a large amount (25 to 50 mL) of contrast material into either the right or the left ventricle (the main pumping chambers of the heart), the aortic root, or the pulmonary vessels. Because the coronary arteries are of small caliber and of low flow rate, administration of contrast media into these structures generally does not require a high-pressure injector. Instead, most physicians opt for manual injection using an angiographic control syringe (see Fig. 27.85).

IMAGING

The imaging equipment found in the cardiac catheterization laboratory is essentially the same as the equipment found in the vascular angiography suite. The catheterization laboratory requires a system capable of producing fluoroscopic images with the greatest amount of recorded detail available. Maximum resolution from the optical system is crucial because of the small size of the cardiac anatomy, which must be imaged while in motion. The imaging used for cardiac studies is typically 15 to 30 frames per second compared with 2 to 6 frames per second used for peripheral imaging. The motion of the heart beating requires this increased frame rate to visualize these small arteries properly. The imaging equipment necessary to produce high-resolution imaging is described in the previous section on DSA procedures.

Patient positioning

Procedures such as selective coronary arteriography and certain pediatric catheterizations require imaging equipment to be positioned to reduce the superimposition created by the cardiac vasculature. Patients are placed on the examination table in the supine position. Moving the patient during catheterization is undesirable, particularly when catheters have been carefully positioned to show specific anatomic structures or to record certain data.

Adult and pediatric coronary anatomy has normal and pathologic variations. Projections for each type of catheterization procedure cannot be specified. Instead, each patient's anatomy must be fluoroscopically evaluated to ascertain the optimal degree of rotation and cranial or caudal angulation necessary to visualize each structure of interest.

Physiologic equipment

The physiologic monitor is essential to cardiac catheterization procedures. It is used to monitor and record vital patient functions, including electrical activity (ECG)[c] within the heart and blood pressure (hemodynamic) within the various intracardiac chambers (Fig. 27.87). The patient's ECG and hemodynamic pressures are continuously displayed throughout the various types of procedures. (Selective samplings of ECG and hemodynamic pressures are recorded for permanent documentation.)

---

[c]Interpretation of ECG is beyond the scope of this chapter.

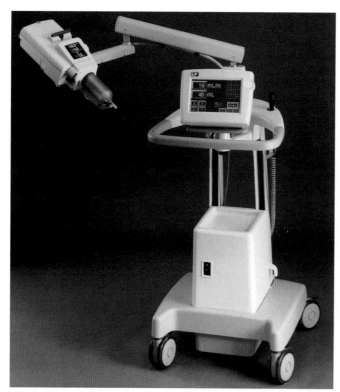

Fig. 27.86 The Angiomat (ILLUMENA) high-pressure injector for radiographic contrast media.

(Courtesy Liebel-Flarsheim, a product of Mallinckrodt, Inc., Cincinnati, OH.)

Fig. 27.87 Computer-based physiologic monitor used to monitor patient ECG and hemodynamic pressures during cardiac catheterization.

(Courtesy GE Medical Systems.)

For the collection of hemodynamic data during catheterization, the physiologic recorder (receiving information in electrical form) must be connected to the catheter (carrying information as physical fluid pressure). Devices called *pressure transducers* are interfaced between the manifold and the physiologic recorder to convert fluid (blood) pressure into an electrical signal.

For a standard cardiac catheterization procedure, four channels of the physiologic recorder are usually prepared: two for ECG recordings and two for pressure recordings. A physiologic recorder can have as many as 32 *channels*.

OTHER EQUIPMENT

Because of the nature of the patient's condition, the inherent risks of cardiac catheterization, and the types of procedures performed, each catheterization room should have the following equipment available:

- A fully equipped emergency cart. The cart typically contains emergency medications, cardiopulmonary resuscitation equipment, intubation equipment, and other related supplies.
- Oxygen and suction.
- Whole-blood oximeters used to determine the oxygen saturation of the blood samples obtained during adult and pediatric catheterizations (Fig. 27.88).
- Defibrillator, used to treat life-threatening arrhythmias. Ideally, the defibrillator would also have external pacemaking capabilities. Some laboratories have two defibrillators available in case one fails.
- Temporary pacemaker to treat potential asystole or symptomatic bradycardia.
- Pulse oximeter to monitor and assess level of oxygenation noninvasively during sedation.
- Noninvasive blood pressure monitoring capabilities.
- Equipment to perform cardiac output studies.
- Intra-aortic balloon pump used to increase myocardial perfusion and cardiac output during interventional procedures.
- Activated clotting time (ACT) used to monitor treatment of high-dose heparin during procedures.

In addition to the basic coronary angiogram and left and right heart studies, many effective tools are available to diagnose and treat coronary artery disease (Table 27.4).

Fig. 27.88 Oximeter used to measure oxygen saturation in blood.

TABLE 27.4

Tools for diagnosis and treatment of coronary artery disease

Equipment	Use	Diagnostic or therapeutic
Pressure wire	Measures blood flow across lesion to determine severity of stenosis	Diagnostic
IVUS	Internal vessel visualization of stenosis, plaque, stent position	Diagnostic
OCT (optical coherence tomography)	Laser light to image the inside of the vessel wall	Diagnostic
Rotablator	Rotational atherectomy of intraluminal plaque or calcium	Therapeutic
Rheolytic thrombectomy	High-velocity saline spray for thrombectomy	Therapeutic
The Crosser	Study device to chronic total occlusions	Therapeutic

PRECATHETERIZATION CARE

Before the catheterization is performed, the procedure is explained, and informed consent is obtained. Testing before catheterization normally includes the following:

- Patient history
- Physical examination
- Chest x-ray examination
- Blood work
- ECG
- Echocardiogram
- Exercise stress test
- Nuclear medicine cardiac perfusion studies

Various medications are frequently administered for sedation and control of nausea. Patients brought to the catheterization laboratory typically are not allowed anything to eat or drink for 4 to 6 hours before the procedure or after midnight. During all catheterizations, a protocol (or detailed record) of the procedure is maintained.

CATHETER INTRODUCTION

After the patient has been transported to the catheterization laboratory, ECG, non-invasive blood pressure monitoring, and *pulse oximetry* are initiated. The appropriate site for catheter introduction must be prepared using aseptic technique to minimize the risk of subsequent infection. The area of the body to be entered is shaved, and an antiseptic solution is applied. Numerous sites can be used for catheter introduction. The specific sites vary according to the age and body habitus of the patient, the preference of the cardiologist, and the procedure attempted. The most frequent sites used for catheterization are the femoral and radial area. The brachial, axillary, jugular (neck), and subclavian (chest) areas may also be chosen.

For catheterization of the artery or vein, the percutaneous approach is employed (see the modified Seldinger technique, which is described and illustrated in Fig. 27.17). On rare occasions, if the percutaneous approach cannot be used, a cutdown technique is employed. This technique requires that a small incision be made in the skin to allow for direct visualization of the artery or vein that the physician wants to catheterize. The skin is aseptically prepared and infiltrated with local anesthetic, and the vessel or vessels are bluntly dissected and exposed. After an opening is created in the desired vessel (arteriotomy or venotomy), the catheter is introduced and advanced toward the heart. Cutdown procedures are performed in the right antecubital fossa to access the basilic vein or brachial artery when this method is used for vascular access.

Diagnostic Cardiac Procedures

LEFT HEART

Catheterization of the left side of the heart is a widely performed basic diagnostic cardiac study. The catheter may be introduced through the radial, brachial, or femoral artery and advanced over a guidewire to the ascending aorta. When in the ascending aorta, the guidewire is removed, and the catheter is aspirated and flushed to prevent migration of any air bubbles.

A normal aortic valve prevents backward flow of contrast media into the left ventricle during injection, whereas an insufficient valve does not (Fig. 27.89). Angiography of the left ventricle is performed in nearly all catheterization studies of the left side of the heart (Fig. 27.90). Left ventriculography provides information about valvular competence, interventricular septal integrity, and the efficiency of the pumping action of the left ventricle (ejection fraction). Mitral regurgitation is another example of valvular incompetence, and angiographically it is seen as the backward flow of contrast media from the left ventricle into the left atrium or pulmonary veins (Fig. 27.91). Computer *planimetry* software calculates how

Fig. 27.89 Aortic root injection showing aortic insufficiency with contrast agent flowing back into left ventricle *(arrowheads)*.

Fig. 27.90 Normal left ventriculogram during diastole.

Fig. 27.91 Left ventriculogram showing mitral valve regurgitation.

well the ventricle functions (Fig. 27.92). After left ventriculography, the presence of aortic valve stenosis is determined as the blood pressure measurements are repeated while the catheter is withdrawn across the aortic valve. Normal flow of blood through the aortic valve allows the systolic pressure in the left ventricle to match the systolic pressure in the aorta. When the systolic blood pressure in the left ventricle is greater than the systolic blood pressure in the aorta, aortic stenosis is present.

SELECTIVE CORONARY ANGIOGRAPHY

Selective angiography of the right coronary artery and left coronary artery is performed, with different projections used for each coronary artery to prevent super-imposition with overlapping structures. Coronary angiography allows the extent of intracoronary stenosis to be evaluated (Figs. 27.93 and 27.94).

Because of the complexity of the anatomy involved, the variations in patient body habitus, and the presence of anomalies, a comprehensive guide for angiographic projections is difficult to establish. Projections commonly used during coronary angiography are listed in Table 27.5. The cardiologist determines the projections that best show the artery of interest. Coronary arteriograms are obtained in nearly all catheterizations of the left side of the heart.

RIGHT HEART

Catheterization of the right side of the heart is another commonly performed procedure. During right heart catheterization, a catheter is inserted into the femoral, antecubital fossa, internal jugular, or subclavian vein, and it is advanced to the vena cava, into the right atrium, across the tricuspid valve, to the right ventricle, and through the pulmonary valve to the pulmonary artery, until it is wedged distally in the pulmonary artery. Pressure measurements and oximetry are performed in each of the heart chambers as the catheter is advanced. The pressure measurements are used to determine the presence of disorders such as valvular heart disease, congestive heart failure, pulmonary hypertension, and certain cardiomyopathies. The oximetry data is used to determine the presence of an intracardiac shunt. DSA is performed as appropriate.

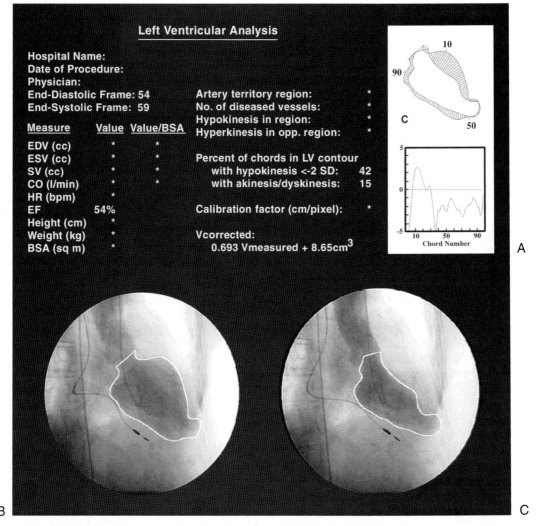

Fig. 27.92 Computerized planimetry for evaluation of left ventricular ejection fraction. (A) Diastolic phase of contraction of the heart. (B) Systolic phase of contraction of the heart. (C) Digital representation of when the diastolic and systolic phases of contraction are superimposed.

Fig. 27.93 Normal right coronary artery.

Fig. 27.94 Normal left coronary artery.

TABLE 27.5

Common angiographic angles for specific coronary arteries

Coronary artery	Vessel segment	Projections
Left coronary artery	Left main	PA or RAO 5–15 degrees
	Left anterior descending	LAO 30–40 degrees, cranial 20–40 degrees
		RAO 5–15 degrees, cranial 15–45 degrees
		RAO 20–40 degrees, caudal 15–30 degrees
		RAO 30–50 degrees
		Lateral
	Circumflex	RAO 20–40 degrees, caudal 15–30 degrees
		LAO 40–55 degrees, caudal 15–30 degrees
		LAO 40–60 degrees
Right coronary artery	Middle right	LAO 20–40 degrees
		RAO 20–40 degrees
	Posterior descending	LAO 5–30 degrees, cranial 15–30 degrees

Exercise hemodynamics are often required in the evaluation of valvular heart disease when symptoms of fatigue and dyspnea are present. In such cases, simultaneous catheterization and pressure measurements of the right and left heart are performed at rest and during peak exercise. Exercise often consists of pedaling a stationary bicycle ergometer that is placed on top of the examination table. During simultaneous catheterization, a catheter is placed in a vein (femoral or basilic) and an artery (femoral or brachial).

ENDOMYOCARDIAL BIOPSY

Endomyocardial biopsy is performed to provide a tissue sample for direct pathologic evaluation of cardiac muscle. A special biopsy catheter with a bioptome tip (Fig. 27.95) is advanced under fluoroscopic control from either the jugular or the femoral vein to the right ventricle (Fig. 27.96). After the bioptome is advanced into the ventricle, the jaws of the device are opened, and the catheter is advanced to the ventricular septum. After the bioptome is in contact with the septum, its jaws are closed, and a gentle tugging motion is applied to retrieve the tissue sample. Several biopsy specimens are acquired in this manner. The specimens are immediately fixed in either glutaraldehyde or buffered formalin before being sent for pathologic evaluation. Endomyocardial biopsy is frequently used to monitor cardiac transplantation patients for early signs of tissue rejection and to differentiate between various types of cardiomyopathies.

Fig. 27.95 (A) Standard biopsy catheters. (B) Bioptome catheter tip used for myocardial biopsy. The jaws on the tip close and take a "bite" from the inside of the heart muscle.

(Courtesy Cordis Corp., Miami, FL.)

Fig. 27.96 Bioptome tip in the right ventricular apex points toward the ventricular septum.

Interventional Cardiac Procedures

Because of the risks associated with mechanical interventions of the vascular system, open-heart surgical facilities must be immediately available. Coronary occlusion is a major complication requiring emergency surgery in patients undergoing catheter-based mechanical interventions.

Interventional pharmacologic procedures in adults consist of the therapeutic administration of medications that may be given before the patient reaches the cardiac catheterization laboratory. A thrombolytic agent can be used in the early hours of an acute MI in an effort to modify its course. Estimates indicate that thrombotic coronary artery occlusion is present in 75% to 85% of patients with acute MI. If reperfusion of the ischemic myocardium is effective, scarring is reduced. Reperfusion in the early stages of MI offers greater potential for heart muscle salvage. ST segment elevation MI is determined from a 12-lead ECG performed in the field or in the emergency department. These patients are the most critical and typically have a complete or almost complete blockage of a coronary artery. Rapid reperfusion to the heart muscle must be performed to minimize damage.

ANGIOPLASTY AND STENT PLACEMENT

Interventional cardiac catheterization techniques requiring special-purpose catheters have expanded significantly since the late 1970s. PTCA is a technique that employs balloon dilation of a coronary artery stenosis to increase blood flow to the heart muscle. Gruentzig performed the first successful PTCA in 1977.

During PTCA, a specially designed guiding catheter is placed into the orifice of the stenotic coronary artery. (Fig. 27.97). A steerable guidewire is inserted into the balloon catheter and advanced within the guiding catheter (Fig. 27.98). The guidewire is advanced across the stenotic area; it serves as a support platform so that the balloon catheter can be advanced and centered across the stenosis. Controlled and precise inflation of the balloon fractures and compresses the fatty deposits into the muscular wall of the artery. This compression, in conjunction with the stretching of the external vessel diameter, is necessary for successful angioplasty. The balloon is deflated to allow rapid reperfusion of blood to the heart muscle. The inflation procedure, followed by arteriography, may be repeated several times until a satisfactory degree of patency is observed (Fig. 27.99). The

limiting factor of PTCA is restenosis, which occurs in approximately 30% to 50% of patients who undergo the procedure. Restenosis of the coronary artery after revascularization is the major factor in failed long-term outcomes. Due to this high restenosis rate, balloon-expandable coronary stent placement, rather than PTCA alone, is now commonly performed. There are several different stent designs. Drug-coated or drug-eluting stents were designed to reduce or inhibit restenosis that occurs after a revascularization procedure. Drugs are chemically bound or coated on a stent. The drug is released in small amounts over time to inhibit restenosis. The various drugs reduce restenosis by limiting the proliferation of smooth muscle cells or reducing the rate at which this occurs. The prevention of restenosis after revascularization remains to be proven.

Bare metal stents are used along with or independently of drug-eluting stents. Patient age, cost, and disease are the determining factors. The procedure is similar to PTCA and is performed in the same manner except that a metallic stent is mounted on the angioplasty balloon (Fig. 27.100). For optimal stent deployment, the stent is centered across the entire length of the stenosis. Deployment of the stent

Fig. 27.97 Stenotic coronary artery before PTCA. *Arrow* indicates the stenotic area, estimated at 95%, with minimum blood flow distal to the lesion.

Fig. 27.98 Catheter system for PTCA. The three sections of the system are the outer guiding catheter *(right)*, central balloon catheter *(middle)*, and internal steerable guidewire *(left)*.

(Courtesy Cordis Corp., Miami, FL.)

Fig. 27.99 Coronary arteriogram after PTCA in the same patient as in Fig. 27.92. Blood flow is estimated to be 100%.

Fig. 27.100 Balloon expandable intracoronary stent. (A) Before stent balloon inflation. (B) After stent balloon inflation.

is achieved with the inflation and deflation of the angioplasty balloon. After the stent is deployed, the angioplasty balloon is removed, and a high-pressure balloon is advanced within the stent. Inflation of the high-pressure balloon is performed to embed the metallic struts of the stent in the walls of the artery. Restenosis rates are lower in patients receiving intracoronary stents than in patients who undergo conventional angioplasty. PTCA and stent interventions constitute the bulk of the coronary interventions being performed at the present time. Of major concern are dissection at the proximal and distal ends of the stent and complete apposition of the stent against the vessel wall.

ATHERECTOMY

Atherectomy devices are used in the treatment of coronary artery disease. In contrast to angioplasty balloons, atherectomy devices remove the fatty deposit or thrombus material from within the artery (Fig. 27.101).

A device called Rotablator has been indicated in the use of atherosclerotic coronary artery disease. Commonly referred to as percutaneous transluminal coronary rotational atherectomy (PTCRA), this procedure can be used in conjunction with PTCA or stenting. The tip of the catheter (1.25 to 2.5 mm in diameter) resembles a football and is embedded with microscopic diamond particles on the front half and is rotated on a special torque guidewire between 160,000 rpm and 200,000 rpm (Figs. 27.102 and 27.103).

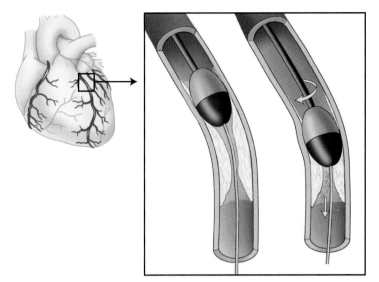

Fig. 27.101 Coronary atherectomy device.

Fig. 27.102 Rotablator rotational atherectomy catheter with advancer unit. *Insert* shows football-shaped burr.

(Courtesy Boston Scientific.)

Fig. 27.103 Atherectomy catheter burr.

(Courtesy Boston Scientific.)

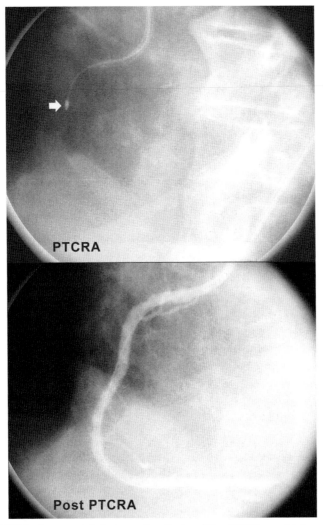

Fig. 27.104 PTCRA. *Arrow* points to burr of catheter. After PTCRA, a widely patent right coronary artery is shown.

Fig. 27.105 IVUS unit. Shown here are the keyboard and monitor.

(Courtesy Volcano.)

Standard angioplasty catheter positioning techniques are used to position a guidewire distal to the targeted lesion. A rotational atherectomy burr size is selected and advanced over the special torque guidewire just proximal to the lesion. At this point, the burr is activated, and the plaque is pulverized and reduced to the size of a blood cell. The pulverized plaque is removed by the reticuloendothelial system. After an adequate amount of plaque is cleared, standard PTCA or stenting techniques are employed to maintain artery patency (Fig. 27.104). PTCRA has proven to be beneficial in the treatment of highly calcified lesions and in-stent restenosis compared with PTCA alone.

INTRAVASCULAR ULTRASOUND

Although coronary angiography remains the gold standard for the diagnosis of coronary artery disease, *intravascular ultrasound* (IVUS) offers further diagnostic and interventional information that cannot be appreciated by angiography alone. IVUS allows a full 360-degree circumference visualization of the vessel wall, permits information regarding vascular pathology and longitudinal and volumetric measurements, and facilitates guidance of catheter-based interventions. The intervention-associated potential of IVUS is the ability to optimize the type and size of device being used and to determine proper apposition of the stent after deployment against the artery wall.

Components consist of the ultrasound unit, recording device (data can be stored on the hard drive, printed on CD-ROM, networked to electronic medical record, or backed up to storage device), printer, transducer, pullback device, and catheter (Fig. 27.105). The intravascular catheters employ 20- to 40-MHz silicon piezoelectric crystals and range in size from 5 Fr on the proximal end of the catheter to 2.9 Fr at the distal end. During the procedure, the IVUS catheter is advanced over the guidewire that was previously placed within the artery being imaged. The IVUS catheter is advanced distal to the targeted lesion, at which time the transducer and recording device are turned on. Slowly, the catheter is withdrawn using the pullback device to maintain a consistent withdrawal of the catheter and to help ascertain the length of the targeted lesion. Documentation of IVUS catheter position can be obtained with angiography. The images are stored on the hard drive of the IVUS system and can be retrieved for the cardiologist to review, take measurements, and print (Figs. 27.106 and 27.107).

At present, IVUS remains an integral part of coronary interventions being performed. With advances in stent designs, brachytherapy, local drug delivery, and future technologies, IVUS will remain a vital source for information in improving the outcomes of percutaneous coronary interventions. The clinical use of IVUS imaging and other improved computerized image enhancements should allow for more precise data collection and more tailored methods of determining the interventional method to use in treating coronary artery disease. The newest diagnostic tool available to visualize intravascular structures is optical coherence tomography (OCT). This technology uses infrared laser light to identify plaque rupture, stent apposition, dissection, and vessel size. This diagnostic tool creates extremely high-resolution images with improved visualization of calcified plaques. The image is obtained while injecting contrast into the vessel of interest, thereby displacing the blood. The only limitation to using this intraprocedure is if a patient has impaired renal function (Fig. 27.108A and B).

Congenital Defects

A primary indication for diagnostic catheterization studies in children is the evaluation and documentation of specific anatomy, hemodynamic data, and selected aspects of cardiac function associated with congenital heart defects. Methods and techniques used for catheterization of the heart vary depending on age, heart size, type and extent of defect, and other coincident pathophysiologic conditions.

Pediatric cardiac catheters are often introduced percutaneously into the femoral vein and, in older children, sometimes into the femoral artery. In very young patients, it may be possible to pass a catheter from the right atrium to the left atrium (allowing access to the left side of the heart) through either a patent foramen ovale (PFO) or a preexisting atrial septal defect. If the atrial septum is intact, temporary access to the left atrium may be obtained using a transseptal catheter system. With the transseptal catheter system, a long introducer and needle are used to puncture the right atrial septum of the heart to gain access to the left atrium if access cannot be attained as previously described.

PATENT DUCTUS ARTERIOSUS CLOSURE

A patent ductus arteriosus is sometimes evident in a newborn. In utero, the pulmonary artery shunts blood flow into the aorta through the ductus arteriosus, which normally closes after birth. Patent ductus arteriosus occurs when this channel fails to close spontaneously. In some instances, closure can be induced with medication. If this measure is unsuccessful, and the residual shunt is deemed significant, surgical closure (ligation) of the vessel is appropriate.

Fig. 27.106 IVUS images shown on the right correlated with angiography images on the left. *Arrows* in B show the echogenicity of the stent struts during IVUS.

Fig. 27.107 IVUS artery images.

Fig. 27.108 (A) OCT demonstrating plaque burden inside a coronary artery. (B) OCT of coronary artery post stent deployment.

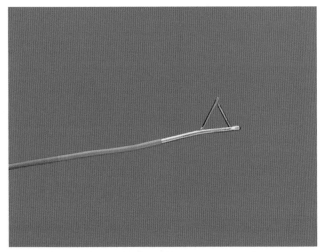

Fig. 27.109 Blade on catheter tip used to incise septal walls in pediatric interventional procedures.

For some patients, occlusion of a patent ductus arteriosus can be accomplished in the catheterization laboratory. A catheter containing an occlusion device, such as an umbrella, is advanced to the ductus. After the position of the lesion is confirmed by angiography, the occluder is released. Subsequent clotting and fibrous infiltration permanently stop the flow and subsequent mixing of blood.

BALLOON SEPTOSTOMY

Balloon septostomy may be used to enlarge a PFO or preexisting *atrial septal defect*. Enlargement of the opening enhances the mixing of right and left atrial blood, thereby improving the level of systemic arterial oxygenation. Transposition of the great arteries is a condition for which atrial septostomy is performed.

Balloon septostomy requires a catheter similar to the type used in PTCA. The balloon is passed through the atrial septal opening into the left atrium, inflated with contrast media, and snapped back through the septal orifice. This maneuver causes the septum to tear. Often the technique must be repeated until the septal opening is sufficiently enlarged to allow the desired level of blood mixing as documented by oximetry, intracardiac pressures, and angiography.

If the atrial septum does not contain a preexisting opening, an artificial defect can be created. A transseptal system approach is employed, and a special catheter containing an internal folding knife-like blade is advanced into the left atrium (Fig. 27.109). After the catheter is inside the left atrium, the blade is advanced out of its protective outer housing and pulled back to the right atrium, creating an incision in the septal wall. This technique may be repeated. A balloon septostomy is performed to widen the new opening, and the condition of the patient is monitored by oximetry, blood pressures, and angiography.

Electrical Conduction System

DIAGNOSTIC PROCEDURES

Electrophysiology procedures involve the collection of sophisticated data to facilitate detailed mapping of the electrical conduction system within the heart. The procedures involve placement of numerous multipolar electrode catheters in areas of the SA node, AV node and/or bundle branches. (Fig. 27.110). Electrophysiology studies are used to analyze the conduction system, induce and evaluate arrhythmias, and determine the effects of therapeutic measures in treating arrhythmias.

Electrode catheters are introduced into the femoral vein, internal jugular vein, or subclavian vein. Because several catheters are used, multiple access sites are needed. It is common to have three introducer sheaths placed within the same vein. The catheters consist of several insulated wires, each of which is attached to an electrode on the catheter tip that serves as an interface with the intracardiac surface. The arrangements of the electrodes on the catheter allow its dual function of recording the electrical signals of the heart (intracardiac electrograms) and pacing the heart. The pacemaker function is performed to introduce premature electrical impulses to determine possible arrhythmias. After the precise defect is characterized, an appropriate course of therapy can be undertaken. Cardiac ablation, pacemaker, and internal cardiac defibrillator are the most common treatments for arrhythmias. In some cases, surgical intervention is required.

INTERVENTIONAL CONDUCTION PROCEDURES

Pacemaker and defibrillator

Permanent implantation of an antiarrhythmic device is another interventional procedure performed in cardiac catheterization laboratories (Fig. 27.111). Antiarrhythmic devices include pacemakers for patients with bradyarrhythmias or disease of the electrical conduction system of the heart and implantable cardioverter defibrillators (ICDs) for patients with lethal ventricular tachyarrhythmias originating from the bottom of the heart.

Pacemaker implantation can be performed successfully under local anesthesia in selected adult and pediatric patients. ICD implantation requires conscious sedation or general anesthesia because of the type of testing required at the time of implantation. Insertion of either a pacemaker or an ICD involves accessing the subclavian or cephalic vein and introducing leads (electrically insulated wires with distal electrodes). The leads are manipulated so that their tips are in direct contact with the right ventricular or right atrial endocardium, or both. The leads are tested for stimulation and sensing properties to ascertain proper functioning before they are attached to the pulse generator. During ICD implantation, defibrillation threshold testing is performed to determine the amount of energy required to defibrillate a patient from ventricular tachycardia or

A

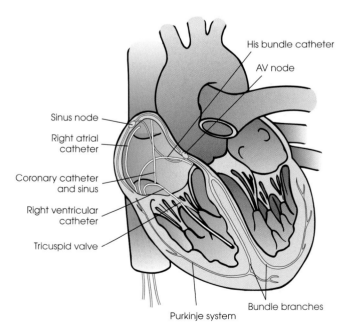

Fig. 27.110 Catheter positions for routine electrophysiologic study. Multipolar catheters are positioned in the high right atrium near the sinus node, in the area of the atrioventricular apex, and in the coronary sinus.

His bundle catheter
AV node
Sinus node
Right atrial catheter
Coronary catheter and sinus
Right ventricular catheter
Tricuspid valve
Bundle branches
Purkinje system

B

Fig. 27.111 (A) Single-chamber ICD. (B) Dual chamber pacemaker.

fibrillation. After testing is completed, the proximal end of the lead is attached to a battery (pacemaker or ICD) and implanted in a subcutaneous or subpectoral pocket created in the thorax (Fig. 27.112). Current pacemakers have longevity of 5 to 10 years, and ICDs have longevity of 6 to 8 years. Newer pacemaker technologies allow the elimination of pacemaker leads, although at present they are only available as an alternative to single lead pacemakers. A small pacemaker device is delivered through a catheter and embedded directly into the right ventricle. This leadless pacemaker is intended for patients with atrial fibrillation or other dangerous arrhythmias, such as bradycardia-tachycardia syndrome.

Radiofrequency ablation

Another interventional procedure to treat disorders of the conduction system is radiofrequency (RF) ablation. Several different arrhythmias previously treated with ICD implantation or drug therapy can now be treated with RF ablation. The procedure is normally performed at the time of the diagnostic electrophysiology study if an underlying mechanism or arrhythmogenic focus is identified.

RF ablation is achieved by delivering a low-voltage, high-frequency alternating current directly to the endocardial tissue through a specially designed ablation catheter. The current desiccates the underlying abnormal myocardial conduction tissue and creates a small, discrete burn lesion. Localized RF lesions create areas of tissue necrosis and scar, subsequently destroying the arrhythmogenic focus. Several RF lesions may be necessary to eliminate the abnormal conduction circuit.

Follow-up electrophysiologic testing is performed to document the resolution of the arrhythmia. RF ablation of the atrioventricular node and pacemaker insertion are quickly becoming the preferred treatment for chronic atrial fibrillation with rapid, irregular responses. The atrioventricular junction is destroyed intentionally; consequently, the rapid, irregular electrical impulses from the atrium are not conducted into the ventricle. A pacemaker is implanted, and a more consistent, regular heart rate is achieved.

POSTCATHETERIZATION CARE

When the catheterization procedure is completed, all catheters are removed. If a cutdown approach was used, the arteriotomy or venotomy is repaired as appropriate. If a percutaneous approach was used, multiple techniques can be employed to obtain hemostasis. Manual pressure is placed on the puncture site until bleeding is controlled. Devices used to close the arteriotomy include collagen seal, suture-mediated devices, or a metal clip. These are deployed under the skin against the artery wall. Wound sites are cleaned and dressed to minimize the risk of infection.

The physician prescribes postcatheterization medications. The puncture site must be observed for hemorrhage or hematoma, and the status of the distal pulse is recorded on the protocol record before the patient leaves the catheterization laboratory. Vital signs should be monitored regularly after the catheterization. The ingestion of fluids should be encouraged, and pain medication may be indicated.

Cardiac catheterization may also be performed on an outpatient or same-day treatment basis. The patient is monitored for 4 to 8 hours in a recovery area and then allowed to go home. Instructions for home care recovery procedures are usually given to the patient or a family member before the patient leaves the recovery area.

CATHETER-BASED THERAPIES

Many procedures previously performed only by cardiothoracic surgeons are presently being done in the catheterization laboratory. These are percutaneous procedures done by specially trained cardiologists and include placement of a device percutaneously to close PFOs and atrioseptal defects, and transcatheter aortic valve replacement (TAVR) (Fig. 27.113).

NOTE: PFO can be the cause of stroke in the adult patient. Occluder devices have shown positive results in treatment of the PFO. This technology is expected to grow in the future.

Fig. 27.112 Chest radiograph of a patient with a permanent pacemaker implanted. Note the pacemaker location in the superior and anterior chest wall, with the distal leads located in the right ventricle and right atrium of the heart.

Magnetic resonance imaging

Techniques and methods for cardiac catheterization continue to be developed and refined. Angiographic imaging and recording devices are becoming even more sophisticated and yielding ever greater resolution and detail. MRI (see Chapter 26) of the cardiovascular system is now a well-recognized investigational technique. Magnetic resonance coronary arteriography is now able to assess anomalous coronary artery anatomy reliably and to identify the presence of calcification in the coronary arteries and bypass grafts.

Many experts believe that the greatest area for growth in the field of cardiac catheterization is in interventional procedures. Despite the use of such techniques as PTCA, intracoronary stenting, and atherectomy in coronary artery disease, restenosis continues to be prevalent and of major concern. Most of the research in interventional procedures is geared toward finding a technique to prevent or limit greatly restenosis after an intervention. Existing and new interventional procedures should continue to provide patients with viable, relatively low-risk, financially reasonable alternatives to open-heart surgery. Current trends indicate that the number and variety of outpatient cardiac catheterizations will continue to increase. The equipment used and procedures performed in the cardiac catheterization laboratories of the future are likely to be significantly different from those associated with existing facilities. Despite changes in cardiovascular technology and medical techniques, cardiac catheterization laboratories will continue to provide the essential patient care services necessary for the diagnosis and treatment of a vast number of cardiovascular-related diseases.

Fig. 27.113 Percutaneous aortic valves: (A) Edwards SAPIEN (Edwards Lifesciences Corp., Irvine, CA). (B) Fluoroscopic image of Edwards SAPIEN device in place. (C) CoreValve (Medtronic, Minneapolis, MN). (D) Aortogram of CoreValve in place.

(From Steinberg DH, Staubach S, Franke J, Sievert H: Defining structural heart disease in the adult patient: current scope, inherent challenges and future directions. *Eur Heart J Suppl* 12(E):E2–E9, 2010.)

Definition of Terms

afferent lymph vessel Vessel carrying lymph toward a lymph vessel.

anastomose Join.

aneurysm Sac formed by local enlargement of a weakened artery wall.

angina pectoris Severe form of chest pain and constriction near the heart; usually caused by a decrease in the blood supply to cardiac tissue; most often associated with stenosis of a coronary artery as a result of atherosclerotic accumulations or spasm. Pain generally lasts for a few minutes and is more likely to occur after stress, exercise, or other activity resulting in increased heart rate.

angiography Radiographic demonstration of blood vessels after the introduction of contrast media.

anomaly Variation from the normal pattern.

aortic dissection Tear in inner lining of the aortic wall that allows blood to enter and track along the muscular coat.

aortography Radiographic examination of the aorta.

arrhythmia Variation from normal heart rhythm.

arrhythmogenic Producing an arrhythmia.

arteriography Radiologic examination of arteries after injection of a radiopaque contrast medium.

arteriole Very small arterial vessel.

arteriosclerotic Indicative of a general pathologic condition characterized by thickening and hardening of arterial walls, leading to general loss of elasticity.

arteriotomy Surgical opening of an artery.

arteriovenous malformation Abnormal anastomosis or communication between an artery and a vein.

artery Large blood vessel carrying blood away from the heart.

atherectomy Excision of atherosclerotic plaque.

atheromatous Characteristic of degenerative change in the inner lining of arteries caused by the deposition of fatty tissue and subsequent thickening of arterial walls that occurs in atherosclerosis.

atherosclerosis Condition in which fibrous and fatty deposits on the luminal wall of an artery may cause obstruction of the vessel.

atrium One of the two upper chambers of the heart.

bifurcation Place where a structure divides into two branches.

biplane Two x-ray exposure planes 90 degrees from one another, usually frontal and lateral.

blood vascular system Vascular system comprising arteries, capillaries, and veins, which convey blood.

bradyarrhythmia Irregular heart rhythm in conjunction with bradycardia.

bradycardia Any heart rhythm with an average heart rate of less than 60 beats/min.

capillary Tiny blood vessel through which blood and tissue cells exchange substances.

cardiac output Amount of blood pumped from the heart per given unit of time; can be calculated by multiplying stroke volume (amount of blood in milliliters ejected from the left ventricle during each heartbeat) by heart rate (number of heartbeats per minute). A normal, resting adult with a stroke volume of 70 mL and a heart rate of 72 beats/min has a cardiac output of approximately 5 L/min.

cardiomyopathies Relatively serious group of heart diseases typically characterized by enlargement of the myocardial layer of the left ventricle and resulting in decreased cardiac output; hypertrophic cardiomyopathy is a condition often studied in the catheterization laboratory.

cardiovascular and interventional technologist Technologists specializing in angiographic and interventional procedures.

cerebral angiography Imaging of vascular system of the brain.

cinefluorography Same as cineradiography; the production of a motion picture record of successive images on a fluoroscopic screen.

claudication Cramping of the leg muscles after physical exertion because of chronically inadequate blood supply.

coagulopathy Any disorder that affects the blood-clotting mechanism.

collateral Secondary or accessory.

diastole Relaxed phase of the atria or ventricles of the heart during which blood enters the chambers; in the cardiac cycle at which the heart is not contracting (at rest).

dyspnea Labored breathing.

efferent lymph vessel Vessel carrying lymph away from a node.

ejection fraction Measurements of ventricular contractility expressed as the percentage of blood pumped out of the left ventricle during contraction; can be estimated by evaluating the left ventriculogram; normal range is 57% to 73% (average 65%). A low ejection fraction indicates failure of the left ventricle to pump effectively.

embolus Foreign material, often thrombus, that detaches and moves freely in the bloodstream.

endocardium Interior lining of heart chambers.

epicardium Exterior layer of heart wall.

ergometer Device used to imitate the muscular, metabolic, and respiratory effects of exercise.

extravasation Escape of fluid from a vessel into the surrounding tissue.

fibrillation Involuntary, chaotic muscular contractions resulting from spontaneous activation of single muscle cells or muscle fibers.

French size Measurement of catheter sizes; 1 French = 0.33 mm; abbreviated Fr.

guidewire Tightly wound metallic wire over which angiographic catheters are placed.

hematoma Collection of extravasated blood in an organ or a tissue space.

hemodynamics Study of factors involved in circulation of blood. Hemodynamic data typically collected during heart catheterization are cardiac output and intracardiac pressures.

hemostasis Stopping of blood flow in a hemorrhage.

iatrogenic Caused by a therapeutic or diagnostic procedure.

innominate or brachiocephalic artery First major artery of the aortic arch supplying the cerebral circulation.

in-stent restenosis Renarrowing of an artery inside a previously placed stent.

intervention Therapeutic modality—mechanical or pharmacologic—used to modify the course of a disease process.

interventional Improving a condition; therapeutic.

interventricular septal integrity Continuity of the membranous partition that separates the right and left ventricles of the heart.

intracoronary stent Metallic device placed within a coronary artery across a region of stenosis.

introducer sheath Plastic tubing placed within the vasculature through which other catheters may be passed.

ischemic Indicative of a local decrease of blood supply to myocardial tissue associated with temporary obstruction of a coronary vessel, typically as a result of thrombus (blood clot).

lesion Injury or other damaging change to an organ or tissue.

lymph Body fluid circulated by the lymphatic vessels and filtered by the lymph nodes.

lymph vessels See *afferent* and *efferent lymph vessel.*

lymphadenography Radiographic study of the lymph nodes.

lymphangiography Radiographic study of the lymph vessels.

lymphography Radiographic evaluation of the lymphatic channels and lymph nodes.

mandrel Inner metallic core of a spiral wound guidewire.

meninges Three membranes that envelop the brain and spinal cord.

misregistration Occurs when the two images used to form a subtraction image are slightly displaced from one another.

myocardial infarction (MI) Acute ischemic episode resulting in myocardial damage and pain; commonly referred to as a heart attack.

myocardium Muscular heart wall.

neointimal hyperplasia Hyperproliferation of smooth muscle cells and extracellular matrix secondary to revascularization.

nephrotoxic Chemically damaging to the kidney cells.

nonocclusive Not completely closed or shut; allowing blood flow.

occlusion Obstruction or closure of a vessel, such as a coronary vessel, as a result of foreign material, thrombus, or spasm.

oximetry Measurement of oxygen saturation in blood.

oxygen saturation Amount of oxygen bound to hemoglobin in blood, expressed as a percentage.

patency State of being open or unobstructed.

patent foramen ovale Opening between the right atrium and left atrium that normally exists in fetal life to allow for the essential mixing of blood. The opening normally closes shortly after birth.

percutaneous Introduced through the skin.

percutaneous transluminal angioplasty (PTA) Surgical correction of a vessel from within the vessel using catheter technology.

percutaneous transluminal coronary angioplasty (PTCA) Manipulative interventional procedure involving the placement and inflation of a balloon catheter in the lumen of a stenosed coronary artery for the purpose of compressing and fracturing the diseased material, allowing subsequent increased distal blood flow to the myocardium.

percutaneous transluminal coronary rotational atherectomy (PTCRA) Manipulative interventional procedure involving a device called a Rotablator to remove atherosclerotic plaque from within the coronary artery using a high-speed rotational burr.

percutaneously Performed through the skin.

pericardium Fibrous sac that surrounds the heart.

planimetry Mechanical tracing to determine the volume of a structure.

pledget Small piece of material used as a dressing or plug.

portal circulation System of vessels carrying blood from the organs of digestion to the liver.

postprocessing Image processing operations performed when reviewing an imaging sequence.

pulmonary circulation System of vessels carrying blood from the heart to the lungs and back to the heart.

pulse Regular expansion and contraction of an artery that is produced by ejection of blood from the heart.

pulse oximetry Measurement of oxygen saturation in the blood via an optic sensor placed on an extremity.

reperfusion Reestablishment of blood flow to the heart muscle through a previously occluded artery.

restenosis Narrowing or constriction of a vessel, orifice, or other type of passageway after interventional correction of primary condition.

rotational burr atherectomy Ablation of atheroma through a percutaneous transcatheter approach using a high-speed rotational burr.

serial imaging Acquisition of images in rapid succession.

stenosis Narrowing or constriction of a vessel, an orifice, or another type of passageway.

stent Wire mesh or plastic conduit placed to maintain flow.

systemic circulation System of vessels carrying blood from the heart out to the body (except the lungs) and back to the heart.

systole Contraction phase of the atria or ventricles of the heart during which blood is ejected from the chambers; point in the cardiac cycle at which the heart is contracting (at work).

tachyarrhythmia Irregular heart rhythm in conjunction with tachycardia.

tachycardia Any heart rhythm having an average heart rate in excess of 100 beats/min.

targeted lesion Area of narrowing within an artery where a revascularization procedure is planned.

thrombogenesis Formation of a blood clot.

thrombolytic Capable of causing the breakup of a thrombus.

thrombosis Formation or existence of a blood clot.

thrombus Blood clot obstructing a blood vessel or cavity of the heart.

transducer Device used to convert one form of energy into another. Transducers used in cardiac catheterization convert fluid (blood) pressure into an electrical signal displayed on a physiologic monitor.

transposition of the great arteries Congenital heart defect requiring interventional therapy. In this defect, the aorta arises from the right side of the heart, and the pulmonary artery arises from the left side of the heart.

umbrella Prosthetic interventional device consisting of two opposing polyurethane disks connected by a central loop mounted on a spring-loaded assembly to provide opposing tension.

valvular competence Ability of the valve to prevent backward flow while not inhibiting forward flow.

varices Irregularly swollen veins.

vasoconstriction Temporary closure of a blood vessel using drug therapy.

vein Vessel that carries blood from the capillaries to the heart.

venography Radiologic study of veins after injection of radiopaque contrast media.

venotomy Surgical opening of a vein.

ventricle One of two larger pumping chambers of the heart.

venule Any of the small blood vessels that collect blood from the capillaries and join to become veins.

References

1. Seldinger SI: Percutaneous selective angiography of the aorta: preliminary report, *Acta Radiol (Stockh)* 45:15, 1956.
2. Egas Moniz AC: L'encéphalographie artérielle, son importance dans la localisation des tumeurs cérébrales, *Rev Neurol* 2:72, 1927.
3. Egas Moniz AC: *L'angiographie cérébrale*, Paris, 1934, Masson & Cie.
4. Greitz T: A radiologic study of the brain circulation by rapid serial angiography of the carotid artery, *Acta Radiol* 46(Suppl 140):1, 1956.
5. Dotter CT, Judkins MP: Transluminal treatment of arteriosclerotic obstruction: description of a new technique and preliminary report of its application, *Circulation* 30:654, 1964.
6. Grüntzig A, Hopff H: Perkutane rekanalisation chronischer arterieller verschlüsse mit einem neuen dilatationskatheter; modifikation der dotter-technik, *Deutsch Med Wochenschr* 99:2502, 1974.
7. Molnar W, Stockum AE: Transhepatic dilatation of choledochoenterostomy strictures, *Radiology* 129:59, 1978.
8. Brooks B: The treatment of traumatic arteriovenous fistula, *South Med J* 23:100, 1930.
9. Brooks B: Discussion. In Nolan L, Taylor AS: pulsating exophthalmos, *Trans South Surg Assoc* 43:176, 1931.
10. Kaufman J, Lee M: *Vascular and interventional radiology: the requisites*, ed 2, Philadelphia, 2014, Elsevier.
11. Scanlon PJ, et al: ACC/AHA guidelines for coronary angiography: a report of the American college of cardiology/American heart association task force on practice guidelines (committee on coronary angiography), *J Am Coll Cardiol* 33:1999, 1758.
12. Laskey W, Boyle J, Johnson LW: Multivariable model for prediction of risk of significant complication during diagnostic cardiac catheterization: the registry committee of the society for cardiac angiography and interventions, *Cathet Cardiovasc Diagn* 30:185–190, 1993.

Selected bibliography

Ahn SS, Concepcion B: Current status of atherectomy for peripheral arterial occlusive disease, *World J Surg* 20:635, 1996.

Burke TH, et al: Cardiovascular and interventional technologists: their growing role in the interventional suite, *J Vasc Interv Radiol* 8:720, 1997.

Caldwell DM, et al: Embolotherapy: agents, clinical applications, and techniques, *RadioGraphics* 14:623, 1994.

Colombo A, et al: Intracoronary stenting without anticoagulation accomplished with intravascular ultrasound guidance, *Circulation* 91:1995, 1676.

Dorffner R, et al: Treatment of abdominal aortic aneurysms with transfemoral placement of stent-grafts: complications and secondary radiologic intervention, *Radiology* 204:79, 1997.

Dyet JF: Endovascular stents in the arterial system—current status, *Clin Radiol* 52:83, 1997.

Eustace S, et al: Magnetic resonance angiography in transjugular intrahepatic portosystemic stenting: comparison with contrast hepatic and portal venography, *Eur J Radiol* 19:43, 1994.

Fillmore DJ, et al: Transjugular intrahepatic portosystemic shunt: midterm clinical and angiographic follow-up, *J Vasc Interv Radiol* 7:255, 1996.

Kandarpa K: Technical determinants of success in catheter-directed thrombolysis for peripheral arterial occlusions, *J Vasc Interv Radiol* 6(6 pt 2 Suppl):55S, 1995.

Kandarpa K, Machan L: *Handbook of interventional radiologic procedures*, ed 4, Philadelphia, 2011, Lippincott Williams & Wilkins.

Kaufman J, Lee M: *Vascular and interventional radiology: the requisites*, ed 2, Philadelphia, 2014, Elsevier.

Kern MJ, et al: *The cardiac catheterization handbook*, ed 6, Philadelphia, 2016, Elsevier.

Kern MJ: *The cardiac catheterization handbook*, ed 4, St Louis, 2003, Mosby.

Kerns SR, et al: Current status of carbon dioxide angiography, *Radiol Clin North Am* 33:15, 1995.

Laine C, et al: Combined cardiac catheterization for uncomplicated ischemic heart disease in a Medicare population, *Am J Med* 105:373, 1998.

LeRoux PD, Winn HR: Current management of aneurysms, *Neurosurg Clin N Am* 9:421, 1998.

Nelson PK, Kricheff II: Cerebral angiography, *Neuroimaging Clin N Am* 6:1, 1996.

Norris TG: Principles of cardiac catheterization, *Radiol Technol* 72:109, 2000.

Pieters PC, et al: Evaluation of the portal venous system: complementary roles of invasive and noninvasive imaging strategies, *Radiographics* 17:879, 1997.

Rees CR, et al: Use of carbon dioxide as a contrast medium for transjugular intrahepatic portosystemic shunt procedures, *J Vasc Interv Radiol* 5:383, 1994.

Rogers CG, Jr, et al: Intrahepatic vascular shunting for portal hypertension: early experience with the transjugular intrahepatic porto-systemic shunt, *Am Surg* 60:114, 1994.

Scanlon PJ, et al: ACC/AHA guidelines for coronary angiography: a report of the American college of cardiology/American heart association task force on practice guidelines (committee on coronary angiography), *J Am Coll Cardiol* 33:1999, 1756.

Seldinger SI: Percutaneous selective angiography of the aorta: preliminary report, *Acta Radiol (Stockh)* 45:15, 1956.

Snopek A: *Fundamentals of special radiographic procedures*, ed 5, St. Louis, 2006, Elsevier.

Vinuela F, et al: Guglielmi detachable coil embolization of acute intracranial aneurysm: perioperative anatomical and clinical outcome in 403 patients, *J Neurosurg* 86:475, 1997.

Warner JJ, et al: Recognizing complications of cardiac catheterization, *Emerg Med* 32:12, 2000.

28

DIAGNOSTIC MEDICAL SONOGRAPHY

SUSANNA L. OVEL

GB SAG

Principles of Diagnostic Ultrasound

Diagnostic medical sonography[a] is a general term used to encompass abdominal, breast, cardiac, gynecologic, obstetric, and vascular sonography. *Registered diagnostic medical sonographers* (RDMSs) specialize in abdominal sonography, obstetrics/gynecology imaging, breast sonography, musculoskeletal imaging, or pediatric sonography. *Registered diagnostic cardiac sonographers* (RDCSs) specialize in fetal, pediatric, or adult echocardiography. *Registered vascular technologists* (RVTs) specialize in abdominal vasculature imaging, imaging of arteries and veins of the upper and lower extremities, imaging of extracranial arteries and veins, transcranial duplex sonography, and physiologic vascular testing in pediatric and adult patients. One overall physics examination, encompassing sonographic principles, hemodynamics, and instrumentation, is required for all these specialties.

Diagnostic medical sonography employs high-frequency transducers ranging from 2 to 30 MHz. The transducer emits short pulses of ultrasound (pulse waves) into the human body. The transducer receives real-time reflections or frequency shifts from structures or vessels along the sound waves path, and they are displayed as a grayscale, color Doppler, spectral, or duplex image. Velocity of the red blood cells can be calculated using the Doppler technique. Pulse wave, continuous wave, and color Doppler techniques show blood flow direction, flow resistance and turbulence within the vessel, and regurgitation of the cardiac chamber.

Diagnostic medical sonography has evolved into a unique imaging tool. Sonography was previously thought to be a completely noninvasive technique; however, with the introduction of intracavity and intraluminal transducers, the collection of diagnostic data of the pelvic and cardiovascular regions has been shown to improve patient management and care.

CHARACTERISTICS OF DIAGNOSTIC MEDICAL SONOGRAPHERS

The diagnostic medical sonographer uses complicated equipment, independent judgment, and systematic problem-solving skills to acquire quality images and technical data for assistance in a patient's diagnosis, management, and care. Integrity and honesty are important qualities in all medical professionals. In sonography, these character traits are crucial because almost 90% of observed data is discarded. After each examination, the sonographer provides the reading physician with a technical report detailing the size and description of normal and abnormal anatomy or hemodynamics along with possible differential diagnostic considerations.

Similar to radiography, diagnostic medical sonography has national standardized protocols for each examination. The sonographer has the ability to expand on basic examination protocols when additional information is needed without fear of ionizing radiation. In-depth knowledge of pathophysiology, laboratory values, and other medical imaging modalities (i.e., computed tomography [CT], magnetic resonance imaging [MRI]) are important parts of sonography education.

Physical requirements play an additional role in sonography. Sonographers must be able to aid in moving patients and medical equipment. Attention to the use of proper body mechanics is essential (Fig. 28.1). Repetitive usage injury or syndrome of the neck, shoulder, elbow, wrist, and back has been documented. The sonographer should be in good physical, emotional, and nutritional health and should possess a dedication to continual learning. The career can be exciting and rewarding as well as stressful, demanding, frustrating, and occasionally depressing.

---

[a]Almost all italicized words on the succeeding pages are defined at the end of this chapter.

RESOURCE ORGANIZATIONS

Resource organizations devoted exclusively to ultrasound include the American Society of Echocardiography (ASE), the Society of Diagnostic Medical Sonography (SDMS), the American Institute of Ultrasound in Medicine (AIUM), the Society of Radiologists in Ultrasound (SRU), and the Society of Vascular Ultrasound (SVU). International Foundation for Sonography Education and Research (IFSER) is a unique organization devoted to the educators of ultrasound.

Historical Development

Ultrasound began with the discovery of the piezoelectric effect in 1880 by Jacques and Pierre Curie. This discovery allowed for the future construction of transducers to generate and receive sound waves in water. In 1915, the first sonar type device was developed by Paul Langevin to locate submarines. After World War II, research was conducted on medical applications of ultrasound. Between 1940 and 1962, various medical applications were researched and developed. In 1962, the first compound B-scanner was developed under the support of the US Public Health Services and the University of Colorado.

Medical imaging using ultrasound was launched in 1963 with a handheld articulated arm compound B-mode (brightness mode) scanner. The original imaging was bi-stable (black and white only) until grayscale imaging was developed by a group in Australia in 1973. By 1980, the digital scan converter was developed allowing 64 shades of gray in the ultrasound image. In the mid-1980s, ultrasound could be imaged in real time. Not only could we image more reflected intensities, we could also view the motion of the human anatomy live.

Christian Andreas Doppler described the changes in the frequency of transmitted waves when relative motion occurred between the source of the wave and an observer. The first Doppler ultrasound device for medical use was created in the late 1950s in Japan. A prototype of a continuous wave Doppler soon followed with the reported ability to assess blood flow using the Doppler frequency shift. In the mid-1960s Dr. Eugene Strandness, at the University of Washington began research on the use of Doppler ultrasound to detect vascular disease. The first pulsed Doppler technique was developed in 1974 by an engineer, Donald Baker. Color Doppler was established in 1983 in Japan; however,

it was not until 1987 that color Doppler launched in the United States.

For the present day general sonographer, it may be inconceivable that a diagnosis could be made using only bistable and static grayscale scanners to image human anatomy and the presence of abnormalities. The present day vascular and cardiac sonographers would likely feel the same with the lack of color Doppler to aid in assessing vessel pathology and hemodynamics in vascular and cardiac imaging. Technological advances have benefited medical ultrasound with the use of high-frequency, multi-hertz, intracavity, and intraluminal transducers together with three-dimensional and four-dimensional imaging. New technologies, such as elastography, fusion imaging, and contrast enhanced ultrasound imaging, are allowing the diagnosis of pathology without the risks of ionizing radiation and invasive procedures. Most recently, an ultrasound transducer can be attached to a smart phone or tablet allowing imaging in areas remote from the medical setting.

Diagnostic ultrasound, when used as a clinical imaging tool, has not been associated with any harmful biological effects and is generally accepted as a safe imaging modality.

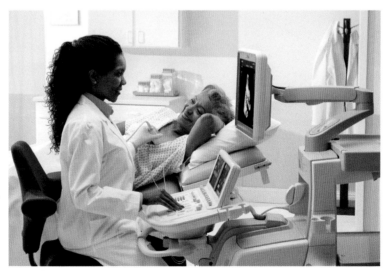

Fig. 28.1 Sonographer performing an ultrasound examination.

(Courtesy Philips Medical Systems.)

Physical Principles

PROPERTIES OF SOUND WAVES

Sound waves are traveling variations of pressure, density, and particle motion. Matter must be present for sound to travel; it cannot travel through a vacuum. Sound carries energy, not matter, from one place to another. Vibrations from one molecule carry to the next molecule along the same axis. These oscillations continue until friction causes the vibrations to cease.

Ultrasound refers to sound waves beyond the audible range (>20 kHz). Diagnostic medical sonography can use frequencies of 2 to 30 MHz.

Acoustic impedance

Sound travels through tissues at different speeds depending on the density and stiffness of the medium. Acoustic impedance of a medium determines how much of the wave transmits to the next medium (Fig. 28.2).

Velocity of sound

Propagation speed is the speed at which a sound wave travels through a medium. It is determined by the density and stiffness of a medium. In soft tissue, the propagation speed of sound is 1540 m/s. Bone shows a very high propagation speed (4080 m/s), whereas air shows the lowest propagation speed (330 m/s).

TRANSDUCER SELECTION

Diagnostic ultrasound transducers operate on the principle of piezoelectricity. The *piezoelectric effect* states that some materials produce a voltage when deformed by an applied pressure. Diagnostic ultrasound transducers convert electrical energy into acoustic energy during transmission, and acoustic energy into electrical energy for reception. Diagnostic imaging transducers routinely operate in a frequency range of 2 to 15 MHz. Transducers may be linear, convex, sector, or vector in construction (Fig. 28.3). Higher frequencies are used in intracavity and intraluminal transducers and for visualizing the extremities or superficial structures. Lower frequencies are needed for deeper structures of the thoracic cavity, abdomen, and pelvis. Lower frequencies provide necessary penetration depth at the expense of *detail resolution.*

Pulse wave transducers transmit pulses of sound and receive returning echoes producing a grayscale ultrasound image. A continuous wave transducer produces a continuous wave of sound and is composed of a separate transmit and receive element within a single transducer assembly. Continuous wave transducers do not produce an image.

VOLUME SCANNING AND THREE-DIMENSIONAL AND FOUR-DIMENSIONAL IMAGING

Volume scanning allows for quick "sweeps" of specific areas of the body or fetus. These sweeps give volume data that can be rendered even after the patient has left the ultrasound department. Three-dimensional imaging systems allow the sonographer to acquire volume data. The sonographer can reconstruct these data into a three-dimensional image on the ultrasound machine or at a workstation. With four-dimensional imaging, the ultrasound system is able to acquire and

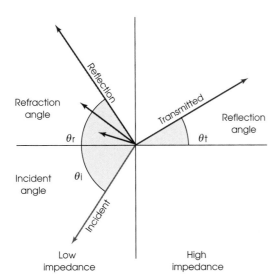

Fig. 28.2 Relationship among incident, reflected, and transmitted waves.

Fig. 28.3 Various ultrasound transducers.

(Courtesy Philips Medical Systems.)

display three-dimensional images in real time.

Anatomic Relationships and Landmarks

The use of anatomic landmarks to define specific areas of the human body is an important part of the imaging and orientation skills of the sonographer. The middle hepatic vein is a sonographic landmark used to locate the division between the left and right hepatic lobes (Fig. 28.4A). The main lobar fissure is used to locate the gallbladder fossa (see Fig. 28.4B). The ovaries are located medial and anterior to the iliac vessels (see Fig. 28.4C). The use of anatomic landmarks is a routine part of many sonographic examinations.

Fig. 28.4 (A) Transverse sonogram of liver showing middle hepatic vein *(MHV)* dividing left and right hepatic lobes. (B) Sagittal image of main lobar fissure *(MLF)* and its relationship to gallbladder *(GB)*. (C) Sagittal color Doppler image of right ovary lying anterior and medial to iliac vessels. *LHV,* Left hepatic vein; *RHV,* right hepatic vein.

(Courtesy Paul Aks, BS, RDMS, RVT.)

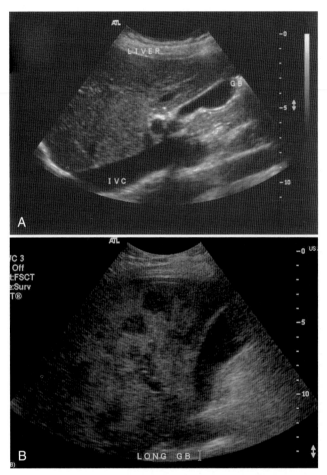

Fig. 28.5 (A) Sagittal sonogram of normal homogeneous liver. (B) Longitudinal sonogram of heterogeneous hepatic lobe in a patient with a history of breast carcinoma.

Clinical Applications
CHARACTERISTICS OF THE SONOGRAPHIC IMAGE

The sonographer uses specific terms to characterize the sonographic image. If the echo pattern is similar throughout a structure or mass, it is termed *homogeneous* (Fig. 28.5A). If the echo pattern is dissimilar throughout a structure or mass, it is termed *heterogeneous* (see Fig. 28.5B). Internal composition of a structure or mass is described using the terms *anechoic* (without internal echoes), *echogenic* (with internal echoes), and *complex* (containing anechoic and echogenic regions) (Fig. 28.6). The sonographer also uses descriptive terms to describe the borders of a mass. Are the borders smooth or irregular, thin or thick, calcified or dilated?

Imaging artifacts are an additional concern for the sonographer. Acoustic artifacts include reflections that are missing; not real; improperly positioned; or of improper brightness, number, shape, or size (Fig. 28.7). Understanding the assumptions of the ultrasound system and the physical principles of sound waves, the sonographer is better able to comprehend the real-time images.

Fig. 28.6 (A) Endovaginal sonogram of anechoic ovarian cyst. (B) Echogenic mass is measured in upper inner quadrant of right breast. (C) Transverse sonogram of complex thyroid mass.

(Courtesy Paul Aks, BS, RDMS, RVT.)

Fig. 28.7 (A) Breast carcinoma showing posterior acoustic shadowing *(arrow)*. (B) Mirror image of anterior tibial artery.

ABDOMEN AND RETROPERITONEUM

The abdominal ultrasound examination generally includes a survey of the liver, pancreas, gallbladder, spleen, great vessels, and kidneys in the sagittal and transverse planes (Figs. 28.8 and 28.9). Specific protocols are followed to image size, shape, and echogenicity of the organ *parenchyma* and anatomic relationships of the surrounding structures. Doppler flow patterns of the upper abdominal blood vessels may be included. Patients are examined in two different body positions (i.e., supine and decubitus). The use of two positions shows the mobility of gallstones and repositions interfering bowel gas. Air reflects most of the sound wave, making visualization of the abdominal and retroperitoneal structures difficult. Abdominal examinations are typically scheduled in the morning with the patient fasting 6 to 8 hours before the sonogram.

The retroperitoneal ultrasound examination includes a survey of the great vessels, kidneys, and bladder in the sagittal and transverse planes before and after voiding. Specific protocols are followed to image the size, shape, cortical thickness, and echogenicity of the renal parenchyma. Anterior–posterior diameters of the inferior vena cava, aorta, and common iliac arteries are measured and documented. Doppler flow patterns of the great vessels and kidneys may be included. Retroperitoneum examinations can be scheduled in the morning or afternoon with the patient drinking 8 to 16 oz. of water 1 hour before the sonogram.

Fig. 28.8 (A) Transverse sonogram of right upper quadrant over right lobe of liver. (B) Line drawing of gross anatomic section. (C) Gross anatomic section at approximately same level as A.

Fig. 28.9 (A) Sagittal sonogram of right upper quadrant over medial segment of left lobe of the liver, hepatic vein, and inferior vena cava. (B) Line drawing of gross anatomic section. (C) Gross anatomic section at approximately same level as A.

Fig. 28.10 (A) Transverse sonogram of liver shows a complex mass in the left lobe. (B) Sonogram of liver shows fatty infiltration with small area of normal liver parenchyma anterior to porta hepatis *(arrow)*.

(A, Courtesy Paul Aks, BS, RDMS, RVT.)

To produce an adequate survey of the abdominal and retroperitoneal cavities, the sonographer must have an understanding of the patient's clinical history. Although ultrasound cannot diagnose the specific pathology of a lesion or condition, a complete clinical picture may lead to more specific differential diagnostic considerations.

Liver and biliary tree

Sonographic examinations of the liver and biliary tree are generally requested in patients with right upper quadrant pain or elevations in liver function laboratory tests. The liver is assessed for size and echogenicity of the parenchyma. Under normal circumstances, the liver parenchyma appears moderately echogenic and homogeneous. Some types of liver pathologies shown on ultrasound include fatty infiltration, cirrhosis, cavernous hemangioma, and hepatoma (Fig. 28.10). Doppler evaluation of the hepatic artery, hepatic veins, and portal veins is included with a patient history or suspicion of cirrhosis, portal hypertension, portal vein thrombosis, and Budd–Chiari syndrome.

The biliary tree includes the gallbladder and the intrahepatic and extrahepatic bile ducts. The gallbladder is evaluated for size, wall thickness, and absence of internal echoes. Under normal circumstances, the gallbladder is a pear-shaped anechoic structure located in the gallbladder fossa on the posterior surface of the liver (Fig. 28.11). The intrahepatic biliary ducts converge near the *porta hepatis* forming the common hepatic duct. The cystic duct joins the common hepatic duct to form the extrahepatic common bile duct. The biliary tree is evaluated for size and evidence of intraductal stones or masses. Some abnormalities of the biliary tree shown on ultrasound include intrahepatic and extrahepatic biliary obstruction, cholelithiasis, and cholecystitis (Fig. 28.12).

Fig. 28.11 Sagittal sonogram of normal gallbladder (*GB*).

Fig. 28.12 (A) Sagittal sonogram of gallbladder showing multiple small gallstones with posterior acoustic shadowing. (B) Transverse sonogram of acute cholecystitis.

Fig. 28.13 Transverse sonogram of normal pancreas. The body of the pancreas lies anterior to splenic vein (*SV*), superior mesenteric artery (*SMA*), and aorta (*AO*).

Fig. 28.14 Transverse sonogram shows hypoechoic mass in head of the pancreas (*arrow*).

Pancreas

The pancreas is an elongated organ oriented in a *transverse oblique plane* in the epigastric and left hypochondriac regions of the retroperitoneal cavity. The head of the pancreas lies in the descending portion of the duodenum and lateral to the superior mesenteric artery. The body is the largest portion, lying anterior to the superior mesenteric artery and splenic vein (Fig. 28.13). The tail is the superiormost portion lying posterior to the antrum of the stomach and generally extends toward the splenic hilum. The echogenicity of the pancreas varies depending on the amount of fat but should appear homogeneous throughout the organ. Ultrasound examinations of the pancreas are requested in patients with a history of unexplained weight loss, epigastric pain, and elevation in pancreatic enzymes or liver function laboratory tests. The pancreas is evaluated for size and echogenicity of the parenchyma. The distal common bile duct is routinely measured in the posterior lateral portion of the head of the pancreas. Some abnormalities of the pancreas shown on ultrasound include inflammation, calcifications, tumor, or abscess formation (Fig. 28.14).

Spleen

The spleen is the predominant organ in the left upper quadrant located inferior to the diaphragm and anterior to the left kidney. Ultrasound examinations of the spleen are requested in patients with a history of abdominal trauma, chronic liver disease, and leukocytosis. An increase in hepatic pressures from liver disease may cause an abnormal increase in the size of the spleen (Fig. 28.15). The normal spleen appears moderately echogenic, similar to the normal liver parenchyma. The spleen is evaluated for size and echogenicity of the parenchyma. Some abnormalities of the spleen shown on ultrasound include splenomegaly, splenic rupture, calcifications, or abscess formation. Doppler evaluation of the splenic artery and vein is included with a patient history or suspicion of portal hypertension.

Fig. 28.15 Sagittal sonogram of enlarged spleen measuring greater than 15 cm in length (splenomegaly).

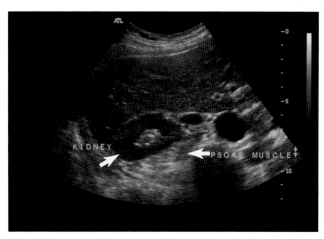

Fig. 28.16 Transverse sonogram of right kidney lying posterior to the liver and lateral to the psoas muscle.

Kidneys and bladder

The kidneys are bean-shaped structures lying in a *sagittal* oblique plane lateral to the psoas muscles in the retroperitoneal cavity (Fig. 28.16). Ultrasound examinations of the kidneys and bladder are requested in patients with a history of urinary tract infection, flank pain, hematuria, and an increase in creatinine levels. The normal adult renal cortex shows a moderate- to low-level echo pattern, *hypoechoic,* to the liver and spleen. The renal sinus is the most echogenic portion of the kidney and considered *hyperechoic* to the surrounding structures. The kidneys are evaluated for contour, size, cortical thickness, dilation of calyces (hydronephrosis), and echogenicity of the renal parenchyma. Ultrasound guidance is used to localize the kidney during renal biopsy procedures and to evaluate for any post-biopsy complications.

Fig. 28.17 (A) Sagittal sonogram shows hypoechoic mass in anterior right kidney. (B) Sagittal sonogram of right kidney shows mild hydronephrosis and hyperechoic kidney stone.

Ultrasound is a useful imaging tool to monitor a renal transplant. The transplant is typically placed superficially in the right iliac fossa. Sonograms of the transplant include grayscale images to evaluate size, contour, echogenicity, and cortical thickness. The renal artery and vein are evaluated with Doppler checking for intimal thickening, stenosis, and thrombosis.

A partially distended urinary bladder is evaluated for wall thickness, contour, and evidence of neoplasm. Post-void imaging is included to evaluate the amount of residual urine and competence of the ureteral valves. Abnormalities of the kidneys and bladder shown on ultrasound include urinary obstruction, nephrolithiasis, abscess formation, cortical thinning, and benign and malignant neoplasms (Fig. 28.17).

MUSCULOSKELETAL STRUCTURES

The musculoskeletal system provides movement of the body parts and organs. Ultrasound examinations of the musculoskeletal structures are requested in patients with a history of trauma, palpable mass, and chronic pain. On ultrasound, normal muscles show a low to medium shade of gray echo pattern with hyperechoic striations throughout. Tendons appear homogeneous with hyperechoic linear bands. Some abnormalities of the musculoskeletal system shown on ultrasound include muscle or tendon tears, inflammation, hematoma, and edema (Fig. 28.18).

SUPERFICIAL STRUCTURES

Superficial structures image well with ultrasound and include soft tissues, thyroid glands, breast, scrotum, and abdominal wall. The echogenicity of the thyroid glands and testes is similar, showing a moderately echogenic parenchymal pattern. Breast tissue varies depending on the amount of fat content. In sonography, all breast tissues are compared with the medium level echo pattern of normal breast fat. Abdominal wall ultrasound examinations may be requested to rule out evidence of herniation or hematoma. Soft tissue ultrasound examinations are generally requested to evaluate a specific mass. Abnormalities of the superficial structures shown on ultrasound include inflammation, herniation, hematomas, and benign and malignant neoplasms (Figs. 28.19 and 28.20).

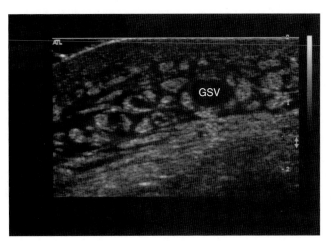

Fig. 28.18 Transverse sonogram of medial thigh shows tissue edema surrounding great saphenous vein (*GSV*).

Fig. 28.19 (A) Breast cyst with debris is shown demonstrating well-defined borders, fluid–fluid level, and increased through transmission. (B) Fibroadenomas (*calipers*) demonstrate well-defined borders and may have some increased transmission; however, the internal echo pattern is solid and homogeneous. Benign lesions typically demonstrate a mass wider rather than tall.

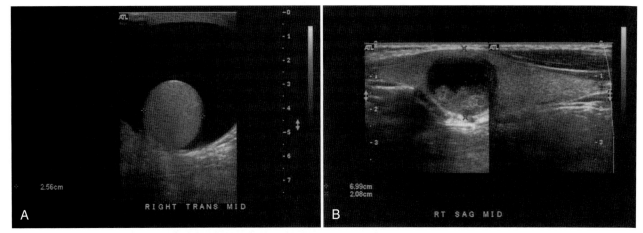

Fig. 28.20 (A) Transverse sonogram of right testis surrounded by anechoic fluid (hydrocele). (B) Sagittal image of complex thyroid mass.

(Courtesy Paul Aks, BS, RDMS, RVT.)

PEDIATRIC SONOGRAPHY

The goal of pediatric imaging is to perform a study with the lowest amount of radiation and the least amount of sedation. Ultrasound is becoming one of the most widely used imaging modalities, and it is frequently the initial imaging modality in infants and children. A specialty examination to include all general pediatric examinations was implemented in 2015 to replace the existing neonatal neurosonography specialty.

Normal sonographic appearance of anatomy in infants and children can differ from that of the adult patient. This new specialty examination covers the abdomen, pelvis, and small parts, along with pediatric-specific examinations. Examples of pediatric-specific examinations include the gastrointestinal tract for pyloric stenosis and intussusception (Fig. 28.21), infant spine for tethered cord, infant hips for developmental dysplasia of the hip (Fig. 28.22), and neonatal brain for hydrocephalus and intraventricular hemorrhage (Fig. 28.23)

Infants and children pose a challenge to the sonographer. A detailed understanding of the normal and abnormal sonographic appearances of pediatric anatomy is necessary to accurately assess and quickly image the pediatric patient.

Fig. 28.21 Sagittal image of the pylorus in a case of pyloric stenosis.

(Courtesy Susanna Ovel, RT, RDMS, RVT.)

Fig. 28.22 Coronal image demonstrating the Graf angles in a normal infant hip.

(Courtesy Susanna Ovel, RT, RDMS, RVT.)

Fig. 28.23 (A) Coronal sonogram in a neonate showing bilateral ventriculomegaly. (B) Sagittal sonogram of left lateral ventricle showing ventriculomegaly.

GYNECOLOGIC APPLICATIONS

Anatomic features of the pelvis

The pelvis is divided into the true and false pelvis by the *iliopectineal line*. The *false pelvis* contains loops of bowel and is bound by the abdominal wall, the ala of the iliac bones, and the base of the sacrum.

The *true pelvis* contains the female reproductive organs, urinary bladder, distal ureters, and bowel (Fig. 28.24). It is bound by the symphysis pubis, sacrum, and coccyx. The pelvic floor is formed by ligaments and the levator ani, piriformis, and coccygeus muscles.

The *retrouterine pouch or pouch of Douglas* lies between the uterus and the rectum. Free fluid routinely accumulates in this area. All pelvic recesses should be imaged on all transabdominal and endovaginal sonograms.

Rectouterine pouch

Rectum

Anus

Uterus

Bladder

Vagina

Fig. 28.24 Sagittal line drawing of female pelvis.

Sonography of the female pelvis

Sonography of the female pelvis is clinically useful in the premenarche, menarche, and postmenopausal periods. Pelvic ultrasound examinations are requested for assessment of a pelvic mass, pelvic pain, or abnormal uterine bleeding; infertility monitoring; and localization of an intrauterine device.

A complete transabdominal examination of the female pelvis includes evaluation and documentation of the distended urinary bladder, uterus, cervix, endometrial canal, vagina, ovaries, adnexal regions, pelvic recesses, and supporting pelvic musculature. The full bladder helps to reposition the intestines laterally into the false pelvis. The urinary bladder serves as an *acoustic window* and anechoic landmark in transabdominal imaging. Real-time imaging allows the sonographer to evaluate the entire pelvic area for pathology and peristalsis of the bowel (Fig. 28.25).

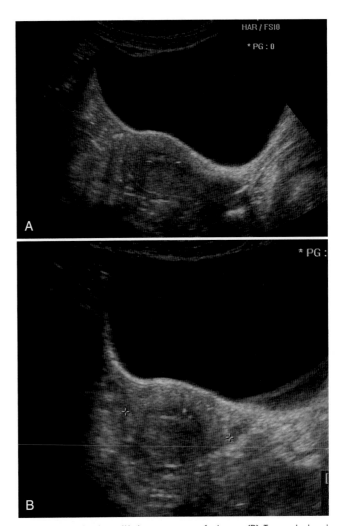

Fig. 28.25 (A) Transabdominal sagittal sonogram of uterus. (B) Transabdominal transverse sonogram of uterus with measurements.

Endovaginal transducers show excellent detail resolution of the uterine endometrium at the expense of penetration depth and acoustic windows (Fig. 28.26). Endovaginal sonography should be used in conjunction with a transabdominal pelvic examination. A high-frequency transducer is inserted into the vaginal canal to evaluate the uterus, endometrium, ovaries, adnexal regions, and pelvic recesses in the sagittal and coronal planes (Fig. 28.27).

The normal adult uterine myometrium appears homogeneous and moderately echogenic on ultrasound. The echogenicity and thickness of the normal endometrium vary with the menstrual cycle but should not exceed 14 mm in anteroposterior diameter. Normal ovaries appear moderately echogenic with small functional cysts (follicles) of varying size and number. Monitoring the number and size of *follicular cysts* is a common practice in infertility treatment. Ultrasound is used to aid the gynecologist in determining when the ovum is ready for stimulation with high doses of human chorionic gonadotropin. Some abnormalities of the female pelvis shown on ultrasound include congenital malformation, leiomyoma, endometrial polyp, ovarian cyst, and tubal ovarian abscess (Fig. 28.28).

OBSTETRIC APPLICATIONS

Obstetric sonography is probably the most well-known ultrasound examination. An obstetric sonogram allows the obstetrician to view and monitor the developing *embryo* and *fetus*. Routine screening examinations are requested between 16 and 24 *gestational weeks* to measure *gestational age,* evaluate fetal anatomy, localize placental placement, assess amniotic fluid, and evaluate cervical competence. Evaluation of the fetus is relatively easy because the fetus occupies a fluid-filled *gestational sac,* an excellent acoustic window for ultrasound.

In the first trimester, endovaginal imaging is more likely to image an early gestational sac, yolk sac, amniotic cavity, and embryo (Figs. 28.29 and 28.30). The number of viable embryos is easily diagnosed with a first-trimester sonogram. The gestational sac may be visualized at 4.5 gestational weeks, and embryo cardiac activity can be identified at 5.5 gestational weeks with endovaginal sonography. By the ninth gestational week, the cerebral hemispheres and limb buds are evident. By the 12th gestational week, the fetus has a skeletal body.

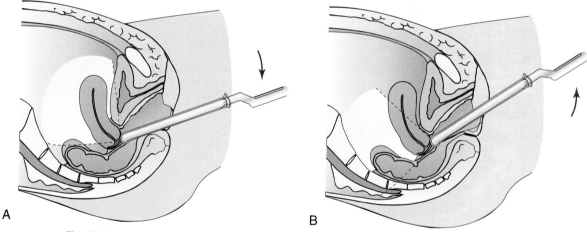

Fig. 28.26 (A) Transvaginal sagittal scan with anterior angulation to visualize better the fundus of normal anteflexed uterus. (B) Transvaginal sagittal scan with posterior angulation to visualize better cervix and rectouterine recess.

Fig. 28.27 (A) Endovaginal sagittal sonogram of uterus. (B) Coronal sonogram of uterus.

A COR ENDO

B 1.62cm UTERUS TRANS

C 5.97cm 3.87cm LT OVARY

Fig. 28.28 (A) Volumetric coronal sonogram of uterine cervix showing improper location of an intrauterine device. (B) Coronal image of the endometrium showing a hyperechoic neoplasm (calipers). (C) Sagittal image of complex left ovarian mass.

(A and C, Courtesy Paul Aks, BS, RDMS, RVT.)

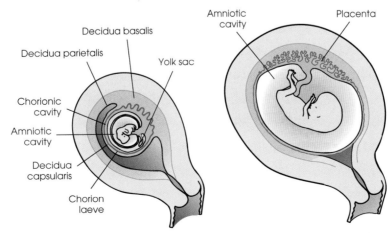

Fig. 28.29 First-trimester representations of developing embryo and yolk sac within amniotic and chorionic cavities of the uterus.

Fig. 28.30 Endovaginal sonogram of first-trimester pregnancy. Yolk sac *(YS)*, embryo, and amnion are easily visualized within fluid-filled gestational sac.

(Courtesy Sharon Ballestero, RT, RDMS.)

During the second trimester (13 to 28 gestational weeks), detailed anatomy of the fetus is identified. Structures such as the brain, face, limbs, spine, abdominal wall, stomach, kidneys, bladder, and heart are evaluated and documented. Measurements of the biparietal diameter, circumference of the fetal head, abdominal circumference, and femur length are used to determine gestational age and are termed *biometric measurements* (Fig. 28.31). Documentation of the placenta, amniotic fluid, and fetal position is also included.

In the third trimester (29 to 40 gestational weeks), the fetus grows an additional 4 inches in length and gains 2000 to 2800 g in weight (4 to 6 lb). Third-trimester ultrasound examinations are generally requested

Fig. 28.31 (A) Biparietal diameter *(BPD)* is measured perpendicular to falx cerebri in a plane that passes through the third ventricle and thalami. (B) Fetal head circumference is measured in a plane that must include the cavum septi pellucidi *(CSP)* and tentorial hiatus. (C) Abdominal circumference is a cross-sectional measurement slightly superior to cord insertion at junction of left and right portal veins and shows a short length of umbilical vein and left portal vein. (D) Femur length *(FL)* is measured parallel to femoral shaft at level of femoral head cartilage and distal femoral condyle.

(Courtesy Sharon Ballestero, RT, RDMS.)

Fig. 28.32 (A) Early second-trimester sonogram of the fetal face showing anencephaly (frog-face). (B) Sagittal image of early second-trimester fetus showing gastroschisis. (C) Sagittal image of second-trimester fetus showing sacral teratoma *(arrow)*. (D) Sagittal image of left kidney showing hydronephrosis.

(B, Courtesy Sharon Ballestero, RT, RDMS; C, courtesy B. Alex Stewart, RT, RDMS.)

to evaluate fetal growth and position, amniotic fluid volume, and placental placement.

Obstetric sonography is a safe imaging modality for evaluating normal and abnormal development of embryologic and fetal anatomy. A detailed ultrasound examination can assess complications of pregnancy, such as ectopic pregnancy, fetal demise, neural tube defects, nuchal cord, skeletal or limb anomalies, cardiac defects, gastrointestinal and genitourinary defects, and head anomalies (Fig. 28.32). Evaluation of the fetus using three-dimensional and four-dimensional imaging is not presently a routine part of obstetric screening examinations (Fig. 28.33).

Fig. 28.33 Three-dimensional sonogram of second-trimester fetal face.

(Courtesy Jeanette Burlbaw, BS, RDMS, FSDMS, FAIUM.)

Fig. 28.34 Sagittal sonogram of carotid artery and bifurcation *(arrow)* into internal and external carotid arteries.

VASCULAR APPLICATIONS

Sonography applications for evaluating the hemodynamics and anatomy of vascular structures continue to increase. Color Doppler imaging and spectral analysis can evaluate blood flow characteristics of the vascular structures in the neck, upper and lower extremities, abdomen, and pelvis. RVTs have specialized education and training in arterial and venous anatomy, hemodynamics, arterial and venous abnormalities, and additional physiologic vascular testing (i.e., pulse volume recording).

Abdominal duplex examinations are requested in patients with a history or suspicion of portal hypertension, mesenteric ischemia, renal artery stenosis, and portal vein thrombosis. Spectral analysis of blood flow velocity and direction is evaluated and documented. Specific criteria are used to diagnose the degree of arterial narrowing shown on the spectral analysis.

The extracranial carotid arteries are evaluated using duplex sonography (Fig. 28.34). Arterial patency, blood flow velocity, resistance, direction, and evidence of turbulence are evaluated with color Doppler and spectral analysis. The highest flow velocities in the common carotid, internal carotid, external carotid, vertebral, and subclavian arteries are recorded. The velocity difference between the common and internal carotid arteries is used to diagnose the degree or percentage of stenosis (i.e., 50%) (Fig. 28.35).

Fig. 28.35 (A) Sagittal image of carotid artery with high-grade stenosis in proximal internal carotid artery. (B) Color Doppler and spectral analysis show increases in flow velocity in stenotic internal carotid artery.

Duplex sonograms of the lower extremity arterial arteries are requested in patients with symptoms of claudication, rest pain, a decrease in palpable pedal pulse, and bypass graft surveillance. Patients with a clinical history of hypertension, cigarette smoking, and diabetes mellitus have an increased risk of developing peripheral arterial disease. Duplex examination of the lower extremities begins at the distal aorta. The common and external iliac arteries are examined for any inflow abnormalities. The common femoral, deep femoral, femoral, popliteal, anterior tibial, posterior tibial, and peroneal arteries are evaluated in grayscale, with color Doppler and spectral analysis for patency, plaque formation, increases in flow velocity, and, when applicable, degree of stenosis. Upper extremity arterial duplex examinations are requested in patients with arm or hand pain, asymmetric blood pressures, and changes in skin pallor. Using duplex sonography, the subclavian, axillary, brachial, ulnar, and radial arteries are evaluated for patency, plaque formation, increase in flow velocities, and, when applicable, degree of stenosis.

Duplex sonographic examination of the lower extremity veins is an inexpensive imaging modality to evaluate for deep vein thrombosis and venous insufficiency. Acute or chronic leg pain, edema, changes in skin pigmentation, and varicose veins are indications for a lower extremity venous duplex sonogram.

When evaluating for deep vein thrombosis, the deep system is evaluated for patency and phasic flow. Incompetence of the venous valve is the most common cause of varicose vein development. When evaluating for venous insufficiency, the deep venous system is evaluated for patency and valve competency. The small and great saphenous veins are measured and evaluated for patency, valve competency, and association with varicosities. Visible perforator veins are also evaluated for patency and valve competency. The sonographer provides a technical report to the reading physician detailing the findings regarding evidence of lower extremity deep vein thrombosis, venous insufficiency, and possible source of varicosities (Fig. 28.36). Upper extremity venous examinations are requested in patients with indwelling catheters, arm or hand swelling, and arm pain. The internal jugular, subclavian, axillary, brachial, cephalic, and basilic veins are evaluated for patency and *phasic flow*.

Additional physiologic testing is used to evaluate peripheral arterial and venous flow. The ankle/brachial index (ABI), venous return time, and pulse volume recording are examples of nonimaging vascular testing.

Cardiologic Applications

Real-time echocardiography of the fetal, neonatal, pediatric, and adult heart has proven to be a tremendous diagnostic aid for the cardiologist and internist. Multiple imaging windows are used to image cardiac anatomy in detail, including the four chambers of the heart, four heart valves (mitral, tricuspid, aortic, and pulmonic), interventricular and interatrial septa, muscular wall of the ventricles, papillary muscles, and chordae tendineae cordis. Difficult cases can be imaged using a transesophageal technique in which the transducer is passed from the mouth, through the esophagus, to the orifice of the stomach.

PROCEDURE FOR ECHOCARDIOGRAPHY

The echocardiographic examination begins with the patient in a left lateral decubitus position. This position allows the heart to move away from the sternum and fall closer to the chest wall, providing a better cardiac "window," or open area, for the sonographer to image. The transducer is placed in the third, fourth, or fifth intercostal space to the left of the sternum. The protocol for a complete echocardiographic examination includes images in the long axis, short axis, apical, and suprasternal windows (Fig. 28.37). Contrast agents improve visualization of viable myocardial tissue.

CARDIAC PATHOLOGY

Echocardiography is used to evaluate many cardiac conditions. Atherosclerosis or previous rheumatic fever may lead to scarring, calcification, and thickening of the valve leaflets. With these conditions, valve tissue destruction continues, causing stenosis and regurgitation of the leaflets and subsequent chamber enlargement.

The effects of sub-bacterial endocarditis can also be evaluated with echocardiography. With this infectious process, multiple small vegetations form on the endocardial surface of the valve leaflets, causing the leaflets to tear or thicken, with resultant severe regurgitation into subsequent cardiac chambers. The echocardiogram of a patient with congestive cardiomyopathy shows generalized four-chamber enlargement, valve regurgitation, and the threat of thrombus formation along the nonfunctioning ventricular wall. The pericardial sac surrounds the ventricles and right atrium, and may fill with fluid, impairing normal cardiac function.

Analysis of ventricular function and serial evaluation of patients after a myocardial infarction are accomplished with two-dimensional echocardiography and, in some cases, stress dobutamine echocardiography. Complications of myocardial infarction include rupture of the ventricular septum, development of a left ventricular aneurysm in the weakest area of the wall, and coagulation of thrombus in the akinetic or immobile apex of the left ventricle (Fig. 28.38).

Fig. 28.36 (A) Transverse sonograms of popliteal artery and vein without compression *(left image)* and with compression *(right image)* showing a deep vein thrombosis.
(B) Sagittal sonogram of popliteal vein showing echogenic thrombus *(arrow)*.
(C) Spectral analysis of great saphenous vein shows venous reflux during Valsalva maneuver signifying venous incompetence at this level.

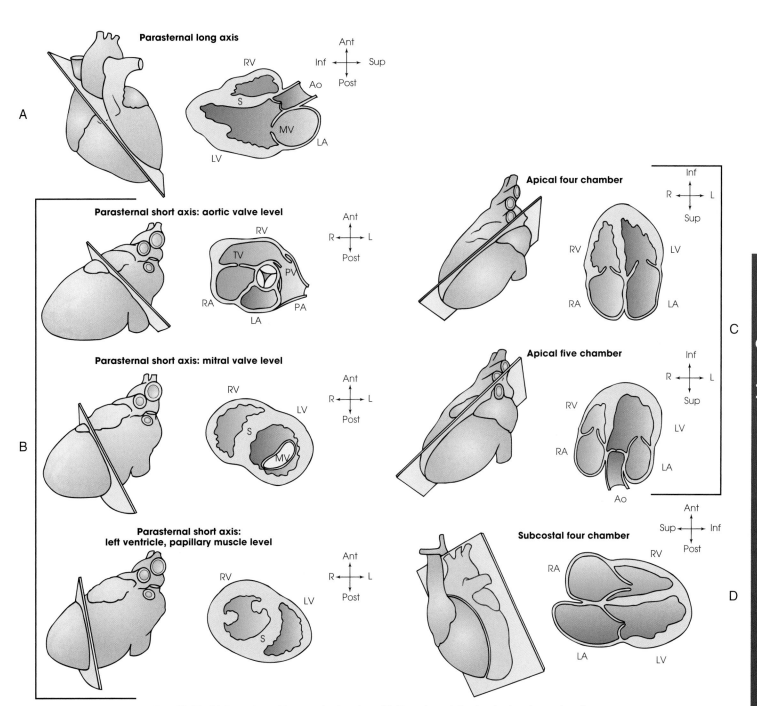

Parasternal long axis

RV
Ao
S
MV
LV
LA

Ant
Inf ←→ Sup
Post

A

Parasternal short axis: aortic valve level

RV
TV
PV
RA
LA
PA

Ant
R ←→ L
Post

Parasternal short axis: mitral valve level

RV
LV
S
MV

Ant
R ←→ L
Post

B

**Parasternal short axis:
left ventricle, papillary muscle level**

RV
LV
S

Ant
R ←→ L
Post

Apical four chamber

RV
LV
RA
LA

Inf
R ←→ L
Sup

C

Apical five chamber

RV
LV
RA
LA
Ao

Inf
R ←→ L
Sup

Subcostal four chamber

RV
RA
LA
LV

Ant
Sup ←→ Inf
Post

D

Fig. 28.37 (A) Parasternal long-axis drawing. (B) Parasternal short-axis drawings at various levels: aortic valve level; mitral valve level; and left ventricle, papillary muscle level. (C) Apical four-chamber image and apical five-chamber image. (D) Subcostal four-chamber image. *Ao,* Aorta; *LA,* left atrium; *LV,* left ventricle; *MV,* mitral valve; *PA,* pulmonary artery; *PV,* pulmonic valve; *RA,* right atrium; *RV,* right ventricle; *S,* septum; *TV,* tricuspid valve.

Congenital heart lesions

Echocardiography has been used to diagnose congenital lesions of the heart in fetuses, neonates, and young children. The cardiac sonographer is able to assess abnormalities of the four cardiac valves, determine the size of the cardiac chambers, assess the interatrial and interventricular septum for the presence of shunt flow, and identify the continuity of the aorta and pulmonary artery with the ventricular chambers to look for abnormal attachment relationships.

A premature infant has an improved chance of survival if the correct diagnosis is made early. If the neonate is cyanotic, congenital heart disease or respiratory failure may be rapidly diagnosed with echocardiography. Critical cyanotic disease in a premature infant may include hypoplastic left heart syndrome, transposition of the great vessels with pulmonary atresia, or severe tetralogy of Fallot.

Conclusion

The contribution of diagnostic ultrasound to clinical medicine has been assisted by technologic advances in instrumentation and transducer design, an increased ability to process the returned echo information, and an improved methodology for three-dimensional reconstruction of images. The development of high-frequency *endovaginal, endorectal,* and *transesophageal transducers* with endoscopic imaging has aided the visualization of previously difficult areas. Improved computer capabilities and advances in teleradiography have enabled the sonographer to obtain more information and process multiple data points to obtain a comprehensive report from the ultrasound study. Color-flow Doppler has made it possible for the sonographer to distinguish the direction and velocity of arterial and venous blood flow from vascular and other pathologic structures in the body. Doppler has allowed the sonographer to determine the exact area of obstruction or leakage present, and to determine precisely the degree of turbulence within a vessel or cardiac chamber.

Modifications in transducer design have improved resolution in superficial structures, muscles, and tendons. Advancements in equipment and transducer design have also improved the results of ultrasound examinations in neonates and children. Increased sensitivity allows the sonographer to define the texture of organs and glands with more detail and greater tissue differentiation. Improvements in resolution have aided the visualization of small cleft palate defects, abnormal development of fingers and toes, and small spinal defects. The ability to image the detail of the fetal heart has assisted the early diagnosis of congenital heart disease.

Advanced research and development of computer analysis and tissue characterization of echo reflections should contribute further to the total diagnostic approach using ultrasound. Various abdominal contrast agents continue to be investigated to improve visualization of the stomach, the pancreas, and the small and large intestines. Cardiac contrast agents are already being used to improve the visualization of viable myocardial tissue within the heart. Saline and other contrast agents are being injected into the endometrial cavity to outline the lining of the endometrium for the purpose of distinguishing polyps and other lesions from the normal endometrium.

Ultrasound has rapidly emerged as a powerful, inexpensive, diagnostic imaging modality with various applications in patient management and care. Expected advancements include further developments in transducer design, image resolution, tissue characterization applications, color-flow sensitivity, and four-dimensional reconstruction of images.

Fig. 28.38 Apical four-chamber image with large apical thrombus. This thrombus *(arrows)*, which is distinguished from an artifact because it is located in a region with abnormal wall motion, is attached to the apical endocardium, has well-defined borders, and moves in the same direction as the apex. *LA,* Left atrium; *LV,* left ventricle; *RA,* right atrium; *RV,* right ventricle.

Definition of Terms

acoustic impedance Resistance of sound as it propagates through a medium.

acoustic window Ability of sonography to visualize a particular area. The full urinary bladder is a good acoustic window to image the uterus and ovaries in a transabdominal sonogram. The intercostal margins may be a good acoustic window to image the liver parenchyma.

anechoic Property of being free of echoes or without echoes.

angle of incidence Angle at which the ultrasound beam strikes an interface with respect to normal (perpendicular) incidence.

ankle/brachial index (ABI) Ratio of ankle pressure to brachial pressure to provide a general guide to help determine the degree of disability of the lower extremity.

attenuation Weakening of the sound wave as it propagates through a medium.

axial resolution Ability to distinguish two structures along a path parallel to the sound beam.

biparietal diameter (BPD) Largest dimension of the fetal head perpendicular to the midsagittal plane; measured by ultrasonic visualization and used to measure fetal development.

color-flow Doppler Velocity in each direction is quantified by allocating a pixel to each area; each velocity frequency change is allocated a color.

complex Containing anechoic and echogenic areas.

continuous wave ultrasound Wave in which cycles repeat indefinitely; consists of a separate transmit and receive transducer housed within one assembly.

coronal image plane Anatomic term used to describe a plane perpendicular to the sagittal and transverse planes of the body.

detail resolution Includes axial and lateral resolution.

Doppler effect Shift in frequency or wavelength, depending on the conditions of observation; caused by relative motions among sources, receivers, and medium.

Doppler ultrasound Application of Doppler effect to ultrasound to detect movement of a reflecting boundary relative to the source, resulting in a change of the wavelength of the reflected wave.

duplex imaging Combination of grayscale real-time imaging and color or spectral Doppler.

echogenic Refers to a medium that contains echo-producing structures.

embryo Term used for a developing zygote through the 10th week of gestation.

endometrium Inner layer of the uterine canal.

endorectal transducer High-frequency transducer that can be inserted into the rectum to visualize the bladder and prostate gland.

endovaginal transducer High-frequency transducer (and decreased penetration) that can be inserted into the vagina to obtain high-resolution images of the pelvic structures.

false pelvis Region above the pelvic brim.

fetus Term used for the developing embryo from the 11th gestational week until birth.

follicular cyst Functional or physiologic ovulatory cyst consisting of an ovum surrounded by a layer of cells.

frequency Number of cycles per unit of time, usually expressed in Hertz (Hz) or megahertz (MHz) (a million cycles per second).

gestational age Length of time calculated from the first day of the last menstrual period; also known as gestational weeks.

gestational sac Fluid-filled structure normally found in the uterus containing the pregnancy.

grayscale Range of amplitudes (brightness) between white and black.

heterogeneous Having a mixed composition.

homogeneous Having a uniform composition.

hyperechoic Producing more echoes than normal.

hypoechoic Producing less echoes than normal.

iliopectineal line Bony ridge on the inner surface of the ileum and pubic bones that divides the true and false pelvis.

intima Inner layer of the vessel; the middle layer is the media and the outer layer is the adventitia.

ischemia Area of the cardiac myocardium that has been damaged by disruption of the blood supply by the coronary arteries.

isoechoic Having a texture nearly the same as that of the surrounding parenchyma.

lateral resolution Ability to distinguish two structures lying perpendicular to the sound beam.

leiomyoma Most common benign tumor of the uterine myometrium.

myometrium Thick middle layer of the uterine wall.

noninvasive technique Procedure that does not require the skin to be broken or an organ or cavity to be entered (e.g., taking the pulse).

oblique plane Slanting direction or any variation that is not starting at a right angle to any axis.

parenchyma Functional tissue or cells of an organ or gland.

phasic flow Normal venous respiratory variations.

piezoelectric effect Conversion of pressure to electrical voltage or conversion of electrical voltage to mechanical pressure.

porta hepatis Region in hepatic hilum containing common duct, proper hepatic artery, and main portal vein.

posterior acoustic enhancement Increase in reflection amplitude from structures that lie behind a weakly attenuating structure (i.e., cyst).

posterior acoustic shadowing Reduction in reflection amplitude from reflectors lying behind a strongly reflecting or attenuating structure.

pulse wave ultrasound A transducer emits short pulses of ultrasound into the human body and receives reflections from the body before emitting another pulse of sound.

real-time imaging Imaging with rapid frame rate visualizing moving structures or scan planes continuously.

reflection Redirection (return) of a portion of the sound beam back to the transducer.

refraction Phenomenon of bending wave fronts as the acoustic energy propagates from the medium of one acoustic velocity to a second medium of differing acoustic velocity.

regurgitation Occurs when blood leaks from one high-pressure chamber to a chamber of lower pressure.

resolution Measure of ability to display two closely spaced structures as discrete targets.

retroperitoneal cavity Area posterior to the peritoneal cavity that contains the aorta, inferior vena cava, pancreas, part of the duodenum and colon, kidneys, and adrenal glands.

retrouterine pouch Pelvic space located anterior to the rectum and posterior to the uterus; also known as pouch of Douglas.

sagittal Plane that travels vertically from the top to the bottom of the body along the *y* axis.

scattering Diffusion or redirection of sound in several directions on encountering a particle suspension or rough surface.

sonar Instrument used to discover objects under the water and to show their location.

sound wave Longitudinal waves of mechanical energy propagated through a medium.

transducer Device that converts energy from one form to another.

transverse Plane that passes through the width of the body in a horizontal direction.

ultrasound Sound with a frequency greater than 20 kHz.

velocity of sound Speed with direction of motion specified.

Selected bibliography

Callen PW: *Ultrasonography in obstetrics and gynecology*, ed 6, Philadelphia, 2017, Saunders.

Curry RA, Tempkin BB: *Ultrasonography: an introduction to normal structure and function*, ed 4, Philadelphia, 2016, Saunders.

Hagen-Ansert SL: *Textbook of diagnostic ultrasonography* (vol I and II). ed 7, St Louis, 2012, Elsevier Mosby.

Henningsen C, Kuntz K, Youngs D: *Clinical guide to ultrasonography*, ed 2, St Louis, 2014, Mosby.

Kremkau FW: *Diagnostic ultrasound principles and instrumentation*, ed 9, St Louis, 2016, Saunders.

Ovel S: *Sonography exam review: physics, abdomen, obstetrics and gynecology*, ed 2, St Louis, 2014, Mosby.

Rumack CM, et al: *Diagnostic ultrasound*, ed 4, St Louis, 2011, Elsevier Mosby.

Zweibel WJ, Pellerito J, editors: *Introduction to vascular ultrasonography*, ed 6, St Louis, 2012.

29

NUCLEAR MEDICINE AND MOLECULAR IMAGING

RAYMOND J. JOHNSON

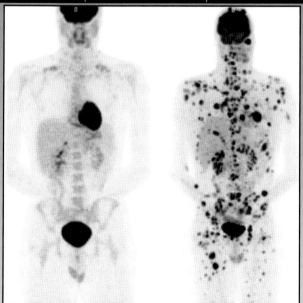

Principles of Nuclear Medicine

Nuclear medicine is a medical specialty that focuses on the use of radioactive materials called *radiopharmaceuticals*.[a] Radiopharmaceuticals are used for diagnosis, therapy, and medical research. In contrast to typical radiographic procedures that determine the presence of disease based on structural appearance, nuclear medicine determines the cause of a medical problem based on the physiologic function of organs or tissues.

For a nuclear medicine procedure, the radiopharmaceutical, commonly referred to as a *radiotracer* or *tracer,* is primarily introduced into the body through a multitude of ways. These include but are not limited to, injection (intravenous, intradermal, or intrathecal), ingestion, or inhalation. Different radiotracers are used to study different parts of the body. Specific tracers are selected based on their ability to localize in specific organs or tissues. Radiotracers undergo radioactive decay to produce gamma-ray emissions that allow for the detection of the tracer's presence. A special piece of equipment, known as a *gamma* or *scintillation camera,* is used to transform these emissions into images that provide information about the function (primarily) and anatomy of the organ or system being studied. Physicians attempt to prescribe the lowest amount of radiotracer in each exam to reduce the radiation exposure to the patient without compromising image quality.

Nuclear medicine procedures are performed by a team of specially educated professionals: a nuclear medicine physician, a specialist with extensive education in the basic and clinical science of medicine who is licensed to use radioactive materials; a nuclear medicine technologist who performs the tests and is educated in the theory and practice of nuclear medicine procedures; a physicist who is experienced in the technology of nuclear medicine and the care of the equipment; and a radiopharmacist who is qualified to prepare the necessary radioactive pharmaceuticals.

Historical Development

John Dalton is considered the father of the modern theory of atoms and molecules. In 1803, Dalton, an English schoolteacher, stated that all atoms of a given element are chemically identical, unchanged by chemical reaction, and combine in a ratio of simple numbers. Dalton measured atomic weights in reference to hydrogen, to which he assigned the value of 1 (the atomic number of this element).

The discovery of x-rays by Wilhelm Conrad Roentgen in 1895 was a great contribution to physics and the care of the sick. A few months later, another physicist, Antoine Henri Becquerel, discovered naturally occurring radioactive substances. In 1898, Marie Curie discovered two new elements in the uranium ore pitchblende. Curie named these trace elements polonium (after her homeland, Poland) and radium. Curie also coined the terms *radioactive* and *radioactivity*.

GENERAL NUCLEAR MEDICINE

In 1923, George de Hevesy, often called the "father of nuclear medicine," developed the tracer principle. He coined the term "radioindicator" and extended his studies from inorganic to organic chemistry. The first radioindicators were naturally occurring substances such as radium and radon. The invention of the *cyclotron* by Ernest Lawrence in 1931 made it possible for de Hevesy to expand his studies to a broader spectrum of biologic processes by using ^{32}P (phosphorus-32), ^{22}Na (sodium-22), and other cyclotron-produced (synthetic) radioactive tracers.

Radioactive elements began to be produced in *nuclear reactors* developed by Enrico Fermi and colleagues in 1946. The nuclear reactor greatly extended the ability of the cyclotron to produce radioactive tracers. A key development was the introduction of the *gamma camera* by Hal Anger in 1958. In the early 1960s, Edwards and Kuhl made the next advance in nuclear medicine with the development of a crude single photon emission computed tomography (SPECT) camera known as the MARK IV. With this new technology, it was possible to create three-dimensional images of organ function instead of the two-dimensional images created previously. It was not until the early 1980s, when computers became fast enough to acquire and process all of the information successfully, that SPECT imaging could become standard practice.

One of the first organs to be examined by nuclear medicine studies using *external radiation detectors* was the thyroid.

In the 1940s, investigators found that the rate of incorporation of radioactive iodine by the thyroid gland was greatly increased in hyperthyroidism (the overproduction of thyroid hormones) and greatly decreased in hypothyroidism (the underproduction of thyroid hormones). Over the years, tracers and instruments were developed to allow almost every major organ of the body to be studied by application of the tracer principle. Subsequently, images were made of structures such as the liver, spleen, brain, and kidneys. Currently, the emphasis of nuclear medicine studies is more on function and chemistry than anatomic structure.

Positron Emission Tomography

With the development of more suitable *scintillators,* such as sodium iodide (NaI), and more sophisticated nuclear counting electronics, positron coincidence localization became possible. In 1951, Wrenn demonstrated the use of positron-emitting radioisotopes for the localization of brain tumors. Gordon Brownell further developed instrumentation for similar studies. The next major advancement came in 1967, when Sir Godfrey Hounsfield demonstrated the clinical use of computed tomography (CT). The mathematics of positron emission tomography (PET) image *reconstruction* is similar to that used for CT reconstruction techniques. Instead of x-rays from a point source traversing the body and being detected by a single or multiple detectors as in CT, PET imaging uses two opposing detectors to count pairs of 511-KeV photons simultaneously that originate from a single positron–electron annihilation event.

From 1967 to 1974, significant developments occurred in computer technology, scintillator materials, and *photomultiplier tube* (PMT) design. In 1975, the first closed-ring transverse positron emission tomograph was built for PET imaging by Michel M. Ter-Pogossian and Michael E. Phelps.

Developments now continue on two fronts that have accelerated the use of PET. First, scientists are approaching the theoretic limits (1 to 2 mm) of PET scanner resolution by employing smaller, more efficient, scintillators and PMTs. Microprocessors tune and adjust the entire ring of *detectors* that surround the patient. Each ring in the PET tomograph

---

[a]Almost all italicized words on the succeeding pages are defined at the end of this chapter.

may contain 1000 detectors, and the tomograph may be composed of 30 to 60 rings. The second major area of development is in the design of new radiopharmaceuticals. Agents are being developed to measure blood flow, metabolism, protein synthesis, lipid content, receptor binding, and many other physiologic parameters and processes.

During the mid-1980s, PET was used predominantly as a research tool. However, by the early 1990s, clinical PET centers had been established, and PET was routinely used for diagnostic procedures on the brain, heart, and tumors. In the mid- to late-1990s, three-dimensional PET systems that eliminated the use of interdetector *septa* were developed. This development allowed the injected dose of the radiopharmaceutical to be reduced by approximately 6- to 10-fold. New image reconstruction methods have been developed to better characterize the distribution of annihilation photons from these three-dimensional systems.

HYBRID IMAGING: PET/CT, AND PET/MRI

Beginning in 2000, major nuclear medicine camera manufacturers developed combined PET and CT systems that can simultaneously acquire PET functional images and CT anatomic images. Both modalities are coregistered or exactly matched in size and position. The success of these camera systems led to the development of combined SPECT and CT systems, as well. Significant benefits are expected for diagnosing metastatic disease because precise localization of the tumor site and function can now be determined. In addition to anatomic registration, CT has allowed for improved attenuation correction (AC) in PET and SPECT. By more accurately mapping the different densities in the body, more accurate correction of the different gamma attenuators can be applied to PET and SPECT image data. Rapid enhancements and developments are anticipated to continue with this technology over the next several years.

In addition to the hybrid fusion of PET and CT, the first PET/magnetic resonance imaging (MRI) system was approved by the U.S. Food and Drug Administration (FDA) for customer purchase in 2011. The integration of PET and MRI is not straightforward and challenges the technical design of both systems. PET/MRI merges the metabolic ability of PET imaging with the morphologic imaging of MRI (see Chapter 26) to generate diagnostic images for oncologic, cardiologic, and neurologic purposes. With only a few PET/MRI systems installed throughout the United States, growth in this area is anxiously anticipated.

Comparison With Other Modalities

Nuclear medicine is predominantly used to measure human cellular, organ, or system function. A parameter that characterizes a particular aspect of human physiology is determined from the measurement of the radioactivity emitted by a radiopharmaceutical in a given volume of tissue. In contrast, conventional radiography measures the structure, size, and position of organs or human anatomy by determining x-ray transmission through a given volume of tissue. X-ray attenuation by structures interposed between the x-ray source and the radiographic image receptor provides the contrast necessary to visualize an organ. CT creates cross-sectional images by computer reconstruction of multiple x-ray transmissions (see Chapter 25). The characteristics of radiologic imaging modalities are compared in Table 29.1.

TABLE 29.1

Comparison of imaging modalities

Modality information	PET	SPECT	MRI	CT
Measures	Physiology	Physiology	Anatomy (physiology)[a]	Anatomy
Resolution	3–5 mm	8–10 mm	0.5–1 mm	1–1.5 mm
Technique	Positron annihilation	Gamma emission	Nuclear magnetic resonance	Absorption of x-rays
Harmful	Radiation exposure	Radiation exposure	None known	Radiation effects exposure
Use	Research and clinical	Clinical	Clinical (research)[a]	Clinical
No. examinations per day	4–12	5–10	10–15	15–20

[a]Secondary function.

SPECT is a conventional nuclear imaging technique that is used to determine tissue function. Because SPECT employs collimators and lower energy photons, it is less sensitive (by 10^1 to 10^5) and less accurate than PET. Generally, PET resolution is better than SPECT resolution by a factor of 2 to 10. PET easily accounts for photon loss through attenuation by performing a *transmission scan*. This is difficult to achieve and not routinely done with SPECT imaging; however, newly designed SPECT instrumentation that couples a low-output x-ray CT to the gamma camera for the collection of attenuation information is now being used to correct for gamma attenuation. Software approaches are also being investigated that assign known *attenuation coefficients* for specific tissues to segmented regions of images for analytic AC of SPECT imaging data.

The differences between the various imaging modalities can be highlighted using a study of brain blood flow as an example. Without an intact circulatory system, an intravenously injected radiotracer cannot make its way into the brain for distribution throughout the brain's capillary network, ultimately diffusing into cells that are well perfused.

For radiographic procedures, such as CT, structures within the brain may be intact, but there may be impaired or limited blood flow to and through major vessels within the brain. Under these circumstances, the CT scan may appear almost normal despite reduced blood flow to the brain. If the circulatory system at the level of the capillaries is not intact, a PET scan can be performed, but no perfusion information is obtained because the radioactive water used to measure blood flow is not transported through the capillaries and diffused into the brain cells.

The image-enhancing contrast agents used in many radiographic studies may cause a toxic reaction (a warm uncomfortable feeling all over the body or even a severe allergic reaction). The x-ray dose to the patient in these radiographic studies is greater than the radiation dose in nuclear imaging studies. The radiotracers used in PET studies are similar to the body's own biochemical constituents and are administered in very small amounts. This biochemical compatibility of the tracers within the body minimizes the risks to the patient because the tracers are not found to be toxic. At the same time, trace amounts minimize any alterations of the body's *homeostasis*.

An imaging technique that augments CT and PET is MRI (see Chapter 26). Images obtained with PET and MRI are shown in Fig. 29.1. MRI is used primarily to measure anatomy or morphology. In contrast to CT, which derives its greatest image contrast from varying tissue densities (bone from soft tissue), MRI better differentiates tissues by their proton content and the degree to which the protons are bound in lattice structures. The tightly bound protons of bone make it virtually transparent to MRI.

CT, MRI, and other anatomic imaging modalities provide complementary information to nuclear medicine imaging and PET. These imaging modalities benefit from *image coregistration* with CT and MRI by pinpointing physiologic function with precise anatomic locations. Greater emphasis is being placed on multimodality image coregistration between PET, CT, SPECT, and MRI for brain research and tumor localization throughout the body (Fig. 29.2). All new PET imaging systems are fused with a CT scanner for AC and anatomic positioning information. Many SPECT imaging systems incorporate CT technology for the same purposes.

Fig. 29.1 Coregistered MRI and PET scans. *Arrows* indicate an abnormality on the anatomic image (A, MRI scan) and the functional image (B, PET scan). ^{18}F-FDG PET image depicts hypometabolic area of seizure focus *(arrow)* in a patient with a diagnosis of epilepsy.

Physical Principles of Nuclear Medicine

An understanding of radioactivity must precede an attempt to grasp the principles of nuclear medicine and how images are created using radioactive compounds. The term *radiation* is taken from the Latin word *radii,* which refers to the spokes of a wheel leading out from a central point. The term *radioactivity* is used to describe the radiation of energy in the form of high-speed *alpha* or *beta particles* or waves (gamma rays) from the nucleus of an atom.

BASIC NUCLEAR PHYSICS

The basic components of an atom include the nucleus (which is composed of varying numbers of protons, and neutrons) and the orbiting electrons (which revolve around the nucleus in discrete energy levels). Protons have a positive electrical charge, electrons have a negative charge, and neutrons are electrically neutral. Protons and neutrons have masses nearly 2000 times the mass of the electron; thus the nucleus is responsible for most of the mass of an atom (~99%). The Bohr atomic model (Fig. 29.3) can describe this configuration. The total number of protons, neutrons, and electrons in an atom determines its characteristics, including its stability.

The term *nuclide* is used to describe an atomic species with a particular arrangement of protons and neutrons within the nucleus. Elements with the same number of protons but a different number of neutrons are referred to as *isotopes.* Isotopes have the same chemical properties as one another because the total number of protons and electrons is the same. They differ simply in the total number of neutrons contained in the nucleus. The neutron-to-proton ratio in the nucleus determines the stability of the atom. At certain ratios, atoms may become unstable, and a process known as spontaneous *decay* can occur as the atom attempts to regain stability. Energy is released in various ways during this decay process, or as it returns to its *ground state.*

Radionuclides decay by the emission of alpha, beta, and/or gamma radiation. For most radionuclides to reach their ground state, it usually requires multiple steps and various decay processes. This can include any array of the following; alpha, beta, or positron emission; *electron capture;* and several other methods. These decay methods determine the type of particles or gamma rays given off as the radionuclide decays.

To explain this process better, investigators have created decay schemes to show the details of how a *parent* nuclide decays to its *daughter* or ground state (Fig. 29.4A). A decay scheme is a simple illustration depicting how a radionuclide decays. Each radionuclide has its own unique decay scheme, similar to a fingerprint, which identifies the type(s) of decay, the energy associated with each process, the probability of a particular process, the probability of a particular

decay process occurring, and the rate of change into the ground state element (see Fig. 29.4B).

Radioactive decay is considered a purely random and spontaneous process that can be mathematically defined by complex equations and represented by average decay rates. The term *half-life* is used to describe the time it takes for a quantity of a particular radionuclide to decay to one half of its original activity or one half of the original number of atoms through spontaneous disintegration. The rate of decay has an exponential function, which can be plotted on a linear scale (see Fig. 29.4C). If plotted on a semilogarithmic scale, the decay rate would be represented as a straight line. Radionuclide half-lives can range anywhere from milliseconds to years. The half-lives of most radionuclides used in nuclear medicine range from several seconds to several days.

NUCLEAR PHARMACY (RADIOPHARMACY)

Naturally occurring radionuclides have very long half-lives (i.e., thousands of years). These natural radionuclides are unsuitable for nuclear medicine imaging because of limited availability and the high-absorbed dose the patient would receive. The radionuclides used in nuclear medicine (general and PET) are produced in nuclear reactors' generators, or *particle accelerators.* Radionuclides can be created in nuclear reactors

Fig. 29.2 Combined single photon emission computed tomography/computed tomography camera for a blending of imaging function and form.

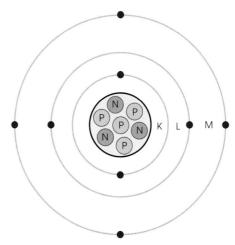

Fig. 29.3 Diagram of Bohr atom containing a single nucleus of protons (*P*) and neutrons (*N*) with surrounding orbital electrons of varying energy levels (e.g., *K, L, M*).

either by inserting a target element into the reactor core where it is irradiated or by separating and collecting the *fission* byproducts. One of these byproducts is molybdenum-99 (^{99}Mo), which is used in the production of technetium-99m (^{99m}Tc) through a *generator system*. The radionuclides for nuclear medicine are produced in a particle accelerator or cyclotron through nuclear reactions created between a specific target chemical and high-speed charged particles. The number of protons in the target nuclei is changed when the nuclei are bombarded by the high-speed charged particles, and a new element or radionuclide is produced.

Radionuclides used for general nuclear medicine procedures include ^{99m}Tc, ^{123}I (iodine), ^{131}I (iodine), ^{111}In (indium), ^{201}Tl (thallium), and ^{67}Ga (gallium). Labeled compounds with these high atomic weight radionuclides often do not mimic the physiologic properties of natural occurring substances found in the body. This is due to their size, mass, and different chemical properties. Compounds labeled with traditional nuclear medicine radionuclides are also found to be poor radioactive *analogs* for other natural substances. Imaging studies with these agents are qualitative and emphasize nonbiochemical properties.

Radionuclides used in PET include ^{11}C (carbon), ^{13}N (nitrogen), and ^{15}O (oxygen). The elements hydrogen, carbon, nitrogen, and oxygen are the predominant constituents of natural compounds found in the body. Different from common nuclear medicine radionuclides, these emit positrons, have low atomic weight, and can directly replace their stable isotopes in substrates, metabolites, drugs, and other biologically active compounds. This is also achieved without disrupting any bodily biochemical mechanisms and processes. For example, the most commonly used PET radionuclide, ^{18}F (fluorine), can replace hydrogen in many molecules,

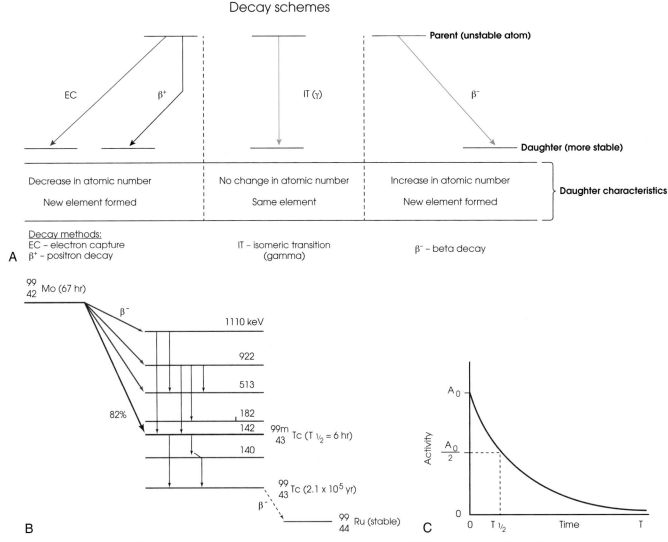

Fig. 29.4 (A) Four types of decay schemes and pathways. (B) Decay scheme illustrating the method by which radioactive molybdenum (^{99}Mo) decays to radioactive technetium (^{99m}Tc), one of the most commonly used radiopharmaceuticals in nuclear medicine. (C) Graphic representation showing the rate of physical decay of a radionuclide. The y (*vertical*) axis represents the amount of radioactivity, and the x (*horizontal*) axis represents the time at which a specific amount of activity has decreased to one-half of its initial value. Every radionuclide has an associated half-life that is representative of its rate of decay.

providing an even greater assortment of biologic analogs.

The most commonly used radionuclide in nuclear medicine is ^{99m}Tc, which is produced in a generator system. This apparatus makes available desirable short-lived radionuclides (the *daughters*), which are formed by the decay of relatively longer lived radionuclides (the *parents*). The generator system uses ^{99}Mo as the parent; ^{99}Mo has a half-life of 66.7 hours and decays (86% of the time) to a daughter product known as *metastable* ^{99m}Tc. Because ^{99m}Tc and ^{99}Mo are chemically different, they can easily be separated through an ion-exchange column. ^{99m}Tc exhibits nearly ideal characteristics for use in nuclear medicine examinations, including a relatively short physical half-life

of 6.04 hours and a high-yield yield of low-energy gamma photons (98.6% at 140-keV) (see Fig. 29.4B).

A radiopharmaceutical generally has two components: a radionuclide and a *pharmaceutical.* The pharmaceutical is a biologically active compound chosen on the basis of its preferential localization or participation in the physiologic function of a given organ. A radionuclide is the radioactive material used to tag the pharmaceutical, which allows for the localization of the compound within the body (Fig. 29.5). After the radiopharmaceutical is administered, the target organ is localized by means of the physiologic pharmaceutical distribution, and the radiation emitted from it can be detected by imaging instruments, or gamma cameras.

The following characteristics are desirable in an imaging radiopharmaceutical:
- Ease of production, low cost, and readily available
- Lowest possible radiation dose to the patient
- Primary photon energy between 100 keV and 400 keV
- Physical half-life greater than the time required to prepare the material, deliver it, and use it
- Effective half-life longer than the examination time
- Suitable chemical forms for rapid localization
- Different uptake in the structure to be detected than in the surrounding tissue
- Low toxicity in the chemical form administered to the patient
- Stability or near-stability

Because most radiopharmaceuticals are administered intravenously, they need to be sterile and *pyrogen-free.* They also need to undergo all of the quality control measures required of conventional drugs.

A commonly used radiopharmaceutical is ^{99m}Tc tagged to a macroaggregated albumin (MAA). After intravenous injection, this substance follows the pathway of blood flow to the lungs, where it is distributed throughout and trapped in the small pulmonary capillaries (Fig. 29.6).

Radionuclide + Pharmaceutical = Radiopharmaceutical

Fig. 29.5 A radionuclide is chosen based on the characteristics of its gamma emission and ability to tag to a specific pharmaceutical; the pharmaceutical is chosen based on its ability to localize to a specific organ or function. When combined, a radiopharmaceutical, *or tracer,* is formed.

POSTERIOR   RPO   RT. LATERAL   LPO

PERFUSION LUNG SCAN

LT. LATERAL   ANTERIOR

DIACAM

MATRIX: 128 X 128

DOSE: 3 mCi 99mTc-MAA

COUNTS: 500K / VIEW

H: 46 YEAR OLD FEMALE
HISTORY OF SHORTNESS OF BREATH

D: NORMAL LUNG STUDY

Fig. 29.6 Normal perfusion lung scan using 3 mCi of ^{99m}Tc tagged to a macroaggregated albumin (^{99m}Tc MAA) on a large field-of-view gamma camera approximately 5 minutes after injection of the radiopharmaceutical. *LPO,* left posterior oblique; *RPO,* right posterior oblique.

(Courtesy Siemens Medical Systems, Iselin, NJ.)

Blood clots along the pathway prevent this radiopharmaceutical from distributing in the area beyond the clot. As a result, the image shows a void or clear area, often described as *photopenia* or a *cold spot*. More than 30 different radiopharmaceuticals are used in nuclear medicine (Table 29.2).

Radioactivity is measured using either the *becquerel* (Bq), which corresponds to the decay rate, expressed as 1 disintegration per second (dps), or as the *curie* (Ci), which equals 3.73×10^{10} dps, relative to the number of decaying atoms in 1 g of radium.

TABLE 29.2
Radiopharmaceuticals used in nuclear medicine

Radionuclide	Symbol	Physical half-life	Chemical form	Diagnostic use
Carbon	^{11}C	20.4 min	Sodium acetate	Oncology and myocardial imaging
			Choline	Oncology imaging
Fluorine	^{18}F	110 min	Fluorodeoxyglucose	Oncology and myocardial hibernation
			Sodium fluoride	Bone imaging
Gallium	^{67}Ga	77 h	Gallium citrate	Inflammatory process and tumor imaging
Indium	^{111}In	67.4 h	DTPA	Cerebrospinal fluid imaging
			Ibritumomab tiuxetan	Localization of tumor
			OctreoScan (pentetreotide)	Neuroendocrine tumors
			ProstaScint (capromab pendetide)	Prostate cancer
			Oxine	White blood cell/abscess imaging
Iodine	^{123}I	13.3 h	Sodium iodide	Thyroid function and imaging
			Human serum albumin	Plasma volume
	^{131}I	8 days	Sodium iodide	Thyroid function, imaging, and therapy
			Hippurate	Renal function
Nitrogen	^{13}N	10 min	Ammonia	Myocardial perfusion
Oxygen	^{15}O	2.03 min	Water $(^{15}O)H_2O$	Oncology and myocardial blood flow agent
			Gas	Cerebral blood flow imaging
Rubidium	^{82}Rb	75 s	Rubidium chloride	Cardiovascular imaging
Technetium	^{99m}Tc	6 h	Sodium pertechnetate	Imaging of brain, thyroid, scrotum, salivary glands, renal perfusion, and pericardial effusion; evaluation of left-to-right cardiac shunts
			Sulfur colloid	Imaging of liver and spleen and renal transplants, lymphoscintigraphy
			Macroaggregated albumin	Lung imaging
			Sestamibi	Cardiovascular imaging, myocardial perfusion
			DTPA	Brain and renal imaging
			DMSA	Renal imaging
			MAG3	Renal imaging
			Diphosphonate	Bone imaging
			Pyrophosphate	Bone and myocardial imaging
			Red blood cells	Cardiac function imaging
			HMPAO	Functional brain imaging and white blood cell/abscess imaging
			Iminodiacetic derivations	Liver function imaging
			Neurolite (Bicisate)	Brain imaging
			Myoview (Tetrofosmin)	Myocardial perfusion
			Cardiolite (Sestamibi)	Myocardial perfusion
Thallium	^{201}Tl	73.5 h	Thallous chloride	Myocardial imaging
Xenon	^{133}Xe	5.3 days	Xenon gas	Lung ventilation imaging

DMSA, Dimercaptosuccinic acid; *DTPA,* diethylenetriamine pentaacetic acid; *HMPAO,* hexamethylpropyleneamine oxime; *MAG3,* mertiatide.

Radiopharmaceutical Dosing

Prescribed radiopharmaceutical doses vary depending on the radionuclide used, the examination to be performed, the pathology involved, the size (kg), and the age of the patient. A radiologist will usually set an acceptable dose range to administer an adult patient based on the factors listed above. Pediatric patients only receive a fraction of the adult dose. Currently, there are several formulas used to calculate an appropriate pediatric dose (Fig. 29.7). All pediatric doses provided in this chapter reference the *North American Consensus Guidelines for Pediatric Administered Radiopharmaceutical Activities*.

Pediatric dose formulas:

A) North American Consensus Guidelines*:

    mCi / kg (with min and max)

B) European Association of Nuclear Medicine (EANM):**

    Activity to be administered = baseline activity × multiplier

C) Body weight:

    mCi / kg (with min and max)

D) Body surface area (BSA):

$$\frac{\sqrt{Mass\ (kg) \times height\ (cm)}}{3600} = BSA$$

E) Clark's rule (assumes adult weight of 70 kg):

$$\frac{(Adult\ dose) \times (Child's\ weight\ (kg))}{70\ kg} = Activity\ to\ be\ administered$$

F) Webster's rule (age based):

$$\frac{(Adult\ dose) \times (Patient's\ age + 1)}{Age + 7} = Activity\ to\ be\ administered$$

G) Young's rule (age based):

$$\frac{(Adult\ dose) \times (Patient's\ age)}{Age + 12} = Activity\ to\ be\ administered$$

H) Fried's rule (age based):

$$\frac{(Adult\ dose) \times (Patient's\ age\ (in\ months))}{150} = Activity\ to\ be\ administered$$

*The North American Consensus Guidelines has created a weight-based table (mCi/kg) identifying pediatric doses based on the isotope, radiopharmaceutical (RP), and exam.

**The EANM created a dosing reference card. Depending on the isotope and RP, a *Class* (A, B, or C) and *Baseline Activity* are assigned. Using the card, the patient's weight is referenced against the class, providing a *multiplier*. This is then multiplied by the Baseline Activity to identify the prescribed dose.

Fig. 29.7 Pediatric dose formulas.

Radiation Safety in Nuclear Medicine

The radiation protection requirements in nuclear medicine differ from the general radiation safety measures used for diagnostic radiography. The radionuclides employed in nuclear medicine are in liquid, solid, or gaseous form. Because of the nature of radioactive decay, these radionuclides continuously emit radiation (in contrast to diagnostic x-rays, which can be turned on and off mechanically). Thus, special radiation safety precautions are required.

Technologists and nuclear pharmacists are required to wear appropriate radiation monitoring (dosimetry) devices, such as radiation badges and thermoluminescent dosimetry (TLD) rings, to monitor radiation exposure to the body and hands. The *ALARA* (as low as reasonably achievable) principle/program applies to all nuclear medicine personnel at all times.

Generally, the quantities of radioactive tracers used in nuclear medicine present no significant hazard. Nonetheless, care must be taken to reduce unnecessary exposure. The high concentrations or activities of the radionuclides used in a nuclear pharmacy necessitate the establishment of a designated preparation area. These elected rooms are called *hot labs* and usually contain isolated ventilation, protective lead or leaded glass shielding for vials and syringes, absorbent materials, and gloves. The handling and administration of diagnostic doses to patients warrants the use of gloves and a lead or tungsten syringe shield, which is especially effective for reduction of exposure to the technologist's hands and fingers (Fig. 29.8).

Any spilled radioactive material continues to emit radiation and must be cleaned up and contained immediately. Because radioactive material that contacts the skin can be absorbed and may not be easily washed off, it is very important to wear appropriate personal protective equipment (e.g., lab coat and gloves) when handling radiopharmaceuticals.

Fig. 29.8 (A) Area in a radiopharmacy in which doses of radiopharmaceuticals are prepared in a clean and protected environment. (B) Nuclear medicine technologist administering a radiopharmaceutical intravenously using appropriate radiation safety precautions, including gloves and a syringe shield.

Instrumentation in Nuclear Medicine

MODERN-DAY GAMMA CAMERA

The term *scintillate* means to emit light photons. Becquerel discovered that ionizing radiation caused certain materials to glow. A scintillation material is a sensitive element that emits light photons after being exposed to ionizing radiation. When a light-sensitive device is affixed to this material, the flash of light can be converted into small electrical impulses.

Together, this is known as a *scintillation detector*. The electrical impulses are amplified and counted to determine the amount and nature of radiation striking the scintillating materials. Scintillation detectors were used in the development of the first-generation nuclear medicine scanner—the rectilinear scanner—which was built in 1950.

Scanners have evolved into complex imaging systems known today as *gamma cameras* (because they detect gamma rays). The gamma camera has many components that work together to produce an image (Fig. 29.9). These cameras are scintillation detectors that use a thallium-activated sodium iodide crystal to detect and transform radioactive emissions into light photons. Through a complex process, these light photons are amplified, and their locations are electronically recorded to produce an image that is displayed on computer output systems. Scintillation cameras today use single or multiple crystals.

Fig. 29.9 Typical gamma camera system, which includes complex computers and electronic mechanical components for acquiring, processing, displaying, and analyzing nuclear medicine images.

Collimator

Located at the face of the detector, where photons from radioactive sources first enter the camera, is the *collimator*. The collimator is used to filter gamma rays not perpendicular to the camera and keep scattered rays from reaching the scintillation crystal. *Resolution* and *sensitivity* are terms used to describe the physical characteristics of collimators. Collimator sensitivity is determined by the fraction of photons that are transmitted through the collimator and strike the face of the camera crystal. Spatial resolution refers to the system's ability to separate two points on an image.

Collimators are usually made of a material with a high atomic number, such as lead, which absorbs scattered gamma rays. Depending on the desired level of sensitivity and resolution, different collimators are used for different types of examinations (Fig. 29.10).

Crystal, light pipe, and PMT

The scintillation crystals commonly used in gamma cameras are made of sodium iodide with trace quantities of thallium added to increase light production. This crystal composition is effective for stopping most common gamma rays emitted from the radiopharmaceuticals used in nuclear medicine.

The thickness of the crystal varies from a quarter inch to a half inch (0.6 to 1.3 cm). Thicker crystals are better for imaging radiopharmaceuticals with higher energies (>180 keV) but have decreased resolution because of the decreased ability of the electronics to localize the exact location of the photon absorption within the thicker crystal. Thinner crystals provide improved resolution but cannot efficiently image photons with a higher kiloelectron voltage because of the inability of the thinner crystals to stop the higher-energy photons from passing through the crystal without being absorbed.

A *light pipe* may be used to attach the crystal to the PMTs. The light pipe is a disk of optically transparent material that helps direct photons from the crystal into the PMTs.

Attached to the back of the crystal or light pipe is an array of PMTs that are used to detect and convert light photons emitted from the crystal into an electronic signal. The PMT also amplifies the original photon signal by a factor of up to 10^7. A typical gamma camera detector head contains 80 to 100 PMTs. The PMTs send the detected signal through a series of processing steps, which include determining the location *(x, y)* of the original photon and its amplitude or energy *(z)*. The *x* and *y* values are determined by where the photon strikes the face of the crystal. Electronic circuitry known as a *pulse height analyzer* is used to eliminate the *z* signals that are of the appropriate energy based on the particular radionuclide being used. It is also used for rejecting photons not within the desired energy range. This helps reduce scattered lower energy, unwanted photons ("noise") that generally would degrade the resolution of the image. When the information has been processed, the signals are transmitted to the display system.

Multihead gamma camera systems

The original gamma camera was a single detector that could be moved in various positions around the patient. Today,

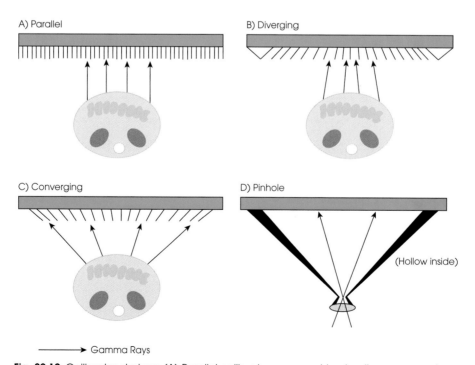

➡ Gamma Rays

Fig. 29.10 Collimator designs: (A) Parallel collimators are used to visualize organs as is, usually with no or very little zoom. (B) Diverging collimators are used to shrink or minimize large organs or organ systems. (C and D) Converging and pinhole collimators magnify small organs so they can be better visualized.

gamma camera systems may include up to three detectors (heads). Dual-head gamma camera systems are the most common, allowing for simultaneous anterior and posterior planar imaging, and are ideal for SPECT. Triple-head systems are not as popular as dual-head systems and are generally used for brain and heart studies. Although the triple-head systems are primarily suited for SPECT, they can also provide multiplanar images (see the section on imaging methods presented later in this chapter).

COMPUTERS

Computers have become an integral part of the nuclear medicine imaging system. Computer systems are used to acquire and process data from gamma cameras. They allow data to be collected over a specific time frame or to a specified number of counts; the data can be analyzed to determine functional changes occurring over time (Fig. 29.11A and B). A common example is the renal study, in which the radiopharmaceutical that is administered is cleared by normally func-

tioning kidneys in about 20 minutes. The computer can collect several images of the kidney during this period and analyze them to determine how effectively the kidneys clear the radiopharmaceutical. It does this by creating a time activity curve (see Fig. 29.11C–E). The computer also allows the operator to enhance a particular structure by adjusting the contrast and brightness of the image.

Computerization of the nuclear pharmacy operation also has become an important means of record keeping and

Fig. 29.11 (A) Posterior renal blood flow in an adult patient using 10 mCi of ^{99m}Tc with DTPA imaged at 3 seconds per frame. The image in the *lower right corner* is a blood-pool image taken immediately after the initial flow sequence. Together the images show normal renal blood flow to both kidneys. (B) Normal, sequential dynamic 20-minute ^{99m}Tc with mertiatide (MAG3) images. (C) Renal arterial perfusion curves showing minor renal blood flow asymmetry. (D) Renal cortical analysis curves showing rapid uptake and prompt parenchymal clearance. (E) Quantitative renal cortical analysis indices showing normal values.

quality control. Radioactive dosages and dose volumes can be calculated more quickly by computer than by hand. A nuclear pharmacy computer system may be used to provide reminders and keep records as required by the Nuclear Regulatory Commission (NRC), the FDA, and individual state regulatory agencies. Computers also assist in the scheduling of patients, based on dose availability and department policies.

Computers are necessary to acquire and process SPECT images (see the next section). SPECT uses a scintillation camera that moves around the patient to obtain images from multiple angles for tomographic image reconstruction. SPECT studies are complex and, similar to MRI studies, require a great deal of computer processing to create images in transaxial, sagittal, and coronal planes. Rotating three-dimensional images can also be generated from SPECT data (Fig. 29.12).

Computer networks are an integral part of the way a department communicates information within and among institutions. In a network, several or many computers are connected so that they all have access to the same files, programs, and printers. Networking allows the movement of image-based and text-based data to any computer or printer in the network. Networking improves the efficiency of a nuclear medicine department. A computer network can serve as a vital component, reducing the time expended on menial tasks while allowing retrieval and transfer of information. Consolidation of all reporting functions in one area eliminates the need for the nuclear medicine physician to travel between departments to read studies. Centralized archiving, printing, and retrieval of most image-based and

non-image-based data have increased the efficiency of data analysis, reduced the cost of image hard copy, and permitted more sophisticated analysis of image data than would routinely be possible.

Electronically stored records can decrease the reporting turnaround time, the physical image storage requirements, and the use of personnel for record maintenance and retrieval. Long-term computerized records can also form the basis for statistical analysis to improve testing methods and predict disease courses. Most institutions now use some form of picture archiving and communication systems (PACS) to organize all of the imaging that is done. PACS are the foundation of a digital department, allowing for easy transfer, retrieval, and archiving of all imaging done in the nuclear medicine department.

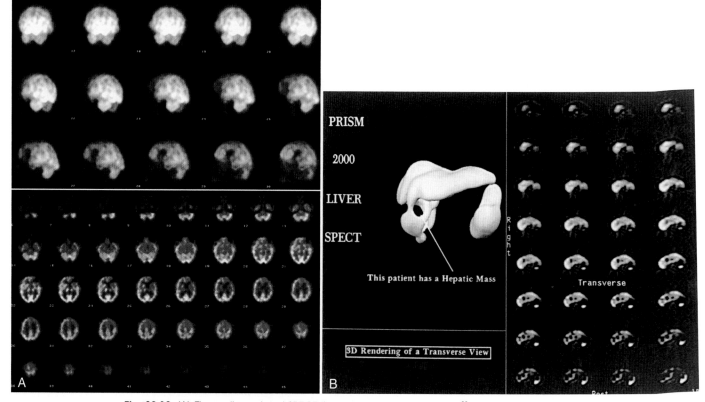

Fig. 29.12 (A) Three-dimensional SPECT brain study using 20 mCi of ^{99m}Tc ethylcysteinate dimer showing a patient with a left frontal lobe brain infarct *(top)*. Baseline and Diamox challenge transaxial, coronal, and sagittal images of the same patient, showing the left frontal lobe brain infarct *(bottom)*. (B) Three-dimensional SPECT liver study using 8 mCi of ^{99m}Tc sulfur colloid. A mass is seen on the three-dimensional image *(left)* and transaxial images *(right)*.

QUANTITATIVE ANALYSIS

Many nuclear medicine procedures require some form of quantitative analysis to provide physicians with numeric or statistical results based on, and depicting, organ function. Specialized software allows computers to collect, process, and analyze functional information obtained from nuclear medicine imaging systems. Cardiac left ventricular ejection fraction is a common quantitation study (Fig. 29.13). In this dynamic study of the heart's contractions and expansions, the computer accurately determines the ejection fraction, or the percent of blood pumped out of the left ventricle with each contraction.

Imaging Methods

A wide variety of diagnostic imaging examinations are performed in nuclear medicine. These examinations can be described on the basis of the imaging method used: static/planar, whole-body, dynamic, SPECT, and PET.

STATIC/PLANAR IMAGING

Static imaging is the acquisition of a single two-dimensional image of a particular structure. This image can be thought of as a snapshot of the radiopharmaceutical distribution within the body. Examples of static imaging used in general nuclear medicine include lung scans, limited bone scans, and thyroid imaging. Static images are usually obtained in various orientations around a particular structure to show multiple aspects of the region in question. Anterior, posterior, and oblique images are often obtained.

In static imaging, low radiopharmaceutical activity levels are used to minimize radiation exposure to the patients. Because of these low activity levels, images must be acquired for a preset time or a minimum number of counts or radioactive emissions. This time frame may vary from a few seconds to several minutes to acquire 100,000 to more than 1 million counts.

Fig. 29.13 Normal multigated acquisition scan. (A) Left anterior oblique (LAO) image of the left ventricle at end-diastole (relaxed phase), with a region of interest drawn around the left ventricle. (B) Same view showing end-systole (contracted phase). (C) Curve representing the volume change in the left ventricle of the heart before, during, and after contraction. This volume change is referred to as the ejection fraction *(EF)*; normal value is approximately 52%. (D) LAO view with regional ejection fractions displayed.

WHOLE-BODY IMAGING

Whole-body imaging uses a specially designed moving detector system to produce an image of the entire body or a large body section. In this type of imaging, the gamma camera collects data as it passes over the body. Earlier detector systems were smaller and required two or three incremental passes to encompass the entire width of the body. Others took multiple static images and "zipped" them together to form one whole body image.

Nearly all camera systems used for whole-body imaging incorporate a dual-head design for simultaneous anterior and posterior acquisitions. Whole-body imaging systems are used primarily for whole-body bone, tumor, or infection imaging along with other clinical and research applications (Fig. 29.14).

DYNAMIC IMAGING

Dynamic images display the distribution of a particular radiopharmaceutical over a specific period of time. Very similar to filming a movie, a series of sequential images are collected and aligned together to show function over time. A dynamic or "flow" study of a particular structure is generally used to evaluate blood perfusion to the tissue. Images may be acquired and displayed in time sequences from one-tenth of a second to longer than 10 minutes per image. Dynamic imaging is commonly used for three-phase bone scans, hepatobiliary studies, and renal exams. (Fig. 29.15)

Anterior　　　　Posterior　　　　Anterior　　　　Posterior

A　　　　　　　　　　　　　　　　　　　　　　　　　　　　　　B

Fig. 29.14 Whole-body scan performed using 25 mCi ^{99m}Tc HDP in a 25-year-old man. The study was normal. (A) Anterior and posterior whole-body view in linear gray scale. (B) Anterior and posterior whole-body view in square-root grayscale, to enhance soft tissue.

(Courtesy General Electric.)

SPECT IMAGING

With SPECT, typically, two gamma detectors are used to produce tomographic images (Fig. 29.16). Tomographic systems are designed to allow the detector heads to rotate 360 degrees around a patient's body to collect "projection" image data. The image data is restructured by a computer using reconstruction algorithms that populate all acquired projections to display the radiopharmaceutical distribution of the object into several formats including transaxial, sagittal, coronal, planar, and three-dimensional representations.

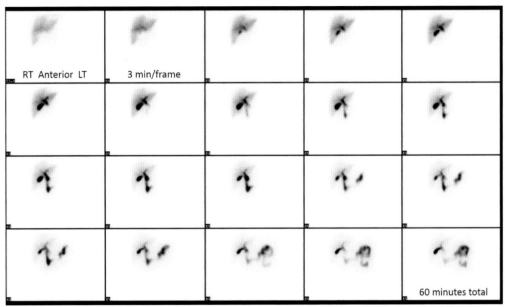

Hepatobiliary Scan, 5 mCi Mebrofenin

Fig. 29.15 Example of a dynamic hepatobiliary scan using 5 mCi of ^{99m}Tc mebrofenin. Imaging was acquired for 60 minutes and displayed over 20 frames (3 min/frame). Normal visualization of the liver, gallbladder, and small bowel is seen within the allotted time.

Fig. 29.16 SPECT camera systems. (A) Dual-headed SPECT/CT system. (B) Triple-headed system.

(B, Courtesy Marconi Medical Systems.)

The reconstruction of SPECT data produces image projections similar to those obtained by CT or MRI. This reconstruction technique is used to create thin slices through a particular organ from different angles, or planes, to help delineate small lesions within tissues. These images can be created for virtually any structure or organ that is acquired using SPECT. Improved clinical results with SPECT are due to improved target-to-background ratios. Planar images record and show all radioactive emissions from the patient within the region of interest (ROI) as well as above and below the ROI, causing degradation of the image. In contrast, SPECT eliminates the unnecessary information.

The most common uses of SPECT include cardiac perfusion, brain, liver (see Fig. 29.12B), tumor, and bone studies. An example of a SPECT study is the myocardial perfusion thallium (^{201}Tl) study, which is used to identify perfusion defects in the left ventricular wall. The ^{201}Tl is injected intravenously while the patient is being physically stressed on a treadmill or is being infused with a vasodilator. The radiopharmaceutical distributes in the heart muscle in the same fashion as blood flowing to the tissue. An initial set of images is acquired immediately after the stress test. A second set is obtained several hours later when the patient is rested (when the ^{201}Tl has redistributed to viable tissue) to determine whether any blood perfusion defects that were seen on the initial images have resolved. By comparing the two image sets, the physician may be able to tell whether the patient has damaged heart tissue resulting from a myocardial infarction or ischemia (Fig. 29.17).

Fig. 29.17 ^{201}Tl myocardial perfusion study comparing stress and redistribution (resting) images in various planes of the heart (short axis and long axis). Perfusion defect is identified in stress images but not seen in redistribution (rest) images. This finding is indicative of ischemia.

COMBINED SPECT AND CT IMAGING

By merging or "fusing" the functional imaging of SPECT with the anatomic landmarks of CT, more powerful diagnostic information is obtainable (Fig. 29.18). This combination has a significant impact on diagnosing and staging malignant disease and on identifying and localizing metastases. This new technology can also be used for AC. According to manufacturers, statistics show that adding CT (for AC and anatomic definition) changes the patient course of treatment 25% to 30% of the time, when compared to medical management based on interpreting the functional image alone. SPECT/CT is discussed further later in this chapter.

Clinical Nuclear Medicine

The term *in vivo* means "within the living body." Because all diagnostic nuclear medicine imaging procedures are based on the distribution of radiopharmaceuticals within the body, they are classified as in vivo examinations.

Patient preparation for nuclear medicine procedures is minimal, with most tests requiring no special preparation. Patients usually remain in their own clothing. All metal objects outside or inside the clothing must be removed because they may attenuate anatomic or pathologic conditions on nuclear medicine imaging. The waiting time(s) between dose administration and imaging varies with each study. After completion of a routine procedure, patients may resume all normal activities.

Technical summaries of commonly performed nuclear medicine procedures follow. After each procedure summary is a list, by organ or system, of many common studies that may be done in an average nuclear medicine department.

BONE SCINTIGRAPHY

Bone scintigraphy is generally a survey procedure to evaluate patients with malignancies, diffuse musculoskeletal symptoms, abnormal laboratory results, osteomyelitis, and hereditary or metabolic disorders. Tracer techniques have been used for many years to study the exchange between bone and blood. Radionuclides have played an important role in understanding normal bone metabolism and the metabolic effects of pathologic involvement of bone. Radio-pharmaceuticals used for bone imaging can localize in bone and in soft tissue structures. Skeletal areas of increased uptake are commonly a result of tumor, infection, or fracture.

Bone scan
Principle

It is unclear how ^{99m}Tc-labeled diphosphonates are incorporated into bone at the molecular level; however, regional blood flow, osteoblastic activity, and extraction efficiency seem to be the major factors that influence the uptake. In areas in which osteoblastic activity is increased, active hydroxyapatite crystals with large surface areas seem to be the most suitable sites for the uptake of the diphosphonate portion of the radiopharmaceutical.

Radiopharmaceutical

Adult dose (intravenous injection):
- 20 mCi (740 MBq) of ^{99m}Tc hydroxy-methylene diphosphonate (HDP) or
- 20 mCi (740 MBq) of ^{99m}Tc methylene diphosphonate (MDP)

Pediatric dose (weight-based intravenous injection) (see Fig. 29.7):
- 0.25 mCi/kg (9.3 MBq/kg) of ^{99m}Tc MDP

Fig. 29.18 ^{111}In-Octreotide SPECT/CT fusion images showing numerous foci of increased uptake within the liver. This is consistent with the patient's known hepatic metastases. Very small focus of increased uptake is also seen in the inferior abdomen, near midline, anterior to the lumbar spine, and is consistent with nodal metastasis. These findings are indicative of somatostatin-avid hepatic and probable nodal metastases.

Scanning

A routine survey (whole-body, static views, or SPECT) begins about 3 hours after radiopharmaceutical injection and takes 30 to 60 minutes. A flow study would begin immediately after the injection, and extremity imaging may be needed 4 to 5 hours later. The number of camera images acquired depends on the indication for the examination.

Bone (skeletal) studies

Skeletal studies include bone scans, three-phase bone scans, and bone marrow scans.

NUCLEAR CARDIOLOGY

Nuclear cardiology has experienced rapid growth in recent years and currently constitutes a significant portion of daily nuclear medicine procedures. These noninvasive studies assess cardiac performance, evaluate myocardial perfusion, and measure viability and metabolism. Advances in camera technology have facilitated the development of a quantitative cardiac evaluation unequaled by any other noninvasive or invasive methods. Stress tests can be performed with the patient walking on a treadmill or by infusing a pharmacologic stress agent. Once the stress test has begun, the patient's heart rate, electrocardiogram (ECG), blood pressure, and symptoms are continuously monitored and recorded. Some patients cannot exercise because of peripheral vascular disease, neurologic problems, or musculoskeletal abnormalities. In these cases, a pharmacologic intervention can be used in place of the exercise stress test to alter the blood flow to the heart in a way that simulates exercise, allowing the detection of myocardial ischemia.

Radionuclide angiography
Principle

Gated radionuclide angiography (RNA) can be used to measure left ventricular ejection fraction and evaluate left ventricular regional wall motion. RNA requires that the blood be labeled with an appropriate tracer such as ^{99m}Tc. The technique is based on imaging using a multigated acquisition (MUGA) format. During a gated acquisition, the cardiac cycle is divided into 16 to 20 frames. The R wave of each cycle resets the gate so that each count is added to each frame, until there are adequate count statistics for analysis. RNA requires simultaneous acquisition of the patient's ECG and images of the left

ventricle. The *ejection fraction* and wall motion analysis are measured at rest (see Fig. 29.13).

Radiopharmaceutical

Adult dose (intravenous injection):
- 25 to 30 mCi (925 to 1110 MBq) of ^{99m}Tc-labeled red blood cells.

Pediatric dose (weight-based intravenous injection) (see Fig. 29.7):
- 0.32 mCi/kg (11.8 MBq/kg) of ^{99m}Tc-labeled red blood cells

Scanning

Imaging can begin immediately after the injection and takes about 1 hour. For a rest MUGA, imaging of the heart should be obtained in the anterior, left lateral, and left anterior oblique positions. For an ejection fraction–only MUGA, only the left anterior oblique is necessary.

Technetium-99m sestamibi and technetium-99m tetrofosmin MPI
Principle

^{99m}Tc sestamibi and ^{99m}Tc tetrafosmin are radiopharmaceuticals that both have favorable biologic properties for myocardial perfusion imaging (MPI). They are used to assess myocardial salvage resulting from therapeutic intervention in acute infarction; to determine the myocardial blood flow during periods of spontaneous chest pain; and to diagnose coronary artery disease in obese patients. Both ^{99m}Tc sestamibi and ^{99m}Tc tetrofosmin localize in the heart wall based on regional blood flow. Thus, areas of the heart that suffer from reduced flow due to coronary artery disease will have decreased or no activity (photopenia) on the images. By injecting and imaging patients under rest (baseline) and stress (treadmill or pharmacologic) conditions helps to illustrate the severity of their situation (normal/ischemic/infarct). Gating (refer to MUGA) the exam can be performed at stress only, or both rest and stress, to obtain an ejection fraction and evaluate wall motion.

Radiopharmaceutical

Adult dose (intravenous injection):
- At peak stress: 20 to 30 mCi (740 to 1110 MBq) for 2-day MPI and 30 to 36 mCi (1110 to 1332 MBq) for 1-day MPI
- At rest: 8 to 12 mCi (296 to 444 MBq) for a 1-day MPI and 20 to 30 mCi (740 to 1110 MBq) for a 2-day MPI

Scanning

SPECT imaging at 180 degrees (45 degrees right anterior oblique to 45 degrees left posterior oblique) is normally performed 30 to 60 minutes after the injection of the radiotracer for both stress and rest studies. When needed, delayed images can be obtained up to 4 to 6 hours after injection based on the tracer used. A 2-day protocol provides optimal image quality, but the 1-day protocol is more convenient for patients, technologists, and physicians.

Thallium-201 MPI and viability studies
Principle

^{201}Tl is sometimes used in MPI studies and has a high sensitivity (about 90%) and specificity (about 75%) for the diagnosis of coronary artery disease, but currently sestamibi and tetrofosmin are used more often due to their better imaging properties. ^{201}Tl also has been useful for assessing myocardial viability in patients with known coronary artery disease and for evaluating patients after revascularization

^{201}Tl is an analog of potassium and has a high rate of extraction by the myocardium over a wide range of metabolic and physiologic conditions. It is distributed in the myocardium in proportion to regional blood flow and myocardial cell viability. Regions of the heart that are infarcted or hypoperfused at the time of injection appear as areas of decreased activity (photopenia).

Radiopharmaceutical

Adult MPI dose (intravenous injection):
- At peak stress:3 mCi (111 MBq) of ^{201}Tl thallous chloride
- A rest: 1 mCi (37 MBq) of ^{201}Tl Thallous chloride (generally 3 to 4 hours after stress)

Adult viability dose (intravenous injection):
- One dose given at rest: 4 mCi (148 MBq) of ^{201}Tl Thallous chloride

NOTE: In obese patients ^{99m}Tc sestamibi (adult peak stress dose) can be used in place of ^{201}Tl so that a higher dose may be administered for clearer imaging results.

Scanning

Imaging for a ^{201}Tl MPI study includes a 180-degree SPECT study (45 degrees right anterior oblique to 45 degrees left posterior oblique) approximately 10 minutes after the peak stress injection has occurred. Due to ^{201}Tl's high redistribution rate the patient must be scanned very close to their injection time. Rest 180-degree SPECT imaging usually takes place 4 hours after stress imaging and 15 to 30 minutes after the rest injection.

For a viability study a 180-degree SPECT imaging usually takes place 15 minutes post injection and 4 to 6 hours post injection. The 4 to 6 hours delay allows the ^{201}Tl to redistribute to regions of the heart that do not have direct blood flow but are viable.

Cardiovascular studies

Cardiovascular studies include cardiac shunt study, MUGA (dobutamine, exercise, and rest), MPI (^{99m}Tc sestamibi, ^{99m}Tc Tetrofosmin, ^{201}Tl Thallous chloride), viability imaging (^{99m}Tc sestamibi and ^{201}Tl Thallous chloride), and ^{99m}Tc pyrophosphate (PYP) myocardial infarct scan.

CENTRAL NERVOUS SYSTEM IMAGING

The central nervous system consists of the brain and spinal cord. For patients with diseases of the central or peripheral nervous systems, nuclear medicine techniques can be used to assess the effectiveness of surgery or radiation therapy, document the extent of involvement of the brain by tumors, and determine the progression or regression of lesions in response to different forms of treatment. Brain perfusion imaging is useful in the evaluation of patients with stroke, transient ischemia, and other neurologic disorders, such as Alzheimer disease (AD), epilepsy, and Parkinson disease. Radionuclide cisternography is particularly useful in facilitating the diagnosis of cerebrospinal fluid leakage after trauma or surgery and normal-pressure hydrocephalus. More recent studies indicate that documented lack of cerebral blood flow should be the criterion of choice to confirm brain death when clinical criteria are equivocal; a complete neurologic examination cannot be performed; or patients are younger than 1 year.

Brain SPECT study
Principle

Some imaging agents are capable of penetrating the intact *blood-brain barrier*. After a radiopharmaceutical crosses the blood-brain barrier, it becomes trapped inside the brain. The regional uptake and retention of the tracer are related to the regional perfusion.

Radiopharmaceutical

Adult dose (intravenous injection):
- 20 mCi (740 MBq) of ^{99m}Tc ethylcysteinate dimer (ECD) or
- 20 mCi (740 MBq) of ^{99m}Tc hexamethylpropyleneamine oxime (HMPAO).

Pediatric dose (weight-based intravenous injection) (see Fig 29.7)
- 0.3 mCi/kg (11.1 MBq/kg), minimum of 5 mCi (185 MBq)

Scanning

Before the tracer is injected, the patient is placed in a quiet, darkened area and instructed to close their eyes. These measures are helpful in reducing uptake of the tracer in the visual cortex (occipital lobe). Imaging begins 30 to 90 minutes after ^{99m}Tc ECD injection or ^{99m}Tc HMPAO injection. Tomographic images of the brain are obtained.

Dopamine transporter study
Principle

A reduction of dopaminergic neurons in the striatal region of the brain is a characteristic of Parkinson disease, parkinsonian syndromes, multiple system atrophy, and progressive supranuclear palsy. ^{123}I ioflupane has a high binding affinity for presynaptic dopamine transporters in the striatal region of the brain.

Radiopharmaceutical

Adult dose (intravenous injection):
- A slow infusion of 3 to 5 mCi (111 to 185 MBq) of ^{123}I ioflupane.

Scanning

Prior to the administration of ^{123}I Ioflupane, a thyroid blocking agent such as Lugol's solution should be given to the patient. This will prevent the iodine from being absorbed by the thyroid, thus protecting it from any unnecessary exposure. Imaging begins 3 to 6 hours after injection. Tomographic images of the brain are obtained.

Central nervous system studies

Central nervous system studies include brain perfusion imaging–SPECT study, brain imaging–acetazolamide challenge study, central nervous system shunt patency, cerebrospinal fluid imaging–cisternography/ventriculography, and ^{99m}Tc HMPAO scan for determination of brain death.

ENDOCRINE SYSTEM IMAGING

The endocrine system organs, located throughout the body, secrete hormones into the bloodstream. Hormones have profound effects on overall body function and metabolism. The endocrine system consists of the thyroid, parathyroid, pituitary, adrenal glands, the islet cells of the pancreas, and the gonads. Nuclear medicine procedures have played a significant part in the current understanding of the function of the endocrine glands and their role in health and disease. These procedures are useful for monitoring the treatment of endocrine disorders, especially in the thyroid gland.

Thyroid scan
Principle

Thyroid imaging is performed to evaluate the size, shape, nodularity, and functional status of the thyroid gland. Imaging is used to determine the relative function in different regions within the thyroid, to screen for thyroid cancer, and to differentiate hyperthyroidism, nodular goiter, solitary thyroid nodule, and thyroiditis. Scanning can also determine the presence and site of thyroid tissue in unusual areas of the body, such as the tongue and anterior chest (ectopic tissue).

^{99m}Tc pertechnetate or ^{123}I can be used to image the thyroid gland. ^{99m}Tc pertechnetate is trapped by the thyroid gland but, in contrast to ^{123}I, is not *organified*. ^{123}I is organified into the gland and trapped until it is metabolized into thyroid hormones. These agents offer the advantages of a low radiation dose to the patient and well-resolved images.

Radiopharmaceutical

Adult dose:
- 5 mCi (185 MBq) of ^{99m}Tc pertechnetate (intravenous injection)
- 0.2 to 0.3 mCi of ^{123}I (administered orally, pill)

Pediatric dose (see Fig. 29.7):
- 0.03 mCi/kg (1.1 MBq/kg) of ^{99m}Tc pertechnetate (weight-based intravenous injection), minimum of 2.5 mCi (93 MBq)
- 0.0075 mCi/kg (0.28 MBq/kg) of ^{123}I (weight based, administered orally, pill), minimum of 0.027 mCi (1 MBq)

NOTE: *Uptake may be affected by thyroid medication and by foods or drugs, including some iodine-containing contrast agents.*

Scanning

Imaging should start 20 minutes after the injection of ^{99m}Tc pertechnetate, or

24 hours after the administration of ^{123}I. A gamma camera with a pinhole collimator is used to obtain anterior, left anterior oblique, and right anterior oblique statics of the thyroid. The pinhole collimator is a thick, conical collimator that allows for magnification of the thyroid (see Fig. 29.10).

Iodine-123 thyroid uptake measurement
Principle

Radioiodine is concentrated by the thyroid gland in a manner that reflects the ability of the gland to handle stable dietary iodine. ^{123}I uptake is used to estimate the function of the thyroid gland by measuring its avidity for administered radioiodine. The higher the uptake of ^{123}I, the more active the thyroid; conversely, the lower the uptake, the less functional the gland. Uptake conventionally is expressed as the percentage of the dose in the thyroid gland at a given time after administration. Measurement of ^{123}I uptake is valuable in distinguishing between thyroiditis (significantly reduced uptake) and Graves disease and toxic nodular goiter (Plummer disease), which have an increased uptake. It is also used to determine the appropriateness of a therapeutic dose of ^{131}I in patients with Graves disease.

Radiopharmaceutical

The adult and pediatric doses are the same as listed earlier in the Thyroid Scan section. A standard dose is counted with the thyroid probe the morning of the procedure and is used as the 100% uptake

value. The patient's total count is compared with the standard count to obtain the patient percent uptake.

Measurements are obtained using an uptake probe consisting of a 2 × 2 inch (5 × 5 cm) sodium iodide/PMT assembly fitted with a flat-field lead collimator (Fig. 29.19). Uptake readings are generally acquired at 6 hours, at 24 hours, or both.

Total-body iodine-123/ iodine-131 scan
Principle

A total-body ^{123}I/^{131}I (TBI) scan is recommended for locating residual thyroid tissue or recurrent thyroid cancer cells in patients with thyroid carcinoma. Most follicular or papillary thyroid cancers concentrate radioiodine; other types of thyroid cancer do not. A TBI scan is usually performed 1 to 3 months after a thyroidectomy to check for residual normal thyroid tissue and the metastatic spread of the cancer before ^{131}I ablation therapy. After the residual thyroid tissue has been ablated (destroyed), another ^{123}I/^{131}I TBI scan may be performed to check for residual disease.

Radiopharmaceutical

Adult dose (administered orally)
- 2 to 5 mCi (74 to 185 MBq) of ^{123}I

Scanning

Total-body imaging begins 24 to 72 hours after dose administration (depending on the radiopharmaceutical used). Images are obtained of the anterior and posterior whole body. SPECT imaging can also be

performed to localize any specific areas of interest better.

Endocrine studies

Endocrine studies include the adrenal scan (^{131}I or ^{123}I-labeled MIBG), ectopic thyroid scan (^{131}I or ^{123}I), thyroid scan (^{123}I or ^{99m}Tc pertechnetate), thyroid uptake measurement (^{131}I or ^{123}I), thyroid uptake/ scan (^{123}I), total body iodine scan (^{131}I or ^{123}I), parathyroid scan, and ^{111}In pentetreotide scan.

IMAGING OF THE GASTROINTESTINAL SYSTEM

The gastrointestinal system, or alimentary canal, consists of the mouth, oropharynx, esophagus, stomach, small bowel, colon, and several accessory organs (salivary glands, pancreas, liver, and gallbladder). The liver is the largest internal organ of the body. The portal venous system brings blood from the stomach, bowel, spleen, and pancreas to the liver.

Liver and spleen scan
Principle

Liver and spleen imaging is used to evaluate the liver for functional disease (e.g., cirrhosis, hepatitis, metastatic disease) and to search for residual splenic tissue after splenectomy or traumatic event. Imaging techniques, such as ultrasound, CT, and MRI, provide excellent information about the anatomy of the liver, but nuclear medicine studies can assess the *functional* status of this organ. Liver and spleen scintigraphy is also useful for detecting hepatic lesions and evaluating hepatic morphology, perfusion, and function. It is also used to determine whether certain lesions found with other methods may be benign (e.g., focal nodular hyperplasia), or obviating the need for biopsy. Uptake of a radiopharmaceutical in the liver, spleen, and bone marrow depends on blood flow and the functional capacity of the phagocytic cells. In normal patients, 80% to 90% of the radiopharmaceutical is localized in the liver, 5% to 10% is localized in the spleen, and the rest is localized in the bone marrow.

Radiopharmaceutical

Adult dose (intravenous injection):
- 6 mCi (222 MBq) of ^{99m}Tc sulfur colloid

Scanning

Imaging sometimes begins with a flow study based on the indication, but usually

Fig. 29.19 Uptake probe used for thyroid uptake measurements over the extended neck area.

planar (anterior, posterior, right and left anterior oblique, right and left lateral, right posterior oblique, and a marker view) are obtained, followed by SPECT if necessary.

Gastrointestinal studies

Gastrointestinal studies include esophageal scintigraphy, gastroesophageal reflux study, gastric emptying study, hepatic artery perfusion scan, hepatobiliary scan, hepatobiliary scan with gallbladder ejection fraction, liver and spleen scan, liver hemangioma study, Meckel diverticulum study, and salivary gland study.

GENITOURINARY NUCLEAR MEDICINE

Genitourinary nuclear medicine studies are recognized as reliable, noninvasive procedures for evaluating the anatomy and function of the renal system (kidneys, ureters, bladder, and urethra). These studies can be accomplished with minimal risk of allergic reactions, unpleasant side effects, or excessive radiation exposure to the organs.

Dynamic renal scan
Principle

Renal imaging is used to assess renal perfusion and function, particularly in renal failure and renovascular hypertension and after renal transplantation. ^{99m}Tc mertiatide (MAG3) is secreted primarily by the proximal renal tubules and is not retained in the parenchyma of normal kidneys.

Radiopharmaceutical
Adult dose (intravenous injection):
• 10 mCi (370 MBq) of ^{99m}Tc MAG3.
Pediatric dose (weight-based intravenous injection) (see Fig. 29.7):
• Without flow study: 0.10 mCi/kg (1.85 MBq/kg), minimum of 1.0 mCi (37 MBq)
• With flow study: 0.15 mCi/kg (5.55 MBq/kg)

Scanning

Dynamic imaging is initiated immediately after radiopharmaceutical injection. Because radiographic contrast media may interfere with kidney function, renal scanning is usually delayed for 24 hours after contrast studies. Images are often taken over the posterior lower back, centered at the level of the 12th rib. Transplanted kidneys are imaged in the anterior pelvis.

Patients need to be well hydrated before all renal studies.

Genitourinary studies

Genitourinary studies include dynamic renal scan (baseline or no pharmaceutical intervention, with furosemide, or with captopril), ^{99m}Tc dimercaptosuccinic acid (DMSA) renal scan, residual urine determination, testicular scan, and voiding cystography.

IMAGING FOR INFECTION

Imaging for infection is another useful nuclear medicine diagnostic tool. Inflammation, infection, and abscess may be found anywhere within the body. ^{67}Ga scans and ^{111}In-labeled white blood cell scans are useful for diagnosis and localization of infection and inflammation.

Infection studies

Infection studies include ^{67}Ga gallium scan, ^{111}In white blood cell scan, ^{99m}Tc HMPAO, and phase bone scans in conjunction with bone marrow exams following joint replacement surgeries.

RESPIRATORY IMAGING

Respiratory imaging commonly involves the comparison of pulmonary perfusion (using limited, transient capillary blockade) and pulmonary ventilation (using an inhaled radioactive gas or aerosol). Lung imaging is most commonly performed to evaluate acute and chronic pulmonary emboli in patients unable to undergo a CT angiography (CTA). It is also used for lung transplant evaluation.

Xenon-133 lung ventilation scan
Principle

Lung ventilation scans are used in combination with lung perfusion scans. The gas used for a ventilation study must be absorbed significantly by the lungs and diffuse easily. ^{133}Xe has adequate imaging properties, and the body usually absorbs less than 15% of the gas.

Radiopharmaceutical
Adult dose (*inhalation*):
• 15 to 30 mCi (555 to 1110 MBq) of ^{133}Xe gas

Scanning
Imaging begins immediately after inhalation of the ^{133}Xe gas within a closed

rebreathing system to which oxygen is added and carbon dioxide is withdrawn. For optimal imaging, the ventilation study must precede the ^{99m}Tc perfusion scan. Anterior and posterior images are obtained for the first breath, equilibrium, and *washout*. If possible, left and right posterior oblique images should be obtained between the first breath and equilibrium.

Technetium-99m MAA lung perfusion scan
Principle

^{99m}Tc MAA is collection of small radioactive particles (~400,000 to 600,000 in a standard dose) that become trapped in the arterioles of the lungs based on blood flow. If a region (lobe or wedge) of the lung is blocked via emboli, the area will not be perfused by the radiotracer creating a photopenic area on the images. The lungs contain millions of arterioles, thus there are no side effects due to the blockade.

Radiopharmaceutical
Adult dose (intravenous injection):
• 5 mCi (185 MBq) of ^{99m}Tc MAA.
Pediatric dose (weight-based intravenous injection) (see Fig. 29.7):
• If ^{133}Xe was used for the ventilation: 0.03 mCi/kg (1.11 MBq/kg), minimum of 0.4 mCi (14.8 MBq)
• If ^{99m}Tc was used for the ventilation: 0.07 mCi/kg (2.59 MBq/kg)

Scanning

Imaging starts approximately 5 minutes after radiopharmaceutical injection. Eight images are obtained: anterior, posterior, right and left lateral, right and left anterior oblique, and right and left posterior oblique. All patients should have a chest radiograph within 24 hours of the lung scan. The chest radiograph is required for accurate interpretation of the lung scans so as to determine the probability for pulmonary embolism.

Respiratory studies

Respiratory studies include the ^{133}Xe lung ventilation scan, ^{99m}Tc MAA lung perfusion scan, and ^{99m}Tc diethylenetriamine pentaacetic acid (DTPA) lung aerosol scan.

SENTINEL NODE IMAGING

Many tumors metastasize via lymphatic channels. Defining the anatomy of lymph nodes that drain from a primary tumor site helps guide surgeons resecting the nodes during surgery. Sentinel node imaging does just this; it maps the routes of lymphatic drainage and permits more effective surgical or radiation treatments. Radionuclide lympho-scintigraphy has been useful in patients in whom the channels are relatively inaccessible. This method is indicated for patients with melanoma and breast cancer.

Principle

Colloidal particles injected intradermally or subcutaneously adjacent to a tumor site show a drainage pattern similar to that of the tumor. Colloidal particles in the 10- to 50-nm range seem to be the most effective for this application. The colloidal particles drain into the sentinel lymph node, where they are trapped by phagocytic activity; this aids in the identification of the lymph nodes most likely to be sites of metastatic deposits from the tumor.

Radiopharmaceutical

Adult dose (intradermal/subcutaneous injection):
• 100 μCi (3.7 MBq) of ^{99m}Tc filtered sulfur colloid in a volume of 0.1 mL per injection site (up to 4 injection sites)

Scanning

Patients with malignant melanoma should be positioned supine or prone on the imaging table based on tumor location, and patients with breast cancer should be positioned supine with their arms extended over their head. Images are acquired immediately after injection, and then every few minutes for the first 15 minutes followed by every 5 minutes for 30 minutes. Additional lateral and oblique views are required after visualization of the sentinel node.

THERAPEUTIC NUCLEAR MEDICINE

The potential that radionuclides have for detecting and treating cancer has been recognized for decades. The most common nuclear medicine therapies use radioiodine (^{131}I) to treat Graves disease. High-dose ^{131}I therapy ($\geq$30 mCi) can be used in patients with residual thyroid cancer or thyroid metastases. ^{131}I is also labeled with monoclonal antibodies (^{131}I-MoAb) to target specific cancers such as non-Hodgkin lymphoma. ^{90}Yttrium (^{90}Y-MoAb) can also be labeled in a similar manner to treat the same cancer. Skeletal metastases occur in more than 50% of patients with breast, lung, or prostate cancer in the end stages of the disease. ^{89}Sr (strontium-89) or ^{153}Sm (samarium-153) ethylene diamine tetramethylene phosphate (EDTMP) is often useful for managing patients with bone pain from metastases when other treatments have failed. ^{90}Y microspheres are a new treatment in nuclear medicine. This therapy involves the embolization of radioactive ^{90}Y microspheres straight into the liver's arterial supply, directly delivering them into primary and secondary hepatic tumors.

SPECIAL IMAGING PROCEDURES

Special imaging procedures include dacryoscintigraphy, the LeVeen shunt patency test, and lymphoscintigraphy of the limbs.

TUMOR IMAGING

Octreoscan
Principle

Somatostatin is a neuroregulatory peptide known to localize on many cells of neuroendocrine origin. Cell membrane receptors with a high affinity for somatostatin have been shown to be present in most neuroendocrine tumors, including carcinoids, islet cell carcinomas, and gonadotropin hormone-producing pituitary adenomas.[111] In pentetreotide (OctreoScan) is a radiolabeled analog of the neuroendocrine peptide somatostatin. This allows it to localize in somatostatin receptor-rich tumors and aid in identifying questionable masses.

Radiopharmaceutical

Adult dose (intravenous injection):
• 6 mCi (222 MBq) of ^{111}In pentetreotide

Scanning

At 4 to 6 hours after injection, anterior and posterior whole-body images should be acquired. At 24 hours, whole-body images should be obtained once more along with anterior and posterior spot views of the chest and abdomen. SPECT imaging is most helpful in the localization of intra-abdominal tumors. SPECT/CT can assist in lesion localization. Additional imaging at 48 and 72 hours is at the discretion of the radiologist interpreting the exam. Images of an octreotide scan can be seen in Fig. 29.18.

Tumor studies

Tumor studies include ^{67}Ga tumor scan, ^{99m}Tc sestamibi breast scan, ^{111}In capromab pendetide (ProstaScint) scan, ^{99m}Tc nofetumomab merpentan (Verluma), and ^{111}In OctreoScan.

Principles and Facilities in Positron Emission Tomography

PET is a noninvasive nuclear imaging technique that involves the administration of a positron-emitting radioactive tracer followed by subsequent imaging of its physiological distribution. PET radiotracers use extremely small molar amounts of the radiopharmaceutical per dose, which means equilibrium conditions within the body are not altered. Currently PET is used to image multiple organs in the body (heart, brain, lungs, and prostate).

Three important factors distinguish PET from all radiologic procedures and from other nuclear imaging procedures. First, the results of the data acquisition and analysis techniques yield an image related to a particular physiologic parameter such as blood flow or metabolism. The ensuing image is aptly called a *functional* or *parametric image.* Second, the images are created by the simultaneous detection of a pair of *annihilation photons* that result from *positron* decay (Fig. 29.20). The third factor that distinguishes PET is the chemical and biologic form of the radiopharmaceutical. The radiotracer is specifically chosen for its similarity to naturally occurring biochemical constituents of the human body. For example, if the radiopharmaceutical is a form of sugar, it behaves much like the natural sugar used by the body. The kinetics or the movement of the radiotracer (such as sugar) within the body is followed by using the PET scanner to acquire multiple images that measure the distribution of the *radioactivity concentration* as a function of time. From this measurement, the local tissue metabolism may be deduced by converting a temporal sequence of images into a single parametric image. PET is a multidisciplinary technique that involves four major processes: radionuclide production, radiopharmaceutical production, data acquisition (PET scanner or tomograph), and image reconstruction and processing. This section of the chapter is focused on these major categories within in PET.

POSITRONS

Positrons (β^+) are the resultant of a radiation decay process (positron decay) in which an unstable *proton-rich* nucleus is attempting to reach its ground state. As the number of protons increases within a nucleus, so does the net positive charge and its instability. Based on *Coulomb forces* inside the nucleus, protons continuously try to push away from one another. To help stabilize these atoms, the nucleus spontaneously converts a proton into a neutron. This then lowers the net positive charge of the nucleus by one, and the neutron acts as a buffer amongst the remaining protons. To account for the loss of the positive charge and energy, a positron is emitted from the nucleus. Positrons are identical to electrons with the exception that they possess a positive charge instead of negative one. The characteristics of positrons are listed in Table 29.3.

For the positron decay process to occur, the nucleus must possess at least an excess of energy greater than 1.022 MeV (equivalent to the mass of two electrons). Positrons are emitted from the nucleus with high velocity and kinetic energy. As mentioned in the Basic Nuclear Physics section of this chapter, each radioisotope releases its own defined amount of energy per decay and decay process (like a fingerprint). This means different radioisotopes that decay by positron emission, emit positrons with different energies. Based on their energy, positrons from different elements can travel farther from the nucleus than others (Fig. 29.21A).

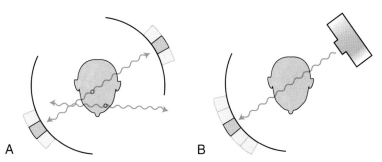

Fig. 29.20 **(A)** PET relies on the simultaneous detection of a pair of annihilation radiations emitted from the body. **(B)** In contrast, CT depends on the detection of x-rays transmitted through the body.

TABLE 29.3
Positron characteristics

Definition	Positively charged electron
Origin	Proton-rich nuclei
Production	Accelerators and Cyclotrons
Nuclide decay	$p = n + \beta^+$ neutrino
Positron decay	Annihilation to two 0.511-MeV photons
Number	About 240 known
Range	Proportional to kinetic energy of β^+
Routine PET nuclides	^{11}C, ^{13}N, ^{15}O, ^{18}F, ^{82}Rb

Proton (+)
Neutron (0)
Electron (–)
Positron (β⁺)

A

An unstable radioactive proton-rich nucleus goes through positron decay by converting a proton into a neutron and emitting a positron. For this decay process to occur the unstable nucleus must contain an excess of energy greater than 1.022 MeV.

B

The emitted positron interacts with surrounding matter (attenuators) slowing it down.

C

As the positron approaches a resting state, the more likely it is to interact with an electron due to the attractive forces between the two. These forces pull them toward one another in a spiraling manner.

D

The positron and electron eventually collide and annihilate. *Annihilation* is a process that consists of a positron and an electron combining and transforming their collective masses completely into energy. The energy is released in the form of 2 gamma rays emitted ˜180° apart from one another.

E

The distance between where the positron was emitted and where the annihilation takes place is known as the *range* (Δd). The range is based on a positron's energy at the time of emission. The more energy, the larger the range. Smaller ranges are better for imaging.

F

Within the PET camera, annihilation photons almost simultaneously strike the Detectors on opposing sides. When both photons of a single annihilation are detected by the camera it is called a *coincidence event*. Calculations are then made to localize where the event took place. The summation of thousands to millions of events are used to construct an image.

Fig. 29.21 (A) An unstable radioactive proton-rich nucleus goes through positron decay by converting a proton into a neutron and emitting a positron. For this decay process to occur the unstable nucleus must contain an excess of energy greater than 1.022 MeV. (B) The emitted positron interacts with surrounding matter (attenuators) slowing it down. (C) As the positron approaches a resting state, the more likely it is to interact with an electron due to the attractive forces between the two. These forces pull them toward one another in a spiraling manner. (D) The positron and electron eventually collide and annihilate. *Annihilation* is a process that consists of a positron and an electron combining and transforming their collective masses completely into energy. The energy is released in the form of 2 gamma rays (511 keV) emitted ~180 degrees apart from one another. (E) The distance between where the positron was emitted and where the annihilation takes place is known as the *range* (Δd). The range is based on a positron's energy at the time of emission. The more energy, the larger the range. Smaller ranges are better for imaging. (F) Within the PET camera, annihilation photons almost simultaneously strike the detectors on opposing sides. When both photons of a single annihilation are detected by the camera it is called a *coincidence event*. Calculations are then made to localize where the event took place. The summation of thousands to millions of events is used to construct an image.

Once the positron has been emitted it begins to rapidly slow due to interactions with surrounding matter (attenuators) (see Fig. 29.21B). As it decreases in speed, the positron becomes more likely to interact with a nearby electron (Coulomb forces, opposite charges attract). When the attraction between the two particles is strong enough to pull them away from their original path, they begin to spiral toward one another (like water circling a drain) (see Fig. 29.21C). Eventually the particles collide and totally *annihilate* or disintegrate. During the annihilation process the combined positron-electron mass (1.022 amu) is completely transformed into two equal-energy photons of 0.511 MeV (annihilation photons/total energy 1.022 MeV), which are emitted approximately 180 degrees (±0.3 degrees) from one another (see Fig. 29.21D). The average distance a positron travels after being ejected from the nucleus to where the annihilation takes place is known as the positron's *range* (see Fig. 29.21E). Specific isotope properties can be reviewed in Table 29.4. The resulting annihilation photons behave like gamma and x-rays: they have sufficient energy to traverse body tissues with only modest attenuation, and they can be detected externally (see Fig. 29.21F).

The positron emitting radioisotopes currently being used in PET are carbon-11 (^{11}C), nitrogen-13 (^{13}N), oxygen-15 (^{15}O), rubidium-82 (^{82}Rb), and fluorine-18 (^{18}F). ^{18}F is the most common used radioisotope because it can be used as a hydrogen substitute in many compounds. This substitution of ^{18}F for hydrogen is successfully accomplished because of its small size and strong bond with carbon.

TABLE 29.4

Characteristics of common PET radionuclides

Nuclide (decay product)	Physical half-life	Decay mode	Maximal and average positron energy (keV)	Maximum and mean range in water (mm)	Production reaction
Carbon-11 (Boron-11)	20.3 min	99.8% positron 0.2% electron capture	960, 320	4.1, 1.1	^{14}N(p,alpha)^{11}C[a]
Nitrogen-13 (Carbon-13)	10 min	100% positron	1198, 432	5.1, 1.5	^{16}O(p,alpha)^{13}N ^{13}C(p,n)^{13}N
Oxygen-15 (Nitrogen-15)	124 s	99.9% positron	1732, 696	7.3, 2.5	^{15}N(p,n)^{15}O ^{14}N(d,n)^{15}O
Fluorine-18 (Oxygen-18)	110 min	97% positron 3% electron capture	634, 202	2.4, 0.6	^{18}O(p,n)^{18}F ^{20}Ne(d,alpha)^{18}F ^{16}O(^{3}He,alpha)^{18}F
Rubidium-82	1.27 min (75 s)	96% positron 4% electron capture	3356, 1385	14.1, 5.9	^{82}Sr generator (T1/2 25.3 days)

[a]This symbolism means that a proton is accelerated into an atom of nitrogen-14, causing ejection of an alpha particle from the nucleus to produce an atom of carbon-11.
From Mettler FA, Guiberteau MJ: *Mettler's essentials of nuclear medicine imaging*, ed 6. Philadelphia, 2012, Elsevier.

RADIONUCLIDE PRODUCTION

Radionuclides used in PET exams are produced using a *nuclear particle accelerator* or cyclotron to bombard appropriate nonradioactive *target* atoms with accelerated charged particles. High energies are necessary to overcome the electrostatic and nuclear forces of the target nuclei so that a nuclear reaction can occur. An example is the production of ^{15}O. *Deuterons* (d), or heavy hydrogen ions are accelerated to approximately 7 MeV. The target material is stable nitrogen gas (N_2). The resultant nuclear reaction yields a neutron and an ^{15}O atom, which can be written in the following form: $^{14}N(d,n)^{15}O$ (^{14}N is the target material, the deuteron (d) is the bombarding charged particle, the neutron (n) is emitted from the nucleus, and ^{15}O is the product). The ^{15}O atom quickly associates with a stable ^{16}O atom that has been intentionally added to the target gas to produce a radioactive ^{15}O-^{16}O molecule in the form of O_2 (oxygen is a diatomic element).

When the unstable or radioactive ^{15}O atom decays via positron emission, the ^{15}O atom becomes a stable ^{15}N atom and forces the O_2 molecule to break apart This process is shown in Fig. 29.22, and the decay schemes for the four routinely produced PET radionuclides are depicted in Fig. 29.23. The common reactions used for the production of positron-emitting forms of carbon, nitrogen, oxygen, and fluorine are given in Table 29.4.

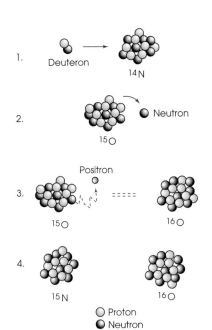

Fig. 29.22 Typical radionuclide production sequence. The $^{14}N(d,n)^{15}O$ reaction is used for making ^{15}O-^{16}O molecules. *1,* A deuteron ion is accelerated to high energy (7 MeV) by a cyclotron and impinges on a stable ^{14}N nucleus. *2,* As a result of the nuclear reaction, a neutron is emitted, leaving a radioactive nucleus of ^{15}O. *3,* ^{15}O atom quickly associates with ^{16}O atom to form O_2 molecule. Later, unstable ^{15}O atom emits a positron. *4,* As a result of positron decay (i.e., positron exits nucleus), ^{15}O atom is transformed into stable ^{15}N atom, and O_2 molecule breaks apart.

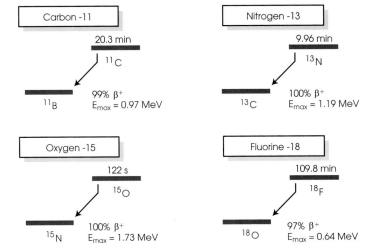

Fig. 29.23 Decay schemes for ^{11}C, ^{13}N, ^{15}O, and ^{18}F. Each positron emitter decays to a stable nuclide by ejecting a positron from the nucleus. E_{max} represents the maximum energy of the emitted positron. Electron capture is a competitive process with positron decay; positron decay is not always 100%.

Because of the very short half-lives of the routinely used positron-emitting radionuclides of oxygen, nitrogen, rubidium, and carbon, nearby access to a nuclear particle accelerator, cyclotron, or generator is necessary to produce sufficient quantities for diagnostic testing. The most common device to achieve nuclide production within reasonable space (250 ft^2 [223 m^2]) and energy (150 kW) constraints is a compact medical cyclotron (Fig. 29.24).

Fig. 29.24 Compact cyclotron (2.2 m high × 1.5 m wide × 1.5 m deep) used for routine production of PET isotopes. Cyclotron can be located in a concrete vault, or it can be self-shielded. Particles are accelerated in vertical orbits and impinge on targets located near the top center of the machine. This is an example of a negative-ion cyclotron.

(Courtesy GE Medical Systems, Milwaukee, WI.)

RADIOPHARMACEUTICAL PRODUCTION

Living organisms are composed primarily of compounds that contain the elements hydrogen, carbon, nitrogen, and oxygen. In PET, radiotracers are made by synthesizing compounds with radioactive isotopes of these elements. Chemically, the radioactive isotope is indistinguishable from its equivalent stable isotope.

Radiopharmaceuticals are synthesized from radionuclides derived from the target material. These agents may be simple, such as the ^{15}O-^{16}O molecules described earlier, or they may be much more complex. Regardless of the chemical complexity of the radioactive molecule, all radiopharmaceuticals must be synthesized rapidly. This entails specialized techniques not only to create the labeled substance but also to verify the purity (chemical, radiochemical, and radionuclide) of the radiotracer.

One of the simplest radiopharmaceuticals used in PET studies is ^{15}O-water ($[^{15}O]$-H_2O), which is produced continuously from the $^{14}N(d,n)^{15}O$ nuclear reaction or in batches from the $^{15}N(p,n)^{15}O$ nuclear reaction. As previously discussed, the radioactive oxygen quickly combines with a stable ^{16}O atom, which has been added to the stable N_2 target gas, to form an oxygen molecule (O_2). The ^{15}O-^{16}O molecule is reduced over a platinum catalyst with small amounts of stable H_2 and N_2 gas. Radioactive water vapor ($[^{15}O]$-H_2O) is produced and collected in sterile saline for injection. It is used primarily for the determination of local cerebral blood flow (LCBF). PET LCBF images from one subject using two different techniques are shown in Fig. 29.25. Blood flow to tumor, heart, kidney, or other tissues also can be measured using $[^{15}O]$-H_2O.

The most common and widely used PET radiopharmaceutical for clinical PET imaging is a little more complex than labeled water and employs ^{18}F-labeled fluoride ions (F–) to form a sugar analog called $[^{18}F]$-2-fluoro-2-deoxy-D-glucose (^{18}F-FDG). This agent is used to determine the local metabolic rate of glucose use in tumor, brain, heart, or other tissues that use glucose at an increased rate. The glucose obtained from food is metabolized by the body's cells via the first stage of cellular respiration (glycolysis) and continues to be broken down, creating large quantities of adenosine triphosphate (ATP). However, in contrast to glucose, ^{18}F-FDG cannot be completely metabolized. Once ^{18}F-FDG is phosphorylated into fluorodeoxyglucose-6-phosphate ($[^{18}F]$-FDG-6-PO_4), the cell can no longer process it. The cell then retains the newly formed $[^{18}F]$-FDG-6-PO_4 for a few hours before breaking it down and filtering it out. This period of retention allows for imaging. These pathways for glucose and ^{18}F-FDG are shown schematically in Fig. 29.26.

The total time for FDG production, which includes target irradiation (1 hour to 90 minutes), radiochemical synthesis (30 minutes to 1 hour), and purity certification (15 minutes), is approximately 2 to 3 hours (depending on the exact synthesis method used). Because of the short half-life of most positron-emitting radioisotopes, radiopharmaceutical production must be closely tied to the clinical patient schedule. Injected doses of ^{18}F-FDG range from 5 to 20 mCi; a standard dose is 15 to 20 mCi. FDG is dissolved in a few milliliters of isotonic saline and is administered intravenously.

Camera design

Scintillators used in PET cameras can be constructed from various materials. Each material has a different set of characteristics that may improve or degrade the quality of the system. The optimal scintillator would have a short decay time, high light output, high-energy resolution, and high stopping power. Characteristics of commercial materials available are listed

Fig. 29.25 PET local cerebral blood flow images. Images in the *top row* were created using a standard filtered back-projection reconstruction technique. An iterative reconstructive method was used to create images in the *bottom row* from the same raw data that were used for upper images. In all images, *dark areas* correspond to high brain blood flow. There is about an 8-mm separation between each brain slice within a row.

Fig. 29.26 Glucose compartmental model *(above dashed line)* compared with the ^{18}F-FDG model *(below dashed line)*. ^{18}F-FDG does not go to complete storage (glycogen) or metabolism (CO_2 + H_2O) as does glucose. The constants (*K*) refer to reaction rates for moving substances from one compartment to another. *Dashed arrow* refers to extremely small *K* value that can usually be neglected.

in Table 29.5. The newest scintillator, lutetium orthosilicate (Lu_2SiO_5:Ce), has a higher light output (approximately four times that of bismuth germanate [BGO]) and faster photofluorescent decay (approximately 7.5 times that of BGO). Scintillator dimensions are also being reduced to improve resolution. At the present time, the resolution within the image plane for PET scanners is between 3 mm and 5 mm full width at half maximum. This means an image of a point source of radioactivity appears to be 3 to 5 mm wide at half the maximum intensity of the source image.

The basic component of the PET scanner is the block. A block is composed of a scintillation crystal coupled with 4 PMTs. The crystal is cut into a matrix (6 × 6, 7 × 8, or 8 × 8) of small rectangular boxes (3 to 6 mm long, 3 to 6 mm wide) with varying depths (10 to 30 mm deep) (Fig. 29.27). These blocks are then organized into a row to form detector modules. Next, the modules are aligned side by side to construct a ring (Fig. 29.28), and to increase the imaging field *(z)*, several rings are combined. Typical new scanners have 800 to 1000 detectors per ring.

The average bore width *(x, y)* of these scanners is approximately 70 cm, with newer scanners being slightly larger in diameter. The radial field of view (FOV) or the imaging dimension parallel to the detector rings for these scanners is approximately 10 inches (24 cm) and 22 inches (55 cm) (Fig. 29.29). The *z* axis or dimension perpendicular to the detector rings is 6 to 20 inches (15 to 50 cm). An actual PET/CT scanner can be seen in Fig. 29.30.

Fig. 29.27 PET scintillation block detector. Many crystal detectors are made from a single block of material and have cuts made to different depths and filled with opaque material. There are often 8 × 8 detector elements made, and the different depths of cuts allow localization with only four PMTs. *A,* If a photon interacts with a central detector element, the shallow cut allows the light from the scintillation to be localized by several PMTs. *B,* A photon interacting with a detector element near the edge of the block may have light that is seen by one PMT only.

(From Mettler FA, Guiberteau MJ: *Mettler's essentials of nuclear medicine imaging,* ed 6, Philadelphia, 2012, Elsevier.)

TABLE 29.5

Properties of PET scintillator materials

Property	NaI	BGO $Bi_4Ge_3O_{12}$	GSO Gd_2SiO_5(Ce)	LSO Lu_2SiO_5(Ce)	LYSO $Lu_{2(1-x)}Y_{2x}SiO_5$(Ce)
Z (atomic number) stopping power	50	74	58	66	65
Density (g/cm³)	3.7	7.1	6.7	7.4	7.1
Light yield	100	15	26	75	80
Decay constant (ns)	230	300	65	40	41
Energy resolution @ 511 keV (%)	6.6	10.2	8.5	10	14
Attenuation length (mm) for 511 keV photons	28.8	10.5	14.3	11.6	12
Attenuation coefficient (cm⁻¹) @ 511 keV	0.34	0.94	0.67	0.87	0.83

BGO, Bismuth germanium oxide; *GSO,* gadolinium oxyorthosilicate; *LSO,* lutetium oxyorthosilicate; *LYSO,* lutetium yttrium orthosilicate; *NAI,* sodium iodide.

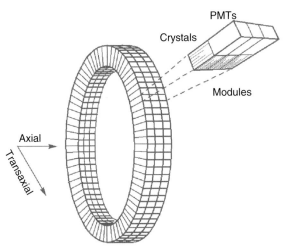

Fig. 29.28 Detector blocks, or modules, are used to construct a ring of detectors around the patient. Hundreds of blocks are used to create 18 to 40 consecutive rings of detectors that for a cylindrical field of view approximately 5 cm long and that can acquire many slices of coincidence data at one time. *PMTs*, Photomultiplier tubes.

(From Waterstram-Rich K, Gilmore D: *Nuclear medicine and PET/CT: technology and techniques*, ed 8, Philadelphia, 2017, Elsevier.)

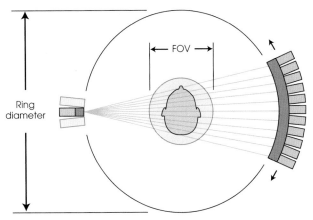

Fig. 29.29 Detector arrangement in neurologic PET ring (head-only scanner). Rays from opposed detector pairs (*lines* between detectors) depict possible coincidence events. The useful field of view *(FOV)* is delineated by the *central circle*.

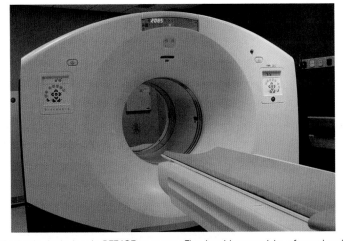

Fig. 29.30 Typical whole-body PET/CT scanner. The bed is capable of moving in and out of the scanner to measure the distribution of PET radiopharmaceuticals throughout the body, and it adjusts to a very low position for easy patient access. Sophisticated computer workstations are required to view and analyze data.

The sensitivity of a PET camera has contributed to not only the scintillator being used but whether or not the camera is using *septa*. PET collimation is the addition of thin lead or tungsten attenuators, placed between the detector elements. The collimation is designed to block annihilation photons not directly in line with the detector. This reduces the sensitivity greatly, requires higher radiopharmaceutical doses to be administered, and requires longer imaging times, but increases the cameras resolution. PET cameras with septa installed are known as *2-Dimensional* or *2D* PET Scanners. With improvements in software reconstruction techniques, current PET scanners have eliminated septa between detector components. These cameras are referred to as *3-Dimensional (3D)* PET scanners. 3D systems allow for first, second, third, fourth, and upward adjacent planes (rings) to be used to produce images all at one time (Fig. 29.31). With the inclusion of the additional cross-plane information, the PET scanner's *sensitivity* is greatly increased. Thus, injected doses of radiopharmaceutical are significantly reduced (50% to 90% less radioactivity given) to yield PET images with a quality equivalent to that of images obtained from the original dose levels used in 2D PET scanners.

Fig. 29.31 (A) Two-dimensional acquisition with septa in position has scanner sensitivity limited by septa. Three-dimensional mode with the septa retracted from the gantry significantly increases the sensitivity. (B) Brain images demonstrate a two-dimensional image *(left)* and a higher-quality three-dimensional image *(right)*.

(From Waterstram-Rich K, Gilmore D: *Nuclear medicine and PET/CT: technology and techniques,* ed 8, Philadelphia, 2017, Elsevier.)

DATA AND IMAGE ACQUISITION

The ring design described above is engineered to capture annihilation photons after they are produced. When two identical or isoenergetic photons are emitted at almost exactly 180 degrees from one another, the nearly simultaneous detection of both photons can define a straight line that passes through the body. The detection of the two annihilation photons is called a *coincidence event*, and the theoretical line that was created is known as the *line-of-response* (LOR). For a coincidence event to occur and be deemed real, the photons must reach the detectors within a specific time frame or the *coincidence time window* (6 to 12 nanoseconds). If one photon is detected and no other photon is observed during that time window, the original event is discarded. This is defined as electronic collimation. If both photons strike opposing detectors it is referred to as a *true* coincidence event, a LOR is generated, and it is used to identify the location of the annihilation. Because each photon travels at the speed of light, coincidence electronics can use simple math to deduce where the event took place based on the time it took each photon to reach the detectors. Multiple true events are summed to formulate an image.

Coincidence events fall into one of three categories; true events, scattered events, or random events. A true event is when the annihilation photon pair, unaffected by any attenuation or scatter, strikes the detectors within the resolving time and is registered as a single count. Scattered events are those in which one of the photons from the annihilation is deflected but not slowed enough to fall outside of the coincidence time frame. This creates a false LOR and increases background noise in the image. A random event is two annihilations taking place in two separate locations, and a single photon from each pair strikes opposing detectors within the coincidence timing window. Again, a false LOR is created, degrading the images. Refer to Fig. 29.32 to get a better understanding of these events.

PET scanners must operate with a high sensitivity, and as a result scanners must also be able to handle very high count rates with minimum *deadtime* losses. Coincidence events are collected not only for detector pairs within each ring (direct-plane information) but also between adjacent rings (cross-plane information) as shown in Fig. 29.33. However, not all photons emitted from the patient can be detected. The emission process is *isotropic*, which means that the annihilation photons are emitted with equal probability in all directions so that only a small fraction of the total number of photons emitted from the patient actually strike two opposing detectors (Fig. 29.34). In most cases, almost 99% of annihilation events are missed or discarded by the camera.

Coincidence Events

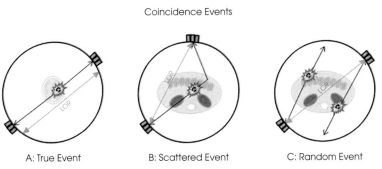

A: True Event   B: Scattered Event   C: Random Event

Fig. 29.32 (A) A *true event* is when annihilation photons from a single annihilation event are detected ~180 degrees apart within the coincidence timing window. This creates correct LOR, increasing the target to background ratio. (B) A *scattered event* occurs due to attenuation deflecting the photon. This results in an incorrect LOR and degrades the image. (C) A *random event* is the resultant of two separate annihilation events striking detectors on opposite sides of the gantry within the same coincidence timing window. This also creates a false LOR and decreases the target to background ratio. *Remember*, all coincidence events are detected and are potentially applied to the final image.

Fig. 29.33 Side-view schematic of a small portion of a multi-ring PET scanner. *Darker green squares* indicate the scintillator-matrix, which is attached to multiple photomultiplier tubes. *Solid lines* indicate the direct planes, and *dashed lines* depict the cross planes. Improvements in PET scanner instrumentation not only permit cross-plane information between adjacent rings to be acquired, but it also allows for expansion to the second, third, fourth, and fifth neighboring rings. This significantly enhances overall scanner sensitivity.

Imaging

The *z*-axis or the imaging dimension parallel to the detector rings for these scanners is approximately 6 to 20 inches (15 to 50 cm). When imaging a patient, the length of the *z*-axis is referred to as the bed. Depending on the imaging being performed, one to several beds may be required. To obtain enough counts to form a diagnostic PET image, the patient must remain in one bed position for a set period of time (~2 to 4 minutes). Once adequate counts have been gathered, the scanner table moves the patient in/out to scan the next section of their body. Because the resolution and sensitivity of PET cameras become increasingly poor as it approaches the edges of the FOV, motion increments are designed to overlap by a few centimeters. This allows for sufficient axial sampling achieved for all but the first and last bed position. Fig. 29.35 illustrates bed and patient positioning.

In PET there are three types of scans. One is brain and cardiac imaging, which only requires one bed. Imaging times vary due to the attenuation (skull) and radiopharmaceutical doses. Brain scans can take up to 10 minutes, while only 5 minutes is required for most heart scans. The second is known as "eye-to-thigh" imaging. Eye-to-thigh imaging is just that; images are obtained from a patient's orbitals to their mid-thighs. A scout or low-grade x-ray image (similar to CT) is taken of the patient to identify these anatomical structures so the technologist can adjust the beginning and ending points. The average eye-to-thigh exam is composed of about seven beds, at 3 minutes per bed. The last scan is the whole body scan. A whole body scan is used in patients with melanoma or cancers that are known to metastasize anywhere in the body. These scans are begun at the top of the head and continued all the way to the tip of the toes. Due to most table constraints, the patients' legs must be scanned separately. Whole body scans consist of 9 to 12 beds, at 1 to 3 minutes per bed.

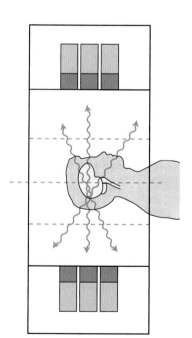

Fig. 29.34 Side view of PET scanner, illustrating possible photon directions. Only 15% of the total number of emitted photons from the patient can be detected in a whole-body tomograph (ring diameter 39 inches (100 cm)). This is increased to 25% for a head tomograph (ring diameter 24 inches (60 cm)). For these estimates, axis coverage was considered to be 6 inches (15 cm). The actual number of detected coincidences would be less than either the 15% or 25% estimate because the detector efficiency is not 100% (typical efficiency 30%).

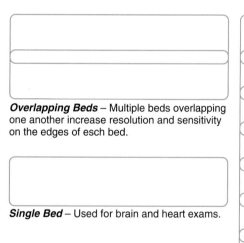

Overlapping Beds – Multiple beds overlapping one another increase resolution and sensitivity on the edges of esch bed.

Single Bed – Used for brain and heart exams.

Example of "Eye to Thigh" exam. The patient is positioned in a manner to be scanned from their orbitals to their mid thighs.

Fig. 29.35 Bed positions during a typical PET scan.

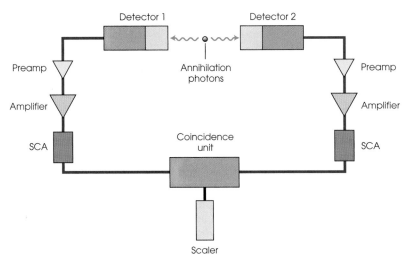

Fig. 29.36 Simplified coincidence electronics for one pair of detectors in a PET tomograph.

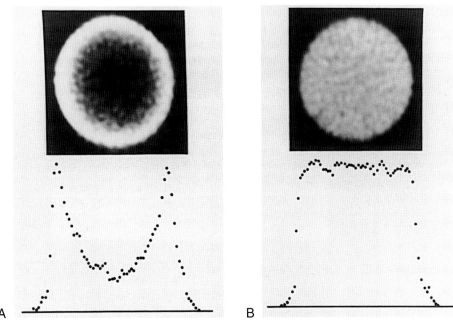

Fig. 29.37 (A) Uncorrected image of a phantom homogeneously filled with water-soluble PET nuclide of ^{68}Ga or ^{18}F. (B) Attenuation-corrected image of same phantom. Cross-sectional cuts through the center of each image are shown in *lower panels.* The attenuation correction for a phantom with a diameter of 8 inches (20 cm) can be 70% in the center of the object.

Fig. 29.38 Typical PET/CT scanner.

(Courtesy GE Medical Systems, Milwaukee, WI.)

IMAGE RECONSTRUCTION AND IMAGE PROCESSING

Array processors are used to perform the maximum likelihood (iterative) reconstruction that converts the raw *sinogram* data into PET images. This technique is similar to the technique employed for CT image reconstruction. Faster and less costly desktop computers are replacing array processor technology and greatly simplifying software requirements for image reconstruction. A simplified block diagram for a single coincidence circuit is shown in Fig. 29.36.

Three important corrections need to be made during image reconstruction to ensure an accurate and interpretable scan. First, the disintegration of radionuclides follows Poisson statistics. As discussed earlier, random and scattered events are registered by the PET scanner as coincidence events, which degrade the overall image quality. A simple approximation allows for the subtraction of the random events after image acquisition and is based on the individual count rates for each detector and the coincidence resolving time (8 to 12 ns) of the tomograph electronics.

Second, photons traversing biologic tissues also undergo absorption and scatter. As shown in Fig. 29.37, an AC is applied to account for photons that should have been detected but were not. AC also identifies events that were registered outside the body and subtracts them from the final images. In the past, the correction was typically based on a transmission scan acquired under computer control using a radioactive rod or pin source of ^{68}Ge (germanium; 271-day half-life) that circumscribed the portion of the patient's body within the PET scanner. At the present time, PET/CT scanners use the CT data to correct for attenuation more accurately (Fig. 29.38).

Lastly, count rates from the detectors also need to be corrected for dead-time losses. At high count rates, detector electronics cannot handle every incoming event; some events are lost because the electronics are busy processing prior events. Measuring the tomograph response to known input count rates allows empiric formulations for the losses to be determined and applied to the reconstructed image data. Valid corrections for deadtime losses can approach 100%.

For PET procedures, data acquisition is not limited to images of tomographic count rates. The creation of *quantitative* parametric images for the measurement of glucose metabolism is used to identify the locations of potential metastases. Cancers known to have high metabolic activity tend to absorb ^{18}F-FDG at a higher rate. By identifying the absorption rates of normal tissues to those of potentially abnormal ones, the physician can gain a better understanding of a patient's condition. This begins with the assessment of the radioactive concentration (mCi/mL) within a specific volume or voxel (cubic pixel) of tissue. This information is then applied to calculate the *standardized uptake value* (SUV). The SUV is a semi-quantitative index used to identify tissues likely of cancer. On average when the SUV is found to be greater than 2.5, the tissue is suggestive of malignancy. SUVs of the brain, heart, kidneys, and liver are already elevated due to their normal high level of glucose metabolism.

Clinical PET

PET is unique in its ability to measure in vivo physiology because its results are quantitative, easily repeatable, and validated against the results of accurate but much more invasive techniques. However, it is relatively costly and best used for answering complex questions that involve locating and quantitatively assessing tissue function (Figs. 29.39 and 29.40). Anatomic imaging, such as CT, is often limited in its ability to determine whether found masses are of malignant or benign etiology. Because PET is a functional modality, it can often be used to determine malignancy, even in very small nodes or masses.

Patient preparation for PET studies can be detailed and is imperative for optimal imaging. In most cases, the area that is to be examined must be free of metallic objects to avoid creating artifacts on the reconstructed images. This is especially important when using a PET/CT scanner because metallic objects may cause false-positive results in the final images due to attenuation overcorrection in that region. The waiting time between dose administration and imaging varies with each study, as does the total imaging time. After completion, patients may resume all normal activities. Technical summaries of commonly performed PET procedures follow.

Fig. 29.39 (A) PET FDG brain imaging with CT fusion shows left subcortical resection site consistent with prior tumor resection. (B) At inferior and lateral margins of resection site, in the adjacent white matter, a hypermetabolic mass is identified. This case represents recurrent high-grade malignancy located in the left periventricular white matter at the frontoparietal junction adjacent to previous resection site.

Fig. 29.40 PET FDG image with CT fusion shows large hypermetabolic right lung mass. Many PET FDG studies are done for lung cancer because of its high glucose metabolism.

A   B

Fig. 29.41 (A) PET image to evaluate a patient with a history of melanoma on the scalp. Scan shows no definite evidence for recurrence. (B) Image 6 months later shows profound and widely disseminated hypermetabolic metastases throughout the body.

PET ONCOLOGY IMAGING

Clinically, 70% to 80% of PET scans are done to diagnose, stage, or restage cancer (Fig. 29.41). ¹⁸F-FDG is the radiopharmaceutical of choice. PET plays an important role in differentiating benign from malignant processes and is used for image-guided biopsies. PET is an important modality for detecting cancer recurrence in patients who have undergone surgery, chemotherapy, or radiation treatments. It is also very effective in monitoring therapeutic interventions by rapidly yet noninvasively assessing the metabolic response of the tissues to drugs.

With new reimbursement policies in effect, most malignant tumors are being imaged with ¹⁸F-FDG in PET. The most common cancers imaged include lung, colorectal, head and neck, lymphoma, thyroid, esophageal, ovarian, and melanoma.

¹⁸F-FDG ONCOLOGIC STUDY

Principle

Even though ¹⁸F-FDG is currently the prevailing radiopharmaceutical in tumor PET imaging, it was initially developed as a tracer to study glucose metabolism in the brain. In the late 1980s, successful reports of ¹⁸F-FDG tumor imaging began to surface. It became apparent that certain tumors had a much greater uptake of ¹⁸F-FDG than surrounding tissues. Tumor cells tend to have a much greater affinity for glucose than cells of surrounding tissues because of their higher glucose metabolism. This distinction is paramount in understanding how ¹⁸F-FDG PET is able to detect metastatic disease.

Although there are many considerations to take into account when performing ¹⁸F-FDG PET, the most important is in the regulation of the patient's blood glucose. Generally, a blood glucose level of less than 180 mg/dL is required for optimal imaging and can be achieved with a 4-hour fast. Patients with high glucose levels generally have poor ¹⁸F-FDG uptake because of the already overabundant presence of glucose in their blood. In cases in which the glucose level is less than 150 mg/dL, it is still important to have the patient fasting for approximately 4 hours before the injection of ¹⁸F-FDG because postprandially the insulin response is still strong enough to push the ¹⁸F-FDG into more soft tissue than is normally seen in a fasting patient. The result is an image that appears to have a low target-to-background ratio. There are several other protocols that various institutions follow to increase ^{18}F-FDG uptake by the tumor, including having the patient eat low-carbohydrate meals the day before and the day of the scan.

^{18}F-FDG studies require a 60- to 90-minute uptake period after injection for the incorporation of the radiopharmaceutical into the body. Some protocols suggest that imaging tumors after 90 minutes of ^{18}F-FDG incorporation may lead to significantly better signal-to-noise values in the tumor compared with surrounding tissues. During the uptake phase of the protocol, it is important that the patient be still and relaxed. Any motion, especially in the area of interest, would cause the muscles in that area to accumulate FDG and make interpretation of the images difficult. No reading, talking on the phone, or other activity is allowed. The patient also must be kept warm. If the patient develops a shiver, muscle uptake also can be increased.

Radiopharmaceutical

Adult dose (intravenous injection):
- 0.214 mCi/kg (7.9 MBq/kg) of ^{18}F-FDG, minimum 10 mCi (370 MBq), maximum 20 mCi (740 MBq)

Pediatric dose (weight-based intravenous injection) (see Fig. 29.7):
- 0.10 to 0.14 mCi/kg (3.7 to 5.2 MBq/kg) of ^{18}F-FDG, minimum of 0.7 mCi (27 MBq)

Scanning

Most oncologic PET exams are eye-to-thigh studies with the exception of melanoma and thyroid cancer (whole-body imaging). Depending on the dose injected and PET scanner sensitivity, approximately 3 minutes per bed position are required for the emission scan to measure the distribution of ^{18}F-FDG glucose metabolism in tissue. When using a CT scan for AC, the total time for the scan is about 25 minutes.

PET NEUROLOGIC IMAGING

Metabolic neurologic study

Principle

Because the brain uses about 25% of the body's total metabolic energy, it provides an excellent gateway for functional imaging of glucose metabolism using ^{18}F-FDG, and this is why most clinical PET brain imaging is currently done with ^{18}F-FDG. PET brain scanning is done to differentiate necrotic tissue from recurrent disease, to facilitate a diagnosis of cognitive status, and to monitor cerebrovascular disease. Another use that is proving to be beneficial is using PET imaging in patients with temporal lobe epilepsy. The identification and location of brain tumors are difficult to assess with ^{18}F-FDG, because of the high metabolic uptake of ^{18}F-FDG in the brain.

When using a PET/CT system, the anatomic information provided by the CT scan can be especially helpful in determining the effects of therapy. The guiding principle in ^{18}F-FDG PET brain imaging is that the healthy brain has high glucose metabolism and high blood flow to the cerebral cortex, which demonstrates the concentration of ^{18}F-FDG within the brain. PET is also routinely used in monitoring the response to therapy and the progression of cognitive disease. With the progression of cognitive decline, glucose metabolism in the brain declines. ^{18}F-FDG assesses temporal lobe epilepsy by evaluating the brain blood flow.

Radiopharmaceutical

Adult dose (intravenous injection):
- 5 to 10 mCi (185 to 370 MBq) of ^{18}F-FDG

Pediatric dose (weight-based intravenous injection) (see Fig. 29.7):
- 0.10 mCi/kg (3.7 MBq/kg) of ^{18}F-FDG, minimum 0.37 mCi (14 MBq)

Scanning

Before and after injection with ^{18}F-FDG, the patient should follow the same procedure as though undergoing an ^{18}F-FDG whole-body scan. The main difference is the importance of having no visual or auditory stimulation if possible. The visual cortex has a high rate of glucose metabolism during stimulation, which can make the images more difficult to interpret. Generally, the patient is injected with ^{18}F-FDG in a darkened room and is given instructions to remain still and to try to stay awake for a 30-minute uptake period. At the end of this period, the scan is performed in three-dimensional mode, with bed time of 8 to 10 minutes. The transmission is generally done for 5 minutes, unless an elliptic or contoured AC is done. When done on a PET/CT scanner, the CT scan is used to determine positioning of the brain and for the attenuation map. The time savings of using the CT scan for the AC can be very helpful, especially in pediatric patients, or claustrophobic patients who may have difficulty staying still for any length of time.

Amyloid neurologic study

Principle

β-amyloid protein is a protein that forms in patients with AD along with other cognitive disorders. Thioflavin binds to beta-amyloid histologically and fluoresces. Amyloid radiotracers are thioflavin derivatives. Patients with AD tend to have a build-up of beta-amyloid proteins between nerve cells that form plaques. Amyloid radiotracers target these plaques and identify their presence. Patients with AD will have increased uptake of ^{18}F-Florbetapir as it targets beta-amyloid plaque.

Radiopharmaceutical

Adult dose (intravenous injection):
- 10 mCi (370 MBq) of ^{18}F-Florbetapir (total volume of 10 mL or less)

Scanning

Because ^{18}F-Florbetapir does not rely on glucose metabolism for distribution, blood glucose does not need to be assessed. A 10-minute, dynamic acquisition should be acquired after a 30- to 50-minute uptake period with the patient laying supine and head positioned in a head holder to help eliminate patient movement. The FOV should include the entire brain.

Other brain studies

Other brain imaging is now being done for Parkinson disease with ^{18}F-fluorodopa, which traces dopamine synthesis in the brain. There are also a few [15]O radiotracers in use, such as $H_2^{15}O$, which are employed to assess cerebral blood flow quantitatively.

PET CARDIOLOGY IMAGING

PET is a highly valuable diagnostic tool in the determination of myocardial viability and coronary flow reserve. Because of its higher temporal and spatial resolution and its built-in AC, PET is able to offer higher diagnostic accuracy than conventional nuclear medicine techniques. Because PET tracers emit higher energy gamma rays (511 keV) compared with conventional nuclear tracers (^{201}Tl at 80 keV and ^{99m}Tc sestamibi at 140 keV), PET is able to measure tracer uptake in the body more accurately. Currently, the clinical application of PET imaging in cardiology can be divided into two main categories: the detection of myocardial viability and the assessment of coronary flow reserve.

Cardiac viability

Principle

PET imaging for cardiac viability is an invaluable tool in the assessment of viable tissue in the left ventricle. The use of ^{18}F-FDG as an indicator of glucose metabolism allows the clinician to assess the likelihood of successful coronary revascularization. Patients with moderate to severe left ventricular dysfunction yet high myocardial viability are the most likely to benefit from revascularization. Patients who are found to have minimally viable tissue would not benefit from revascularization and may undergo the procedure needlessly if no noninvasive testing is done. Normal protocols stipulate that patients undergo a resting cardiac perfusion scan before cardiac ^{18}F-FDG PET. Traditional patterns of myocardial viability include decreased resting blood perfusion in the presence of enhanced metabolic uptake.

Radiopharmaceutical

Adult dose (intravenous injection):
- Viability imaging:
  - 10 mCi of ^{18}F-FDG
- Perfusion (rest imaging)
  - 20 mCi (740 MBq) of ^{13}N-ammonia
  - 30 to 60 mCi (1110 to 2220 MBq) of ^{82}Rb

Scanning

The patient preparation for PET cardiac viability scans is very important in obtaining accurate images. On the day of the scan, all patients are to fast and refrain from caffeine and nicotine intake. Upon arrival, patients have two intravenous lines placed, one in each arm. One line is for the radiopharmaceutical injection; the other is for the insulin and dextrose infusion. A rest perfusion scan with ^{13}N-ammonia or ^{82}Rb is usually performed first. After completion of the scan, the patient is given a combination of dextrose and insulin intravenously to increase the levels of glucose in the bloodstream. This converts the heart from using fatty acids as its primary source of energy to glucose. When the patient's blood glucose level reaches an optimal level, ^{18}F-FDG is injected. Approximately 30 minutes after injection, the patient is moved onto the scanner and positioned for the transmission scan. A transmission scan of 10 to 15 minutes ensues with a 5- to 10-minute emission scan to follow. When the scan is completed, patients are fed a light lunch,

and their blood glucose levels are monitored until they reach normal levels.

Coronary flow reserve

Principle

PET is now commonly used to facilitate diagnosis of coronary artery disease and to assess coronary flow reserve. It is especially helpful in differentiating between stress-induced coronary ischemia and necrosis. These studies are most often done using ^{13}N-ammonia, but the advantages of other radioisotopes, such as ^{82}Rb and ^{15}O, are making their use more common. The advantage of ^{82}Rb is that it is generator-produced and acts as a potassium analog, similar to ^{201}Tl, but it is expensive and requires a large patient load to make it cost effective. The benefit of ^{15}O is that it is freely diffusible into the myocardium and is independent of metabolism, making it an excellent choice for quantitative studies. However, it does present other problems, because its short half-life and short imaging time can lead to grainy images, making it a poor choice for qualitative studies. The use of ^{13}N-ammonia is most common because of its relatively short half-life (10 minutes) and because it is trapped by the myocardium by means of the glutamine synthesis reaction.

Radiopharmaceutical

Adult dose (intravenous injection):
- 10 to 20 mCi (370 to 740 MBq) of ^{13}N-ammonia
- 30 to 60 mCi (1110 to 2220 MBq) of ^{82}Rb

NOTE: *Rest and stress doses are the same.*

Scanning

Patients are asked to eat a light meal approximately 2 hours before the test and to avoid caffeine and nicotine products for 24 hours before the test. This is because caffeine may affect the pharmacologic stress agent used for PET coronary flow reserve studies. The test consists of two portions: rest and stress imaging. The rest imaging is initiated by using the transmission scan to locate and position the heart in the center of the FOV. If the imaging is being done on a PET/CT system, this is done using the CT scan as a scout. When the heart is centered, a transmission scan of 10 to 15 minutes, based on patient girth, is performed for attenuation purposes. On completion of the transmission scan, ^{13}N-ammonia may be injected. The emis-

sion scan generally takes 10 to 15 minutes, and may be done as a gated acquisition if desired. After approximately 50 minutes (five ^{13}N half-lives), the stress study may begin. The stress agent is infused over the appropriate time and ^{13}N-ammonia is injected based on the department protocol. Emission imaging should begin immediately. On completion of the examination, the patient may be discharged and allowed to resume normal activity.

Future of Nuclear Medicine

RADIOIMMUNOTHERAPY

Several radioimmunotherapy protocols have come into clinical use in recent years. Monoclonal antibodies specifically designed to localize on the surface of different types of cancer cells can now be tagged with a radioisotope and then imaged. If the monoclonal antibody successfully localizes on the tumor site, the radioisotope may be replaced with a beta-emitting therapeutic radioisotope such as ^{131}I or ^{90}Y. Current studies are looking to treat refractory low-grade transformed B-cell non-Hodgkin lymphoma with ^{90}Y-ibritumomab tiuxetan (Zevalin) or ^{131}I-tositumomab (Bexxar). These studies provide convincing evidence that more diseases may be treatable in the future using radioimmunotherapy.

HYBRID IMAGING

Considerable research into the fusion of functional (SPECT and PET) and anatomic (CT and MRI) imaging has led to the introduction of dual-modality, or hybrid, imaging systems. This is one of the most exciting developments in the field of nuclear medicine. The combined PET/CT camera shown in Fig. 29.38 couples the functional imaging capabilities of PET with the superb anatomic imaging of CT. Images from each modality are coregistered during the acquisition process and in near-simultaneity. Because the images can be overlaid one on another, the position of suspected tumors can be recognized more easily. Suspicious metabolically active areas can now be identified anatomically from the CT information. These features have improved the reliability of SPECT and PET interpretation. Metabolic and anatomic evaluation after therapy can now be accomplished in one imaging session. For all these reasons, SPECT/CT and

PET/CT are becoming among the most useful diagnostic procedures for staging disease and evaluating the treatment of cancer. All of the advantages of the integration between PET and MRI have not yet been identified. Continued research utilizing PET/MRI in the areas of oncology, neurology, and cardiology will lead radiologic imaging into a new era. With the hybridization of PET/CT and PET/MRI, molecular imaging has made tremendous advancements toward improving diagnostic care for all patients.

PET

PET technology is advancing on many fronts. ^{18}F-FDG is routinely being produced in distribution centers throughout the United States and Europe. One or more cyclotrons at each distribution site are continuously producing ^{18}F-fluoride for incorporation into ^{18}F-FDG. Unit doses are shipped via common commercial carriers, which also include chartered air and special ground couriers from a network of registered pharmacy distribution centers to individual PET centers that do not have cyclotrons. Clinical PET imaging no longer requires the high financial commitment to own and operate a nuclear accelerator to produce PET radiopharmaceuticals at a local site.

New radiopharmaceuticals are also being developed. As PET radiopharmaceutical distribution centers expand and are able to handle the daily demands of providing ^{18}F-FDG to the existing and new PET centers, production of more ^{18}F-labeled radiopharmaceuticals specifically for tumor imaging is likely to become available. FDA approval would be required before clinical imaging, but several PET radiopharmaceutical manufacturers are sponsoring drug clinical trials to accelerate the deployment of new and viable clinical PET imaging agents. Radiolabeled choline, thymidine, fluorodopa, estrogen receptors, and numerous other biomolecules are likely candidates for new PET clinical tracers.

Mobile PET units are a reality, as shown in Figs. 29.42 and 29.43. PET scanner technology has matured to the point that the original frailty of the electronics and detector systems has been eliminated. Robust mobile units travel to community hospitals that need PET imaging but not at the level that necessitates a dedicated in-house PET scanner. By spending 1 or 2 days per week at several different hospitals in smaller communities or rural settings, the mobile PET camera best serves the needs of their oncology patients. The ^{18}F-FDG distribution centers are necessary in this scenario because the mobile PET camera unit needs a supply of radiotracer to carry out PET imaging studies. Until nationwide ^{18}F-FDG distribution centers became a reality, as they now are, the use of mobile PET was extremely limited.

Fig. 29.42 Mobile PET coach showing operator on staff stairs and elevator platform in the elevated position. Elevator used to transport patients from ground level to floor level of the PET scanner unit.

(Courtesy Shared PET Imaging, LLC.)

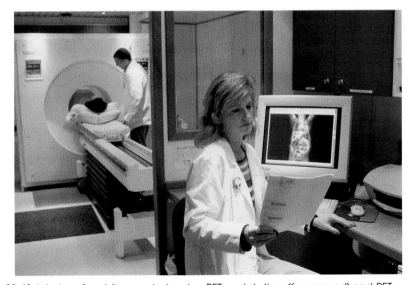

Fig. 29.43 Interior of mobile coach showing PET workstation *(foreground)* and PET scanner *(background)*.

(Courtesy Shared PET Imaging, LLC.)

Conclusion

Nuclear medicine technology is a multidisciplinary field in which medicine is linked to quantitative sciences, including chemistry, radiation biology, physics, and computer technology. Since the early 20th century, nuclear medicine has expanded to include molecular nuclear medicine, in vivo and in vitro chemistry, and physiology. The spectrum of nuclear medicine technology skills and responsibilities varies. The scope of nuclear medicine technology includes patient care, quality control, diagnostic procedures, computer data acquisition and processing, radiopharmaceuticals, radionuclide therapy, and radiation safety. Many clinical procedures are performed in nuclear medicine departments across the United States and throughout the world. Nuclear medicine procedures complement other imaging methods in radiology and pathology departments.

The evolution of PET has provided the nuclear medicine department with complex diagnostic imaging procedures. PET is a useful clinical and research tool, which requires the multidisciplinary support of the physician, physicist, physiologist, chemist, engineer, software programmer, and radiographer. This imaging procedure allows numerous biologic parameters in the working human body to be examined without disturbing normal-equilibrium physiology. PET measures regional function that cannot be determined by any other means, which includes CT and MRI. Current PET studies of the brain involve the imaging of patients with epilepsy, Huntington disease, stroke, schizophrenia, brain tumors, AD, and other disorders of the central nervous system. PET studies of the heart are providing routine diagnostic information on patients with coronary artery disease by identifying viable myocardium for revascularization. The greatest impact PET has made is the ability to identify highly metabolic tumors. PET scanning is critically involved in the determination of the effects of therapeutic drug regimens on tumors and the differentiation of necrosis from viable tumor. Nearly 80% of all PET imaging today is directed at tumor detection and the evaluation of therapeutic intervention. Overall, human physiology will become better understood as the technology advances, yielding higher resolution instruments, new radiopharmaceuticals, and improved analysis of PET data.

The future of nuclear medicine may lie in its unique ability to identify functional or physiologic abnormalities. With the continued development of new radiopharmaceuticals and imaging technology, nuclear medicine will continue to be a unique and valuable tool for diagnosing and treating disease.

Definition of Terms

alpha particle Nucleus of a helium atom, consisting of two protons and two neutrons, having a positive charge of 2.

analog Radiopharmaceutical biochemically equivalent to a naturally occurring compound in the body.

annihilation Total transformation of matter into energy; occurs after the antimatter positron collides with an electron. Two photons are created; each equals the rest mass of the individual particles.

attenuation coefficient Number that represents the statistical reduction in photons that exit a material (N) from the value that entered the material (N_o). The reduced flux is the result of scatter and absorption, which can be expressed in the following equation: $N = N_o e - \mu\chi$, where μ is the attenuation coefficient and l is the distance traversed by the photons.

becquerel (Bq) Unit of activity in the International System of Units; equal to 1 disintegration per second (dps): 1 Bq = 1 dps.

beta particle Electron whose point of origin is the nucleus; electron originating in the nucleus by way of decay of a neutron into a proton and an electron.

blood-brain barrier Anatomic and physiologic feature of the brain thought to consist of walls of capillaries in the central nervous system and surrounding glial membranes. The barrier separates the parenchyma of the central nervous system from blood. The blood–brain barrier prevents or slows the passage of some drugs and other chemical compounds, radioactive ions, and disease-causing organisms, such as viruses from the blood, into the central nervous system.

coincidence event When two annihilation photons strike apposing detectors in a PET scanner

coincidence time window The time in which annihilation photons must strike opposing detectors to be considered coincidence events (6 to 12 nanoseconds).

cold spot Lack of radiation being received or recorded, not producing any image and resulting in an area of no, or very light, density; may be caused by disease or artifact.

collimator Shielding device used to limit the angle of entry of radiation; usually made of lead.

Coulomb forces Forces exerted upon objects with charge. When the charges are the same, the forces repel one another (+, +). If the charges are opposite, the forces attract one another (+, −). Particles without charge (neutrons) are unaffected by these forces.

curie Standard of measurement for radioactive decay; based on the disintegration of 1 g of radium at 3.731010 disintegrations per second.

cyclotron Device for accelerating charged particles to high energies using magnetic and oscillating electrostatic fields. As a result, particles move in a spiral path with increasing energy.

daughter Element that results from the radioactive decay of a parent element.

deadtime Time when the system electronics are already processing information from one photon interaction with a detector and cannot accept new events to be processed from other detectors.

decay Radioactive disintegration of the nucleus of an unstable nuclide.

detector Device that is a combination of a scintillator and photomultiplier tube used to detect x-rays and gamma rays.

deuteron Ionized nucleus of heavy hydrogen (deuterium), which contains one proton and one neutron.

dose Measure of the amount of energy deposited in a known mass of tissue from ionizing radiation. Absorbed dose is described in units of rads; 1 rad is equal to 10^{-2} joules/kg or 100 ergs/g.

ejection fraction (cardiac) Fraction of the total volume of blood of the left ventricle ejected per contraction.

electron capture Radioactive decay process in which a nucleus with an excess of protons brings an electron into the nucleus, creating a neutron out of a proton, decreasing the atomic number by 1. The resulting atom is often unstable and gives off a gamma ray to achieve stability.

external radiation detector Instrument used to determine the presence of radioactivity from the exterior.

¹⁸F-FDG Radioactive analog of naturally available glucose. It follows the same biochemical pathways as glucose; however, in contrast to glucose, it is not totally metabolized to carbon dioxide and water.

fission Splitting of a nucleus into two or more parts with the subsequent release of enormous amounts of energy.

functional image See parametric image.

gamma camera Device that uses the emission of light from a crystal struck by gamma rays to produce an image of the distribution of radioactive material in a body organ.

gamma ray High-energy, short-wavelength electromagnetic radiation emanating from the nucleus of some nuclides.

generator system A piece of equipment used in radiopharmacies to quantitatively separate technetium-99m from its parent radionuclide molybdenum-99.

ground state State of lowest energy of a system.

half-life (T½) Term used to describe the time elapsed until some physical quantity has decreased to half of its original value.

homeostasis State of equilibrium of the body's internal environment.

hot lab Location in a nuclear medicine department or radiopharmacy where radioisotopes are stored before use or compounding.

image coregistration Computer technique that permits realignment of images that have been acquired from different modalities and have different orientations and magnifications. With realignment, images possess the same orientation and size. Images can then be overlaid, one on the other, to show similarities and differences between the images.

in vitro Outside a living organism.

in vivo Within a living organism.

isotope Nuclide of the same element with the same number of protons but a different number of neutrons.

isotropic Referring to uniform emission of radiation or particles in three dimensions.

kinetics Movement of materials into, out of, and through biologic spaces. A mathematic expression is often used to describe and quantify how substances traverse membranes or participate in biochemical reactions.

light pipe Tube-like structure attached to the scintillation crystal to convey the emitted light to the photomultiplier tube.

line of response (LOR) Theoretical line created by the detection of a coincidence event on opposing sides of the PET camera (see Fig. 29.32).

magnetic resonance imaging (MRI) Technique of nuclear magnetic resonance (NMR) as it is applied to medical imaging. Magnetic resonance is abbreviated MR.

metastable Describes the excited state of a nucleus that returns to its ground state by emission of a gamma ray; has a measurable lifetime.

nuclear particle accelerator Device to produce radioactive material by accelerating ions (e.g., electrons, protons, deuterons) to high energies and projecting them toward stable materials. Accelerators include linac, cyclotron, synchrotron, Van de Graaff accelerator, and betatron.

nuclear reactor Device that under controlled conditions is used for supporting a self-sustained nuclear reaction.

nuclide General term applicable to all atomic forms of an element.

organified The ability of the thyroid to absorb and incorporate iodine into thyroid hormone.

parametric image Image that relates anatomic position (the x and y position on an image) to a physiologic parameter such as blood flow (image intensity or color). It may also be referred to as a functional image.

parent Radionuclide that decays to a specific daughter nuclide either directly or as a member of a radioactive series.

particle accelerator Device that provides the energy necessary to enable a nuclear reaction.

pharmaceutical Relating to a medicinal drug.

photomultiplier tube (PMT) Electronic tube that converts light photons to electrical pulses.

photopenia See cold spot.

pixel (picture element) Smallest indivisible part of an image matrix for display on a computer screen. Typical images may be 128×128, 256×256, or 512×512 pixels.

positron Positively charged particle emitted from neutron-deficient radioactive nuclei.

positron emission tomography (PET) Imaging technique that creates transaxial images of organ physiology from the simultaneous detection of positron annihilation photons.

pulse height analyzer Instrument that accepts input from a detector and categorizes the pulses on the basis of signal strength.

pyrogen-free Free of a fever-producing agent of bacterial origin.

quantitative Type of PET study in which the final images are not simply distributions of radioactivity but rather correspond to units of capillary blood flow, glucose metabolism, or receptor density. Studies between individuals and repeat studies in the same individual permit comparison of pixel values on an absolute scale.

radiation Emission of energy; rays of waves.

radioactive Exhibiting the property of spontaneously emitting alpha, beta, and gamma rays by disintegration of the nucleus.

radioactivity Spontaneous disintegration of an unstable atomic nucleus resulting in the emission of ionizing radiation.

radioisotope Synonym for radioactive isotope. Any isotope that is unstable undergoes decay with the emission of characteristic radiation.

radionuclide Unstable nucleus that transmutes via nuclear decay.

radiopharmaceutical Refers to a radioactive drug used for diagnosis or therapy.

radiotracer Synonym for radiopharmaceutical.

random event When two annihilations take place in two separate locations and a single photon from each pair strikes opposing detectors within the coincidence timing window. A false LOR is created, degrading PET images

ray Imaginary line drawn between a pair of detectors in the PET scanner or between the x-ray source and detector in a CT scanner.

reconstruction Mathematic operation that transforms raw data acquired on a PET tomograph (sinogram) into an image with recognizable features.

region of interest (ROI) Area that circumscribes a desired anatomic location on a PET image. Image-processing systems permit drawing of ROI on images. The average parametric value is computed for all pixels within the ROI and returned to the radiographer.

Principles of Radiation Oncology

Radiation oncology,[a] or *radiation therapy*, is one of three principal modalities used in the treatment of cancer. The others are surgery and chemotherapy. In radiation therapy for malignancies, *tumors* or *lesions* are treated with *cancericidal doses* of ionizing radiation as prescribed by a *radiation oncologist*, a physician who specializes in the treatment of malignant disease with radiation. The goals of the treatment are to deliver a cancericidal dose of radiation precisely to the tumor, limiting as much as possible the dose of radiation received by normal, noncancerous tissues. These dual tasks make this form of treatment complex and often challenging. Input from all members of the radiation oncology team is crucial in developing the optimal treatment plan or approach for a patient.

Cancer treatment requires a multidisciplinary approach. First, diagnostic radiologic studies such as radiographs, computed tomography (CT) scans, magnetic resonance imaging (MRI), positron emission tomography (PET) scans, and sonograms are obtained to acquire information about the location and anatomic extent of the tumor. Second, a tissue specimen (*biopsy*) is removed surgically. A *pathologist* examines the tissue to determine whether the lesion is cancerous. When cancer is diagnosed, the plan for the best treatment is determined through consultation with various *oncology* specialists (e.g., surgical *oncologist*, radiation oncologist, medical oncologist).

[a]Almost all italicized words on the succeeding pages are defined at the end of the chapter.

Although radiation oncology may be used as the only method of treatment for malignant disease, a more common approach is to use radiation in conjunction with surgery, chemotherapy, or both. Some patients with cancer may be treated only with surgery or chemotherapy; however, approximately 75% of all diagnosed cancer patients are treated with radiation. The choice of treatment can depend on many patient variables, such as the patient's overall physical and emotional condition, the histologic type of the disease, and the extent and anatomic position of the tumor. If a tumor is small and its margins are well defined, a surgical approach alone may be prescribed. If the disease is *systemic*, a chemotherapeutic approach may be chosen. Most tumors exhibit degrees of size, invasion, and spread, however, and require variations in the treatment approach that are likely to include radiation treatments administered as an adjunct to or in conjunction with surgery or chemotherapy.

Radiation is generally used after surgery when a patient is deemed to be at high risk for tumor recurrence in the *surgical bed.* The risk of recurrence is considered to be increased in the following situations:

- When the surgical margin between normal tissue and cancerous tissue is minimal (<2 cm)
- When the margin is positive for cancer (i.e., when cancerous tissue is not completely removed)
- When the tumor is incompletely resected because of its large size, its relationship with normal vital structures, or both
- When the cancer has spread to adjacent lymph nodes

Radiation can be used as the definitive (primary) cancer treatment or as an adjuvant treatment (i.e., in combination with another form of therapy). It can also be used for *palliation.*

Radiation treatments most often are delivered on a daily basis, Monday through Friday, for 2 to 8 weeks. The length of time and the total dose of radiation delivered depend on the type of cancer being treated and the purpose of treatment (*cure* or palliation). Prescribed dosages of radiation can range from 2000 centigray (cGy) for palliation to 8000 cGy

for curative intent (total doses). The delivery of a small amount of radiation per day (180 to 200 cGy) for a certain number of treatments, instead of one large dose, is termed *fractionation.* Because these smaller doses of radiation are more easily tolerated by normal tissue, fractionation can help minimize the acute toxic effect a patient experiences during treatment and the possible long-term side effects of treatment.

The precision and accuracy necessary to administer high doses of radiation to tumors while not harming normal tissue require the combined effort of all members of the radiation oncology team. Members of this team include the radiation oncologist, a physicist, dosimetrists, radiation therapists, and oncology nurses.

The radiation oncologist prescribes the quantity of radiation and determines the anatomic region or regions to be treated. The *medical physicist* is responsible for calibration and maintenance of the radiation-producing equipment. The physicist also advises the physician about dosage calculations and complex treatment techniques. The *medical dosimetrist* devises a plan for delivering the treatments in a manner to meet best the physician's goals of irradiating the tumor while protecting vital normal structures. The *radiation therapist* is responsible for obtaining radiographs or CT scans that localize the area to be treated, administering the treatments, keeping accurate records of the dose delivered each day, and monitoring the patient's physical and emotional well-being. Educating patients about potential radiation side effects and assisting patients with the management of these side effects are often the responsibilities of the oncology nurse.

The duties and responsibilities of the radiation therapist are more thoroughly described elsewhere in this chapter. In addition, more information is provided about the circumstances in which radiation is used to treat cancer. The steps necessary to prepare a patient for treatment are also described. These steps include (1) simulation, (2) development of the optimal treatment plan in dosimetry, and (3) treatment delivery. Current techniques and future trends are also discussed.

Historical Development

Ionizing radiation was originally used to obtain a radiographic image of internal anatomy for diagnostic purposes. The resultant image depended on many variables, including the energy of the beam, the processing techniques, the material on which the image was recorded, and, most important, the amount of energy absorbed by the various organs of the body. The transfer of energy from the beam of radiation to the biologic system and the observation of the effects of this interaction became the foundation of radiation oncology.

Two of the most obvious and sometimes immediate biologic effects observed during the early diagnostic procedures were epilation (loss of hair) and erythema (reddening of the skin). Epilation and erythema resulted primarily from the great amount of energy absorbed by the skin during radiographic procedures. These short-term, radiation-induced effects afforded radiographic practitioners an opportunity to expand the use of radiation to treat conditions ranging from relatively benign maladies such as hypertrichosis (excessive hair), acne, and boils to grotesque and malignant diseases such as lupus vulgaris and skin cancer.

Ionizing radiation was first applied for the treatment of a more in-depth lesion on January 29, 1896, when Grubbé is reported to have irradiated a woman with carcinoma of the left breast. This event occurred only 3 months after the discovery of x-rays by Röntgen (Table 30.1). Although Grubbé neither expected nor observed any dramatic results from the irradiation, the event is significant simply because it occurred.

In January 1902, Skinner, in New Haven, Connecticut, performed the first reported curative treatment using ionizing radiation. Skinner treated a woman who had a diagnosed malignant fibrosarcoma. Over the next 2 years and 3 months, the woman received 136 applications of the x-rays. In April 1909, 7 years after initial application of the radiation, the woman was free of disease and considered "cured."

As data were collected, the interest in radiation therapy increased. More sophisticated equipment, a greater understanding of the effects of ionizing radiation, an appreciation for time-dose relationships, and numerous other related medical breakthroughs gave impetus to the interest in radiation therapy that led to the evolution of a distinct medical specialty—radiation oncology.

Cancer

Cancer is a disease process that involves an unregulated, uncontrolled replication of cells; put more simply, the cells do not know when to stop dividing. These abnormal cells grow without regard to normal tissue. They invade adjacent tissues, destroy normal tissue, and create a mass of tumor cells. Cancerous cells can spread further by invading the lymph or blood vessels that drain the area. When tumor cells invade the lymphatic or vascular system, they are transported by that system until they become caught or lodged within a lymph node or an organ such as the liver or lungs, where secondary tumors form. The spread of cancer from the original site to different, remote parts of the body is termed *metastasis*. When cancer has spread to a distant site via blood-borne metastasis, the patient is considered incurable. Early detection and diagnosis are the keys to curing cancer.

Cancer was diagnosed in an estimated 1,688,780 individuals in the United States in 2017. This number does not include basal and squamous cell skin cancers, which have high cure rates. These types of cancer are the most common malignant diseases, with more than 5.4 million cases estimated to be diagnosed in 2012. *One in two men will develop or die of cancer in their lifetime. Slightly more than one in three women will develop or die of cancer in their lifetime. Although cancer can occur in persons of any age, it is diagnosed in most patients after age 55 years.*

TABLE 30.1

Significant developments in radiation therapy

Date	Person	Event
1895	Röntgen	Discovery of x-rays
1896	Grubbé	First use of ionizing radiation in treatment of cancer
	Becquerel	Discovery of radioactive emissions by uranium compounds
1898	M. and P. Curie	Discovery of radium
1902	Skinner	First documented case of cancer "cure" using ionizing radiation
1906	Bergonié and Tribondeau	Postulation of first law of radiosensitivity
1932	Lawrence	Invention of cyclotron
1934	Joliot and Joliot-Curie	Production of artificial radioactivity
1939	Lawrence and Stone	Treatment of cancer patient with neutron beam from cyclotron
1940	Kerst	Construction of betatron
1951		Installation of first cobalt-60 teletherapy units
1952		Installation of first linear accelerator (Hammersmith Hospital, London)

The most common cancers that occur in the United States are lung, prostate, breast, and colorectal cancer. Prostate cancer is the most common malignancy in men, and breast cancer is the most common malignancy in women. The second and third most common cancers in men and women are lung and colorectal cancer (Table 30.2).

Cancer is second only to heart disease as the leading cause of death in the United States. Lung cancer is the leading cause of cancer deaths for men and women. In 2017, an estimated 27% of cancer deaths in men and 25% in women were due to lung cancer. The next most common causes of cancer death are colon and rectal cancer in men and breast cancer, which account for 9% and 14% of cancer deaths in the United States.

RISK FACTORS

External factors

Many factors can contribute to a person's potential for the development of a *malignancy*. These factors can be external exposure to chemicals, viruses, or radiation within the environment or internal factors such as hormones, genetic mutations, and disorders of the immune system. Cancer commonly is the result of exposure to a *carcinogen*, which is a substance or material that causes cells to undergo malignant transformation and become cancerous. Some known carcinogenic agents are listed in Table 30.3. Cigarettes and other tobacco products are the principal cause of cancers of the lung, esophagus, oral cavity and pharynx, and bladder. Cigarette smokers are 23 times more likely to develop lung cancer than nonsmokers. Occupational exposure to chemicals such as chromium, nickel, or arsenic can also cause lung cancer. A person who smokes and works with chemical carcinogens is at even greater risk for developing lung cancer than a nonsmoker. In other words, risk factors can have an additive effect, acting together to initiate or promote the development of cancer. Other risk factors that have been identified are obesity, physical inactivity, and poor nutrition.

The human papilloma virus (HPV) is associated with the development of cancer of the uterine cervix, oropharynx, and anus. Infection with the hepatitis B virus (HBV) and hepatitis C virus increase one's risk for the development of hepatocellular carcinoma of the liver. Vaccines do exist to prevent infection with HPV or HBV.

Another carcinogen is *ionizing radiation*. It was responsible for the development of osteogenic sarcoma in radium-dial painters in the 1920s and 1930s, and it caused the development of skin cancers in pioneer radiologists. Early radiation therapy equipment used in the treatment of cancer often induced a second malignancy in the bone. The low-energy x-rays produced by this equipment were within the photoelectric range of interactions with matter, resulting in a 3:1 preferential absorption in bone compared with soft tissue. Some patients with breast cancer who were irradiated developed an osteosarcoma of their ribs after a 15- to 20-year latency period. With advances in diagnostic and therapeutic equipment and improved knowledge of radiation physics, radiobiology, and radiation safety practices, radiation-induced malignancies have become relatively uncommon, although the potential for their development still exists. In keeping with standard radiation safety guidelines, any dose of radiation, no matter how small, significantly increases the chance of a genetic mutation.

Internal factors

Internal factors are causative factors over which persons have no control. Genetic mutations on individual genes and *chromosomes* have been identified as predisposing factors for the development of cancer. Mutations can be sporadic or hereditary, as in colon cancer. Chromosomal defects have also been identified in other cancers, such as leukemia, Wilms tumor, retinoblastoma, and breast cancer. Because of their familial pattern of occurrence, breast, ovarian, and colorectal cancer are three major areas currently under study to obtain earlier diagnosis, which increases the cure rate. Patients with a family history of breast or ovarian cancer can be tested to see whether they have inherited the altered *BRCA-1* and *BRCA-2* genes. Patients with these altered genes are at a significantly higher risk for developing breast and ovarian cancer. Women identified as carriers of the altered genes can benefit from more intensive and early screening programs in which breast cancer may be diagnosed at a much earlier and more curable stage. These patients also have the option of *prophylactic surgery* to remove the breasts or ovaries. Some women still develop cancer, however, in the remaining tissue after surgery.

TABLE 30.2

Top five most common cancers in men and women

Men	Women
1. Prostate	1. Breast
2. Lung and bronchus	2. Lung and bronchus
3. Colon and rectum	3. Colon and rectum
4. Bladder	4. Uterus (endometrium)
5. Melanoma	5. Thyroid

TABLE 30.3

Carcinogenic agents and the cancers they cause

Carcinogen	Resultant cancer
Cigarette smoking	Cancers of lung, esophagus, bladder, and oral cavity/pharynx
Arsenic, chromium, nickel, hydrocarbons	Lung cancer
Ultraviolet light	Melanoma and nonmelanomatous skin cancers
Benzene	Leukemia
Ionizing radiation	Sarcomas of bone and soft tissue, skin cancer, and leukemia

Familial adenomatous polyposis

Familial adenomatous polyposis is a hereditary condition in which the lining of the colon becomes studded with hundreds to thousands of polyps by late adolescence. A mutation in a gene identified as the adenomatous polyposis coli *(APC)* gene is considered the cause of this abnormal growth of polyps. Virtually all people with this condition eventually develop colon cancer. These individuals develop cancer at a much earlier age than the normal population. Treatment involves removal of the entire colon and rectum.

Hereditary nonpolyposis colorectal cancer syndrome

Hereditary nonpolyposis colorectal cancer syndrome is a cancer that develops in the proximal colon in the absence of polyps or with fewer than five polyps. It has a familial distribution, occurring in three first-degree relatives in two generations, with at least one person being diagnosed before age 50 years. Hereditary nonpolyposis colorectal cancer syndrome, also known as Lynch syndrome, has also been associated with the development of cancers of the breast, endometrium, pancreas, and biliary tract.

Familial cancer research

Current research to identify the genes responsible for cancer can assist in detecting cancers at a much earlier stage in high-risk patients. Many institutions have familial cancer programs to provide genetic testing and counseling for persons with strong family histories of cancer. Experts assist in educating individuals about their potential risk for developing cancer and the importance of screening and early detection. Genetic testing remains the patient's option, and many patients prefer not to be tested.

TISSUE ORIGINS OF CANCER

Cancers may arise in any human tissue. Tumors are usually categorized under six general headings according to their tissue of origin (Table 30.4). Of cancers, 90% arise from *epithelial tissue* and are classified as *carcinomas*. Epithelial tissue lines the free internal and external surfaces of the body. Carcinomas are subdivided further into squamous cell carcinomas and adenocarcinomas based on the type of epithelium from which they arise. A squamous cell carcinoma arises from the surface (squamous) epithelium of a structure. Examples of surface epithelium include the oral cavity, pharynx, bronchus, skin, and cervix. An adenocarcinoma is a cancer that develops in glandular epithelium such as in the prostate, colon and rectum, lung, breast, or endometrium.

To facilitate the exchange of patient information from one physician to another, the International Union Against Cancer and the American Joint Committee for Cancer (AJCC) Staging and End Results Reporting designed a system for classifying tumors based on anatomic and histologic considerations. The AJCC TNM classification (Table 30.5) describes a tumor according to the size of the primary lesion or tumor *(T)*, the involvement of the regional lymph nodes *(N)*, and the occurrence of metastasis *(M)*.

TABLE 30.4

Categorization of cancers by tissue of origin

Tissue of origin	Type of tumor
Epithelium	
Surface epithelium	Squamous cell carcinoma
Glandular epithelium	Adenocarcinoma
Connective tissue	
Bone	Osteosarcoma
Fat	Liposarcoma
Lymphoreticular-hematopoietic tissue	
Lymph nodes	Lymphoma
Plasma cells	Multiple myeloma
Blood cells/bone marrow	Leukemia
Nerve tissue	
Glial tissue	Glioma
Neuroectoderm	Neuroblastoma
Tumors of more than one tissue	
Embryonic	Nephroblastoma kidney
Tumors that do not fit into above categories	
Testis	Seminoma
Thymus	Thymoma

TABLE 30.5

Application of TNM classification system

Classification	Description of tumor
Stage 0—$T_0N_0M_0$	Occult lesion; no evidence clinically
Stage I—$T_1N_0M_0$	Small lesion confined to organ of origin with no evidence of vascular and lymphatic spread or metastasis
Stage II—$T_2N_1M_0$	Tumor of <5 cm invading surrounding tissue and first-station lymph nodes but no evidence of metastasis
Stage III—$T_3N_2M_0$	Extensive lesion >5 cm with fixation to deeper structure and lymph invasion but no evidence of metastasis
Stage IV—$T_4N_3M_1$	More extensive lesion than above with invasion of bone or other adjacent structures or with distant metastasis (M_1)

Note: This is a generalization. Variations of the staging system exist for each tumor site.

Theory

The biologic effectiveness of ionizing radiation in living tissue depends partially on the amount of energy that is deposited within the tissue and partially on the condition of the biologic system. The terms used to describe this relationship are *linear energy transfer* (LET) and *relative biologic effectiveness* (RBE).

LET values are expressed in thousands of electron volts deposited per micron of tissue (keV/μm) and vary depending on the type of radiation being considered. Because of their mass and possible charge, particles tend to interact more readily with the material through which they are passing and have a greater LET value. A 5-MeV alpha particle has an LET value of 100 keV/mm in tissue; nonparticulate radiations such as 250-kilovolt (peak) (kVp) x-rays and 1.2-MeV gamma rays have much lower LET values: 2.0 and 0.2 keV/mm.

RBE values are determined by calculating the ratio of the dose from a standard beam of radiation to the dose required of the radiation beam in question to produce a similar biologic effect. The standard beam of radiation is 250-kVp x-rays, and the ratio is set up as follows:

$$RBE = \frac{Standard\ beam\ does\ to\ obtain\ effect}{Similar\ effect\ using\ beam\ in\ question}$$

As the LET increases, so does the RBE. RBE and LET values are listed in Table 30.6.

The effectiveness of ionizing radiation on a biologic system depends not only on the amount of radiation deposited but also on the state of the biologic system. One of the first laws of radiation biology, postulated by Bergonié and Tribondeau, stated in essence that the *radiosensitivity* of a tissue depends on the number of *undifferentiated* cells in the tissue, the degree of mitotic activity of the tissue, and the length of time that cells of the tissue remain in active proliferation. Although exceptions exist, the preceding is true in most tissues. The primary target of ionizing radiation is the DNA molecule, and the human cell is most radiosensitive during mitosis. Current research tends to indicate that all cells are equally radiosensitive; however, the manifestation of the radiation injury occurs at different time frames (i.e., acute versus late effects).

Because tissue cells are composed primarily of water, most of the *ionization* occurs with water molecules. These events are called *indirect effects* and result in the formation of free radicals such as OH, H, and HO_2. These highly reactive free radicals may recombine with no resultant biologic effect, or they may combine with other atoms and molecules to produce biochemical changes that may be deleterious to the cell. The possibility also exists that the radiation may interact with an organic molecule or atom, which may result in the inactivation of the cell; this reaction is called the *direct effect*. Because ionizing radiation is nonspecific (i.e., it interacts with normal cells as readily as with tumor cells), cellular damage occurs in normal and abnormal tissue. The deleterious effects are greater in the tumor cells, however, because a greater percentage of these cells are undergoing mitosis; tumor cells also tend to be more poorly *differentiated*. In addition, normal cells have a greater capability for repairing sublethal damage than tumor cells. Greater cell damage occurs to tumor cells than to normal cells for any given increment of dose. The effects of the interactions in either normal or tumor cells may be expressed by the following descriptions:
- Loss of reproductive ability
- Metabolic changes
- Cell transformation
- Acceleration of the aging process
- Cell mutation

The greater the number of interactions that occur, the greater the possibility of cell death.

The preceding information leads to a categorization of tumors according to their radiosensitivity:
1. *Very radiosensitive*
   - Gonadal germ cell tumors (seminoma of testis, dysgerminoma of ovary)
   - Lymphoproliferative tumors (Hodgkin and non-Hodgkin lymphomas)
   - Embryonal tumors (Wilms tumor of the kidney)
2. *Moderately radiosensitive*
   - Epithelial tumors (squamous and basal cell carcinomas of skin)
   - Glandular tumors (adenocarcinoma of prostate)
3. *Relatively radioresistant*
   - Mesenchymal tumors (sarcomas of bone and connective tissue)
   - Nerve tumors (glioma)

Many concepts that originate in the laboratory have little practical application, but some are beginning to influence the selection of treatment modalities and the techniques of radiation oncology. As cellular function and the effects of radiation on the cell are increasingly understood, attention is being focused on the use of drugs, or simply oxygen, to enhance the effectiveness of radiation treatments.

TABLE 30.6

Relative biologic effectiveness and linear energy transfer values for certain forms of radiation

Radiation	RBE	LET
250-kV x-rays	1	2.0
^{60}Co gamma rays	0.85	0.2
14-MeV neutrons	12	75
5-MeV alpha particles	20	100

LET, Linear energy transfer; *RBE*, relative biologic effectiveness.

Technical Aspects

EXTERNAL-BEAM THERAPY AND BRACHYTHERAPY

Two major categories for the application of radiation for cancer treatment are external-beam therapy and brachytherapy. For *external-beam treatment*, the patient lies underneath a machine that emits radiation or generates a beam of x-rays. Most cancer patients are treated in this fashion. Some patients may also be treated with *brachytherapy*, a technique in which the radioactive material is placed within the patient.

The theory behind brachytherapy is to deliver low-intensity radiation over an extended period to a relatively small volume of tissue. The low-intensity isotopes are placed directly into a tissue or cavity depositing radiation only a short distance, covering the tumor area but sparing surrounding normal tissue. This technique allows a higher total dose of radiation to be delivered to the tumor than is achievable with external-beam radiation alone. Brachytherapy may be accomplished in any of the following ways:

1. Mold technique—placement of a *radioactive* source or sources on or in close proximity to the lesion
2. Intracavitary implant technique—placement of a radioactive source or sources in a body cavity (i.e., uterine canal and vagina)
3. Interstitial implant technique—placement of a radioactive source or sources directly into the tumor site and adjacent tissue (i.e., sarcoma in a muscle)

Most brachytherapy applications tend to be temporary in that the sources are left in the patient until a designated tumor dose has been attained. Two different brachytherapy systems exist. They are *low-dose-rate* (LDR) and *high-dose-rate* (HDR). LDR brachytherapy has been the standard system for many years. A low-activity isotope is used to deliver a dose of radiation at a slow rate of 40 to 500 cGy per hour. This therapy requires that a patient be hospitalized for 3 to 4 days until the desired dose is delivered.

HDR systems are the more standard method of brachytherapy. This system uses a high-activity isotope capable of delivering greater than 1200 cGy per hour. The HDR system allows the prescribed dose to be delivered over minutes, which means this treatment can occur on an outpatient basis. Gynecologic tumors are one of the most common sites to be treated with HDR brachytherapy. HDR systems use a high-activity iridium-192 source.

Permanent implant therapy may also be accomplished. This is the most common type of LDR brachytherapy in practice today. An example of a permanent implant nuclide is iodine-125 and palladium-103 seeds. Permanent implant nuclides have relatively short *half-lives* of days and are left in the patient essentially forever. The amount and distribution of the radionuclide implanted in this manner depends on the total dose that the radiation oncologist is trying to deliver. Early-stage prostate cancer is commonly treated with this technique alone. In some cases of brachytherapy implantation, the implant is applied as part of the patient's overall treatment plan and may be preceded by or followed by additional external-beam radiation therapy.

EQUIPMENT

Most radiation oncology departments use linear accelerators (linacs) as their main treatment unit. Following are treatment units that may be found in a radiation oncology department:

- 120-kVp superficial x-ray unit for treating lesions on or near the surface of the patient
- 250-kVp orthovoltage x-ray unit for moderately superficial tissues
- ^{60}Co (cobalt-60) *gamma ray* source with an average energy of 1.25-MeV; Gamma Knife Unit
- 6-MV to 35-MV *linear accelerator* to serve as a source of high-energy (megavoltage) electrons and x-rays
- TomoTherapy
- CyberKnife

The dose depositions of these units are compared in Fig. 30.1.

The penetrability, or energy, of an x-ray or gamma ray totally depends on its wavelength: The shorter the wavelength, the more penetrating the photon; conversely, the longer the wavelength, the less penetrating the photon. A low-energy beam ($\leq$120 kVp) of radiation tends to deposit all or most of its energy on or near the surface of the patient and is suitable for treating lesions on or near the skin surface. In addition, with the low-energy beam, a greater amount of absorption or dose deposition occurs in bone than in soft tissue.

A high-energy beam of radiation ($\geq$1 MeV) tends to deposit its energy throughout the entire volume of tissue irradiated, with a greater amount of dose deposition occurring at or near the entry port than at the exit port. In this energy range, the dose is deposited about equally in soft tissue and bone. The high-energy (megavoltage) beam is most suitable for tumors deep beneath the body surface.

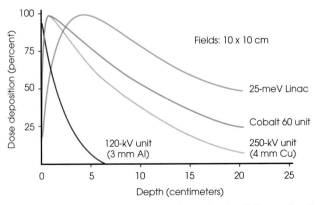

Fig. 30.1 Plot of percent of dose deposition in relation to depth in centimeters of tissue for various energies of photon beams.

The *skin-sparing* effect, a phenomenon that occurs as the energy of a beam of radiation is increased, is valuable from a therapeutic standpoint. In the superficial and orthovoltage energy range, the maximum dose occurs on the surface of the patient, and deposition of the dose decreases as the beam traverses the patient. As the energy of the beam increases into the megavoltage range, the maximum dose absorbed by the patient occurs at some point below the skin surface. The skin-sparing effect is important clinically because the skin is a radiosensitive organ. Excessive dose deposition to the skin can damage the skin, requiring treatments to be stopped and compromising treatment to the underlying tumor. The greater the energy of the beam, the more deeply the maximum dose is deposited (Fig. 30.2).

Cobalt-60 units

The cobalt-60 (^{60}Co) unit was the first skin-sparing machine. It replaced the orthovoltage unit in the early 1950s because of its greater ability to treat tumors located deeper within tissues. ^{60}Co is an artificially produced *isotope* formed in a nuclear *reactor* by the bombardment of stable cobalt-59 with neutrons. ^{60}Co emits two gamma-ray beams with an energy of 1.17 MeV and 1.33 MeV. The unit was known as a "workhorse" because it was extremely reliable, was mechanically simple, and had little downtime. It was the first radiation therapy unit to rotate 360 degrees around a patient. A machine that rotates around a fixed point, or axis, and maintains the same distance from the source of radiation is called an *isocentric machine*. All modern therapeutic units are isocentric machines. This type of machine allows the patient to remain in one position, lessening the chance for patient movement during treatment. Isocentric capabilities also assist in directing the beam precisely at the tumor while sparing normal structures.

Because ^{60}Co is a radioisotope, it constantly emits radiation as it *decays* in an effort to return to a stable state. It has a half-life of 5.26 years (i.e., its activity is reduced by 50% at the end of 5.26 years). Because the source decays at a rate of 1% per month, the radiation treatment time must be adjusted, resulting in longer treatment times as the source decays.

The use of ^{60}Co units has declined significantly since the 1980s, and ^{60}Co is rarely used for conventional external-beam radiation therapy today. This decline has been basically attributed to the introduction of the more sophisticated linac, which has greater skin-sparing capabilities and more sharply defined radiation *fields*. The radiation beam, or field, from a ^{60}Co unit also has large penumbra, which results in fuzzy field edges, another undesirable feature. ^{60}Co is still used in radiation oncology as part of a special procedure called stereotactic radiosurgery (SRS). The treatment unit is called the Gamma Knife. The Gamma Knife consists of 192 to 201 ^{60}Co sources arranged in a hemispherical array with all sources

Fig. 30.2 Three isodose curves showing comparison of percent of dose deposition from three x-ray units of different energies. As the energy of the beam increases, the percentage of dose deposited on the surface of the patient decreases.

converging at a single point (Fig. 30.3). The point where the beams converge forms a treatment area of 4 to 18 mm in diameter.

The Gamma Knife is primarily used to treat small benign or malignant lesions located deep within the brain employing an external rigidly fixed stereotactic head frame. The Gamma Knife does not involve surgery. It is called radiosurgery because the radiation is delivered in such a precise, focused manner that the lesion is ablated as if removed surgically. Adjacent normal tissues receive minimal radiation and are unharmed. The stereotactic head frame provides a coordinate system that allows the lesion to be three-dimensionally localized on MRI, CT scan, or angiography so that the radiation can be planned and targeted directly to the involved area. The Gamma Knife delivers a large dose of radiation in a single treatment to one or more areas in the brain. The types of conditions treated with the Gamma Knife include benign conditions such as acoustic neuromas, pituitary adenomas, arteriovenous malformations, and trigeminal neuralgia. Malignant lesions treated with the Gamma Knife include gliomas, meningiomas, chordoma, and solitary brain metastasis.

There are many advantages of Gamma Knife radiosurgery over conventional neurosurgery. First, the patient does not have to undergo an invasive surgical procedure.

The procedure can be done as an outpatient or may require an overnight stay in the hospital. There is no major recuperation period after a Gamma Knife procedure. The cost of Gamma Knife radiosurgery is much less than the cost of neurosurgery. The Gamma Knife is considered a very effective treatment for small intracranial lesions. One disadvantage of the Gamma Knife is that it can be used only for intracranial lesions. Another disadvantage is that the effects of radiation on the lesion are not immediate but occur over a period of weeks.

Linear accelerators

Linacs are the most commonly used machines for cancer treatment. The first linac was developed in 1952 and first used clinically in the United States in 1956. A linac is capable of producing high-energy beams of photons (x-rays) or electrons in the range of 4 million to 35 million volts. These megavoltage photon beams allow a better distribution of dose to deep-seated tumors with better sparing of normal tissues than their earlier counterparts—the orthovoltage or ^{60}Co units.

The photon beam is produced by accelerating a stream of electrons toward a target. When the electrons hit the target, a beam of x-rays is produced. By removing the target, the linac can also produce a beam of electrons of varying energies.

Typically, a linear accelerator is equipped with two photon energies consisting of one low-energy (6-MeV) and one high-energy (18-MV) photon beam plus a range of electron energies (Fig. 30.4). The dual photon energy machine gives the radiation oncologist more options in prescribing radiation treatments. As the energy of the beam increases, so does its penetrating power. A lower energy beam is used to treat tumors in thinner parts of the body, whereas high-energy beams are prescribed for tumors in thicker parts of the body. A brain tumor or a tumor in a limb would most likely be treated with a 6-MeV beam; conversely, a pelvic malignancy would be better treated with an 18-MeV beam. A small oncology center can serve its patients well by purchasing one dual photon linac for a cost of approximately $1.7 million instead of having to purchase two single energy 6-MeV and 18-MeV machines for almost $2 million.

Electrons are advantageous over photons in that they are a more superficial form of treatment. Electrons are energy dependent, which means that they deposit their energy within a given depth of tissue and go no deeper, depending on the energy selected. An 18-MeV beam has a total penetration depth of 3.5 inches (9 cm). Any structure located deeper than 3.5 inches (9 cm) would not be appreciably affected. This is important when the radiation oncologist is trying to treat a tumor that overlies a critical structure.

Fig. 30.3 Gamma Knife unit without a patient on the treatment table.

(From Washington CM, Leaver DT, editors: *Principles and practice of radiation therapy*, ed 3, St Louis, 2010, Mosby.)

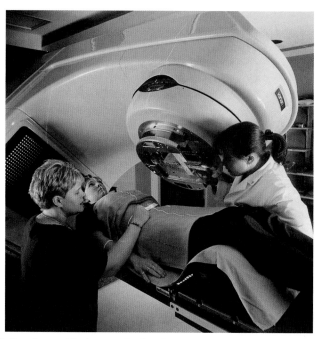

Fig. 30.4 Radiation therapists shown aligning the patient and shielding block in preparation for treatment using a modern linac. X-ray beams of 6 to 25 million V may be produced to treat tumors in the body.

Steering system
Radial and transverse steering coils and a real-time feedback system ensure beam symmetry to within ±2% at all gantry angles.

Focal spot size
Even at maximum dose rate, the circular focal spot remains less than 3 mm, held constant by the achromatic bending magnet. Assures optimum image quality for portal imaging.

Standing wave accelerator guide
Guide maintains optimal bunching for different acceleration conditions, providing high dose rates, stable dosimetry and low-stray radiation. Transport system minimizes power and electron source demands.

Energy switch
Patented switch provides energies within the full therapeutic range, at consistently high, stable dose rates, even with low-energy x-ray beams. Ensures optimum performance and spectral purity at both energies.

Gridded electron gun
Gun controls dose rate rapidly and accurately. Permits precise beam control for dynamic treatments because gun can be gated. Demountable, for cost-effective replacement.

Achromatic dual-plane bending magnet
Unique design with ±3% energy slits ensures exact replication of the input beam for every treatment. Clinac 2300C/D design enhancements allow wider range of beam energies.

10-port carousel with scattering foils/flattening filters
Extra ports allow future specialized beams to be developed. New electron scattering foils provide homogeneous electron beams at therapeutic depths.

Ion chamber
Two independently sealed chambers, impervious to temperature and pressure changes, monitor beam dosimetry to within 2% for long-term consistency and stability.

Asymmetric jaws
Four independent collimators provide flexible beam definition of symmetric or asymmetric fields.

Fig. 30.5 Asymmetric jaws. Note the four independent collimators.

(Courtesy Varian Associates, Palo Alto, CA.)

As with a diagnostic x-ray machine, the irradiated field of a linac is defined by a light field projected onto the patient's skin. This corresponding square or rectangle equals the length and width setting of the x-ray *collimators*. A modern linac is equipped with *asymmetric (independent) jaws;* this allows each of the four collimator blades that define length or width to move independently (Fig. 30.5). The jaw that defines the superior extent of the field may be 2.75 inches (7 cm) from the central axis, whereas the inferior region may be at 4 inches (10 cm). The total length would equal 6.75 inches (17 cm), but it is not divided equally because it is in a diagnostic x-ray collimator. The radiation oncologist is able to design a field that optimally covers the area of interest while sparing normal tissue. Independent collimation can also assist in reducing the total weight of lead shielding blocks generally constructed to protect normal tissues.

Multileaf collimation

Multileaf collimation (MLC) is the newest and most complex beam-defining system. Within the head of the linac, 45 to 80 individual collimator blades, about ⅜ to ¾ inch (1 to 2 cm) wide, are located and can be adjusted to shape the radiation field to conform to the target volume (Fig. 30.6). The design of the field is digitized from a radiograph into a computer software program, which is transferred to the treatment room. The MLC machine receives a code that tells it how to position the individual leaves for the treatment field. Before MLC, custom-made lead blocks, or *cerrobend* blocks, were constructed to shape radiation fields and shield normal tissues from the beam of radiation. Heavy cerrobend blocks were placed within the head of the linac for each treatment field. Linacs equipped with the MLC package now receive a custom-designed field at the stroke of a computer keyboard. Today, multileaf collimators can be programmed to move across the radiation field during a treatment to alter the intensity of the radiation beam. Altering the beam intensity across the radiation field allows a lower dose to be delivered to normal structures and tissues and ensures the tumor or target receives the prescribed dose. This technique is called *intensity modulated radiation therapy* (IMRT). IMRT allows the dose of radiation to be more tightly conformed to the target areas and has greatly reduced the dose to normal tissues and structures. IMRT is widely used and has replaced the conventional treatment field approach for many cancers, such as prostate and gynecologic cancers in the pelvis and cancers of the head and neck. IMRT can be used for almost any anatomic site.

Steps in Radiation Oncology
SIMULATION

The first step of radiation therapy involves determining the volume of tissue that needs to be encompassed within the radiation field. This is done with a *CT simulator*. During simulation, the radiation oncologist uses the patient's CT images or MRI to determine the tumor's precise location and to design a treatment volume, or area. The treatment volume often includes the tumor plus a small margin, the draining lymphatics that are at risk for involvement, and a rim of normal tissue to account for patient movement.

Most centers perform virtual simulations using a CT scanner equipped with radiation oncology software tools (Fig. 30.7). CT simulation is to position the patient in a manner that is stable and reproducible for each of the 28 to 40 radiation treatments. Therapists are responsible for constructing immobilization devices to help patients hold their position. It is crucial for a patient to hold still and maintain the same position. If the patient does not maintain the planned position, critical normal tissues may be irradiated, or the tumor may not be irradiated. Immobilization devices greatly assist the radiation therapist in correctly aligning the patient

Fig. 30.6 Multileaf collimation system on the treatment head.

Fig. 30.7 CT simulator.

Fig. 30.8 Aquaplast mask.

for each treatment, and many patients feel more secure when supported by these devices. Immobilization devices can be constructed for any part of the body but are most important for more mobile parts, such as the head and neck region or the limbs. Many different types of immobilization systems exist. Fig. 30.8 shows a thermoplastic device that secures the head and neck against rotation or flexion-extension. Fig. 30.9 shows a vacuum bag device that may be used to secure upper body or lower extremities.

Contrast material is often administered before or during a simulation to localize the area that needs to be treated or to identify vital normal structures that are to be shielded. A small amount of meglumine diatrizoate (Gastrografin or Gastroview) for CT simulation is injected into the rectum of a patient with rectal cancer to assist in localizing the rectum on the simulation images. Contrast material in the bladder is used to assist in localizing the prostate gland, which lies directly inferior to the bladder. Rectal contrast material is used to show the relationship of the rectum to the prostate to monitor and minimize the dose the rectum receives (Fig. 30.10).

When a CT simulation is performed, a reference isocenter is marked on the patient, and a pilot or scout scan is obtained. The radiation oncologist uses the scout or pilot image to determine the superior and inferior extent of the area to be scanned. The CT data are transferred to the virtual simulation computer workstation. From this limited scan, the physician reviews the CT images and uses imaging tools to outline the target volume and critical normal structures. The physician establishes the actual treatment isocenter. The computer software determines the change in location from the coordinates associated with the reference marks to the newly established treatment isocenter. The radiation therapist adjusts the couch and uses the laser marking system to apply these shifts to mark the treatment isocenter on the patient. The radiation therapist records all details regarding the patient's position in the treatment chart, and the patient is dismissed.

The physician creates treatment fields (length and width) electronically with the CT virtual simulation software (Fig. 30.11). The CT simulation data are transferred to the treatment planning system. In complex cases, the physician communicates preferences for treatment goals to the dosimetrist, who then designs the beam's eye view treatment fields and beam arrangement as part of the three-dimensional planning. A digitally reconstructed radiograph (DRR) for each treatment field is produced. The DRR is analogous to the radiograph taken in the conventional simulator (Fig. 30.12).

Precise measurements and details about the field dimensions, machine position, and patient positioning are recorded in the treatment chart. In some centers, the treatment parameters, such as field length, width, couch, and gantry positions, are electronically captured and transferred to the treatment unit. Recording of this information is crucial so that the radiation therapist performing the treatment can precisely reproduce the exact information.

Fig. 30.9 Vacuum bag immobilization device.

Fig. 30.10 CT simulation digitally reconstructed radiograph of standard PA field.

(From Washington CM, Leaver DT, editors: *Principles and practice of radiation therapy*, ed 4, St Louis, 2016, Mosby.)

Fig. 30.11 Virtual CT simulation. Note divergent radiation beam lines indicating the path of the beam. Target volume, kidneys, and spinal cord have been outlined on CT axial image and reconstructed sagittal and coronal images. Treatment field outline is seen on DRR and coronal image.

Fig. 30.12 DRR PA (A) and lateral (B) pelvis with rectal contrast. Note outline of treatment field.

DOSIMETRY

Dosimetry refers to the measurement of radiation dose, and it shows how the radiation is distributed or *attenuated* throughout the patient's body (absorbing medium). The dosimetrist devises a treatment plan that best fulfills the physician's prescription for the desired dose to the *tumor/target volume*, while minimizing the amount of radiation to critical normal structures or tissues.

Each organ of the body has a tolerance dose to radiation that limits the amount it can receive and still function normally. If an organ receives an excess of the tolerance dose, the organ can fail, resulting in a fatal complication. The kidneys are among the more radiosensitive structures of the body (Table 30.7). A dose greater than 2500 cGy can result in fatal radiation nephritis. The spinal cord has a higher tolerance dose, but many tumors require even higher doses for treatment to be effective.

Precise localization of dose-limiting structures and their relationship with the target volume is crucial for adequate planning. The dosimetrist must devise a plan that delivers a homogeneous dose to the tumor, while not exceeding the tolerance dose of a specific organ. This task can be quite challenging. The radiation oncologist might prescribe 6000 cGy to treat lung cancer located in the mediastinum directly over the spine but must limit the spinal cord dose to 4500 cGy to prevent irreparable damage, which could result in paralysis. The dosimetrist must devise a plan that enables combined treatment and protection to be accomplished.

The first step in dosimetry is to obtain a contour or CT scan of the patient in treatment position. A *contour* is an outline of the external surface of the patient's body at the level of the central axis (center of treatment field). This contour is typically performed in the transverse plane, but other planes may be used. Then the tumor volume and critical dose-limiting internal structures are transferred from the simulation radiographs and drawn onto the contour. CT scans from a CT simulator are more commonly used than contours. With CT scanning, the tumor and internal structures and their relationships are directly visible. These images are interfaced with the treatment planning computer system for development of the plan.

PET and MRI with the patient in treatment position are also obtained sometimes to facilitate the planning process. Fusion of MRI or PET images onto the CT simulation data set allows a more precise delineation of the tumor volume than what would be seen on CT alone. To obtain an even distribution of radiation to the target volume, radiation is delivered from various angles, all focused on the area of interest. Three-dimensional treatment planning allows for the design of a beam that exactly conforms to the shape of the tumor at any plane within the body. The treatment planning computer can digitally reconstruct the anatomy, which allows the dosimetrist to manipulate the image to view the tumor from any angle or plane. Important critical anatomic structures such as the kidneys and spinal cord are also more readily identified. Such a system allows the dosimetrist to plan and design beams that are coplanar and noncoplanar, tightly conforming to the target or tumor volume. This is known as *three-dimensional conformal radiotherapy* (CRT). The beam's eye view obtained by three-dimensional beams allows higher doses of radiation to be administered more safely by treating the cancer through multiple fields (more than four) on different planes, which reduces the amount of dose that normal tissues receive (Fig. 30.13).

The standard approach for a tumor located in the pelvis, such as rectal cancer, is the use of three fields—posteroanterior (PA), right lateral, and left lateral. Using the treatment parameters established in the simulator, the dosimetrist enters this information into the treatment planning computer, designs beam's eye view conformal fields, and obtains an isodose distribution, which shows how the radiation is being deposited. An *isodose line/curve* is a summation of areas of equal radiation dosage and may be stated as percentages of the total prescribed dose or as actual radiation dosages in *gray* (Gy) units.

TABLE 30.7

Tolerance doses to radiation

Structure	Tolerance dose (cGy)
Testes	500
Ovary	500
Lung (whole lung)	1800
Kidney (whole organ)	2300
Liver (whole organ)	3000
Spinal cord (5 cm³)	4500

Fig. 30.13 Dosimetry plan showing nine different radiation fields used to treat pancreatic tumor.

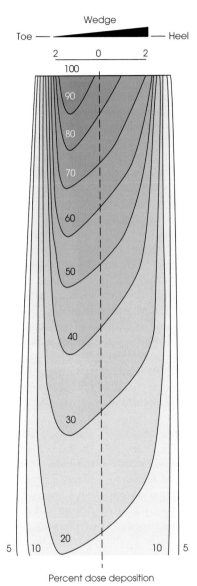

Wedge

Toe — ◣ — Heel

2   0   2

100

90

80

70

60

50

40

30

20

5 | 10   10 | 5

Percent dose deposition

Fig. 30.14 Isodose curve obtained from ⁶⁰Co unit, with wedge placed between the source and absorbing material.

The dosimetrist optimizes the plan by eliminating any areas of dose inhomogeneity (e.g., hot spots). A *hot spot* is an area of excessive radiation dose. One method to adjust for hot spots is to add a *wedge filter*. This wedge-shaped device is made of lead and is placed within the radiation beam to absorb the radiation preferentially, altering the shape of the isodose curve (Fig. 30.14). Another method of reducing hot spots is to change the weighting of the radiation beams by delivering a greater dose of radiation from the anterior field than from the posterior field.

Another major task of the dosimetrist is to monitor the dose that critical structures are receiving and to keep the dose within the established guidelines dictated by the physician. To avoid treating the spinal cord in the aforementioned example, the dosimetrist may angle the entry points of the radiation beams to include the target volume, while not irradiating the spinal cord. The resultant fields might be right anterior oblique and left posterior oblique (RAO/LPO) fields. The dosimetrist evaluates the dose distribution after each modifier is added and looks at different combinations of wedges, beam weighting, and beam entry points until an acceptable plan is produced. This technique is called *forward planning*. The final plan directs the radiation therapist, who treats the patient, how to proceed. For the example presented previously (i.e., lung cancer in the mediastinum directly over the spine), the plan might consist of the following:

1. Do 25 treatments anteroposterior (AP) and PA fields, RAO and LPO, 30 degrees off vertical.
2. Reduce field size to 12 cm long; do five more treatments AP, PA, RAO, and LPO, 30 degrees off vertical.

When the plan is complete, treatment of the patient can begin.

Another type of three-dimensional treatment planning is IMRT. The planning process begins as previously described—the physician identifies target volume and critical structures. Treatment fields are designed and arranged so that the target receives the prescribed dose, and the dose to critical structures is limited. The optimization of the dose distribution is not done, however, by trying different combinations of wedges or dose weighting as in conventional forward planning. IMRT uses a method called inverse planning. The prescribed dose to the target and the dose limit assigned to each critical structure are entered into the inverse planning system. A sophisticated mathematic algorithm creates a dose distribution that conforms to the target area, while sparing critical normal structures. This is achieved by modifying the intensity of radiation within the treatment field. This is accomplished by moving the multileaf collimator across the radiation field during a treatment from open to closed position, modulating the intensity of a beam to obtain the desired dose. The plan is computed by dividing the treatment field beam into hundreds of beamlets. Each beamlet can have an intensity level that measures from 0% to 100%. The intensity of a beamlet is changed by maintaining the multileaf collimator open for a specific amount of time and then closing it.

The IMRT planning process is time intensive and requires a comprehensive physics quality assurance check of multileaf collimator movement and dose verification before treatment is administered for the first time. IMRT has proven to be better at minimizing the dose to normal structures than conventional three-dimensional CRT and has allowed higher doses to be delivered to the target or tumor volume. IMRT was initially used for prostate cancer and cancers of the head and neck region. In prostate cancer treatment, IMRT optimized the dose to the prostate, while substantially minimizing the dose to the rectum. When treating a cancer in the head and neck region (e.g., nasopharynx), IMRT significantly reduced the dose to the parotid gland and spinal cord. IMRT is also used in the treatment of brain tumors, gastrointestinal, gynecologic, lung, breast, and soft tissue sarcomas.

The advantages of IMRT are well known—a method to deliver a highly conformal dose of radiation to the tumor while reducing the dose received by normal tissues. One disadvantage of IMRT is the total time it takes to deliver the daily session of radiation therapy. A patient with head and neck cancer might be on the table for 30 minutes each day to deliver radiation from 10 to 18 different radiation fields. The patient might move between or during the time the radiation beam is on. A new method of delivering IMRT treatment called volumetric modulated arc therapy (VMAT) has been developed. This method involves the linac rotating around the patient while the radiation beam is on and while the MLC leaves are moving for the IMRT delivery. With VMAT, the dose to the target and normal tissues is customized by altering the speed of the rotation, altering the dose rate of the linac, and simultaneously moving the MLC leaves. VMAT results in the delivery of the same highly conformal dose to the target while sparing normal tissues but in about half the time of a traditional IMRT stationary field technique. VMAT is also being used for prostate, lung, gynecologic, gastrointestinal, breast, and brain cancers. VMAT is widely utilized and is a very common form of treatment delivery and has replaced standard IMRT in many cases.

TREATMENT

On completion of the planning stage, including simulation and dosimetry, patient treatment can begin. The radiation therapist positions the patient and aligns the skin marks according to what was recorded in the treatment chart at the time of simulation. Accuracy and attention to detail are crucial for precise administration of the radiation to the patient. The radiation therapist is responsible for interpreting the radiation oncologist's prescription and calculating the correct monitor units, to achieve a desired dose of radiation for each treatment field. This responsibility also involves recording the daily administration of the radiation and the cumulative dose to date.

Precision in positioning the machine, proper selection of treatment field and MLC, accurate placement of cerrobend blocks or wedges, and implementation of any change in a patient's treatment plan are crucial for ensuring optimal treatment. Failure to do any of these may result in an overdose to normal tissue, causing long-term side effects, or underexposure of the tumor, reducing the patient's chance for cure. Most radiation oncology departments use an electronic radiation oncology medical record and computer verification system that ensures a patient's treatment parameters are correct before treatment may begin. The complexity of three-dimensional CRT, IMRT, and VMAT treatments with the numerous positions of the treatment couch, gantry, or collimator necessitates the use of a verification system. The computer verification system compares the machine settings with the information in the patient's electronic radiation chart. If there is a mismatch between any of the parameters in the electronic chart and what is being set up for treatment, the radiation therapist would be unable to initiate treatment. When a mismatch occurs, a computer prompt appears, highlighting the areas of disagreement. The radiation therapist must double-check parameters and patient setup, making corrections before treatment may occur. The verification and record system also records and adds the cumulative radiation doses.

Most linacs are now equipped with electronic portal imaging devices (EPIDs) and a kilovolt (kV) imager. These retractable imaging devices produce a digital image that is displayed immediately on a computer screen adjacent to the linac computer console. The EPID imager uses the 6-MV beam of the linac to obtain an image. Most radiation oncology departments have linacs equipped with a kV x-ray tube and flat panel image detector in addition to EPID. The kV imager, called an on board imager (OBI), provides a better diagnostic quality image with improved skeletal to soft tissue contrast compared with the megavoltage EPID imagers. These images can be viewed before treatment, and adjustments can be made before treating the patient, ensuring accurate and precise treatment. Some systems have computer software that compares the CT simulation image with the EPID or kV image using a registration algorithm. The computer automatically calculates the necessary adjustments (e.g., shift in couch position) to be made. The radiation therapist makes the adjustments and begins treatment.

When this treatment is used in cases of prostate cancer, gold seed markers are injected into the prostate gland before simulation. After the CT simulation is performed, the patient's treatment plan is completed, and treatment begins. The radiation therapist positions the patient, aligns the treatment machine, and takes an anterior and lateral or oblique kV image. The images are analyzed, and the computer generates any necessary shifts. These adjustments in couch or collimator

position are made before initiating treatment. This process is done daily. Many treatment systems or situations also require the radiation therapist to analyze the kV images, compare skeletal anatomy to CT simulation DRR, and make adjustments to the couch position before treating the patient (Fig. 30.15).

If the patient has been positioned correctly, why do these changes or errors in treatment field position occur? Patient movement during treatment has always been a major constraint in providing accurate and precise delivery of radiation treatments. Improvements in immobilization devices have been made; however, they do not prevent internal organ movement. The prostate may move and be in a different position within the treatment field from day to day or even during treatment because of the filling of the rectum or bladder. Tumor or organ movement can also occur because of normal respiration. This movement can result in a geographic miss of the tumor or irradiation of critical normal structures.

Because movement of internal structures does occur, many technologic innovations are being developed to address this issue. Obtaining daily kV or EPID images before treatment is one method. The process of using images such as EPID, kV, to verify the treatment field position daily before treatment is known as *image-guided radiation therapy* (IGRT). Other methods of IGRT involve the use of a CT scan, an infrared camera system, or a sophisticated tracking system that uses two x-ray tubes mounted 90 degrees apart. In addition, there are two newly developed treatment

units, TomoTherapy and the CyberKnife, which combine IGRT and innovative treatment delivery. These various IGRT methods are discussed subsequently.

The use of a CT scan before treatment as a means of IGRT is very common. A CT scan is obtained with the patient in treatment position, immediately before treatment, to verify target, isocenter, and patient position. This method is accomplished in one of two ways. One approach is to equip the linac with a kV x-ray tube and panel detector that obtains a cone-beam CT image when the accelerator gantry rotates a complete 360 degrees. The kV x-ray tube also provides a means of obtaining diagnostic quality images for treatment and patient position verification as previously discussed (Fig. 30.16). Another technique is using the linac's megavoltage beam and EPID imager to acquire a cone-beam CT image. The cone-beam CT image is obtained in the same fashion, by rotating the linac 360 degrees. The kV cone-beam CT image provides better contrast and soft tissue delineation than megavoltage CT. The megavoltage CT images are of a high enough quality to compare target position and related bony anatomy to determine if any adjustments in patient or couch position are necessary before treatment. Another method of CT image guidance is having a CT scanner located in the actual treatment room opposite the linac, near the foot end of the treatment couch. The scanner can be moved into position to obtain a CT scan with the patient positioned for treatment. The most common method is the use of the linac to obtain a cone-beam CT image.

Fig. 30.15 OBI kV image overlaid on CT DRR; therapists shift couch to match skeletal anatomy.

The infrared camera is a complex system that detects respiratory motion during simulation and treatment. This is a technique called *respiratory gating*. A reflective marker box is placed on the external surface of the patient's abdomen during simulation. The infrared camera detects the marker box, and a special computer software program connected to the infrared camera monitors the marker box movement (Fig. 30.17). The movement of the reflective marker is correlated with the patient's diaphragm position during the CT simulation. The respiratory cycle is evaluated relative to the treatment target volume and diaphragm movement. A specific portion of the respiratory cycle that has the least amount of motion is selected as the gated interval. This information is saved as a tolerance or standard to use during treatment. When the patient is treated, the reflective marker box is placed on the same place on the abdomen, and an infrared camera is used to monitor the movement of the box. Pretreatment portal images (AP and lateral) to verify patient position, isocenter location, and gating interval are obtained with the EPID or kV imager. When approved, the radiation therapist initiates treatment. The respiratory gating computer monitors the marker box movement and automatically turns off the radiation beam if the marker moves out of the acceptable gated interval. Treatment automatically begins again when the marker box returns to the acceptable position. Respiratory gating has been done in various ways. One method is to have patients breathe freely, whereas another method is to have patients exhale and hold their breath.

The ExacTrac by Brainlab AG (Heimstetten, Germany) is a system that uses two kV x-ray tubes mounted in the floor 90 degrees apart that project a beam at 45-degree angles to the patient through the linac isocenter. The flat panel detectors are located in the ceiling. This sophisticated system is able to analyze the stereoscopic images and compare bony anatomy or implanted fiducial markers with the digital radiographs from simulation. The computer system calculates shifts in six dimensions rather than using the typical three-dimensional imaging. When the radiation therapist has acknowledged the recommended shifts, the information is sent to the robotic couch, and the adjustments are made automatically from outside the treatment room. The ExacTrac system may be used to take images anytime during treatment for real-time tracking of target motion during treatment as in respiratory gating. ExacTrac is commonly used for the treatment of head and neck cancers, prostate cancer, lung cancer, and small centrally located brain tumors and for stereotactic radiation therapy (SRT).

Fig. 30.16 Linac equipped with kV x-ray tube and flat panel detector. EPID is extended underneath the patient.

Fig. 30.17 (A) Infrared camera system attached to CT simulator. (B) Reflective marker box.

SRT is similar to SRS in that the area being treated is small and surrounded by critical structures. The difference is that SRS is a large dose delivered in one treatment and is typically used for intracranial lesions. SRT is a conventional dose delivered in a fractionated manner using very focused small beams while the patient is rigidly immobilized. This technique is typically for intracranial lesions. SRT has been expanded to include tumors within the body. The treatment involves delivering larger doses of radiation per treatment than conventional treatment with a smaller number of total treatments. A patient may receive only three to five total treatments but the dose may be similar to that of conventional treatment. This new technique is called stereotactic body radiation therapy (SBRT). SBRT is being used for small lesions in the lung, liver, pancreas, other bone metastasis, and spine of patients who cannot undergo surgery.

TomoTherapy

TomoTherapy is a new treatment unit that was developed at the University of Wisconsin in 2001 and was first used clinically in patients in 2004. TomoTherapy combines the principles of helical CT scanning with a 6-MV linac. The TomoTherapy unit resembles a CT scanner and operates in a similar fashion. The 6-MV gantry rotates in a continuous full circle while the couch and patient simultaneously move slowly through the aperture of the machine (Fig. 30.18). The Tomo-Therapy unit is equipped with computer-controlled multileaf collimators that move to modulate the radiation beam intensity. TomoTherapy provides IMRT in a helical pattern delivering highly conformal radiation to the specific prescribed anatomic regions, while sparing normal structures. The TomoTherapy unit also uses daily IGRT. Before initiating treatment, megavoltage CT of the patient is obtained. This newly acquired CT image is compared with the initial CT image used in planning the treatment to verify patient position. Any necessary shifts in isocenter location are made before treatment. TomoTherapy is another option of providing precise and conformal radiation therapy.

Fig. 30.18 TomoTherapy Hi-Art imaging and treatment system, which uses a megavoltage source for CT and for treatment.

(Courtesy TomoTherapy Incorporated. From Washington CM, Leaver DT, editors: *Principles and practice of radiation therapy*, ed 3, St Louis, 2010, Mosby.)

CyberKnife

The CyberKnife (Accuray Inc., Sunnyvale, CA) is a SRS system that uses a precise image guidance system for delivering a single treatment or two to five high-dose treatments called hypofractionated radiotherapy. The CyberKnife is a 6-MV linac housed within a robotic arm. The robotic arm has six different joints or axes that allow the delivery of radiation beams from thousands of angles from any direction around the patient (Fig. 30.19). The CyberKnife provides many more beam options to conform to the target or tumor than a traditional linac. The radiation beams are collimated to range in diameter from 5 to 60 mm. The small beams enter from various angles to conform tightly to the target, while sparing normal tissue, thereby allowing higher doses to be delivered.

The image guidance system consists of two diagnostic x-ray tubes mounted in the ceiling at 45-degree angles, offset 90 degrees from one another with two opposing amorphous silicon detectors located in the floor. The imaging system continually takes a set of images at each treatment angle and analyzes the images during treatment to track target and patient motion. The robotic arm is automatically adjusted to correct for any target or patient motion. The CyberKnife was the first system to use real-time tracking of target motion during treatment. The treatment times for CyberKnife are 30 to 90 minutes. The CyberKnife is used to treat cancers of the lung, pancreas, brain, head and neck, spine, and prostate.

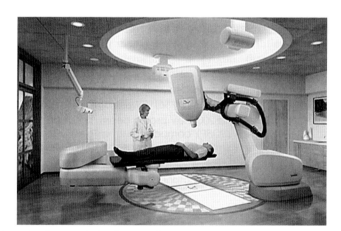

Fig. 30.19 Accelerator on a robotic arm. Two ceiling-mounted x-ray tubes are clearly shown.

(From Washington CM, Leaver DT, editors: *Principles and practice of radiation therapy*, ed 3, St Louis, 2010, Mosby.)

Clinical Applications

The amount of radiation prescribed depends on the type of tumor and the extent of the disease. Following are brief summaries of radiation therapy techniques used in the management of common forms of cancer.

LUNG CANCER

Treatment of lung cancer varies by type and stage. Radiation therapy is often used in conjunction with surgery and chemotherapy. A dose of 5000 to 6000 cGy of 10-MeV photons is often applied via a combination of AP, PA, and off-cord oblique fields. The primary tumor plus draining lymphatics are generally included in the treatment volumes (Fig. 30.23). More recently, the use of multiple oblique IMRT fields, VMAT, or a hybrid technique that incorporates both static fields and VMAT is used to treat lung cancer. These techniques provide a more conformal dose to the target volume while delivering less dose to normal lung and spinal cord than the traditional static AP-PA and oblique fields. SBRT is used for the treatment of medically inoperable patients with stage I non-small-cell lung cancers. One to five treatments with doses in the range of 1000 to 2000 cGy per treatment may be given for a total dose of 5000 to 6000 cGy.

PROSTATE CANCER

Definitive radiation therapy is a standard treatment for prostate cancer. Surgical removal of the prostate gland is another common approach to the management of this disease. Traditionally, a four-field technique of AP, PA, and right and left lateral ports using a megavoltage beam of 10 MV or more is often used to deliver a dose of 7000 to 7600 cGy to the prostate gland. A series of six to eight oblique fields delivered with IMRT or VMAT to a dose of 7600 cGy is a common method of treatment for prostate cancer. Another method of treating limited, early-stage prostate cancer is a brachytherapy procedure known as prostate seed implant. This procedure involves the permanent implantation of 100 or more seeds of the radioisotope iodine-125 or palladium-103 into the prostate gland. A dose of 145 Gy is delivered with iodine-125 and a dose of 125 Gy is delivered with palladium-103.

HDR brachytherapy is another method for treating early-stage prostate cancer. This procedure is done on an outpatient basis and is a temporary implant. The patient has four HDR brachytherapy treatments. The interstitial needles are inserted early in the morning, then the patient has a morning and afternoon treatment. The patient comes back 2 to 3 weeks later for another two HDR treatments. Prostate cancer is one anatomic site that may be treated with protons.

HEAD AND NECK CANCERS

Numerous approaches may be used to treat head and neck cancers, depending on the location, size, and extent of the tumor. The most common method of treating head and neck cancer is with VMAT. VMAT allows a significant reduction in the dose to the parotid gland and spinal cord, while allowing a greater dose to be delivered to the target area. VMAT treatments are shorter in duration than the traditional IMRT technique for head and neck cancer. This makes the treatment more tolerable for the patient, who is held in place on the table by a thermoplastic mask. VMAT is the newest IMRT method for delivering radiation to head and neck cancers.

CERVICAL CANCER

Early diagnosed cervical cancers can be treated with either surgery or radiation therapy. A four-field technique of AP, PA, and right and left lateral ports using a megavoltage unit, preferably 10 MV or greater, delivers 4500 to 5000 cGy in 5 weeks to an area of the primary and regional lymph nodes (Fig. 30.24). IMRT or VMAT are becoming common methods of treating cervical cancer. An intracavitary HDR implant is also included in the standard treatment of cervical cancer.

Fig. 30.23 Digitally reconstructed radiograph for parallel-opposed fields for right lung tumor with extension across the midline.

(Courtesy Bayhealth Medical Center at Kent General Hospital, Dover, DE.)

HODGKIN LYMPHOMA

The age of the patient and extent of the disease may determine treatment and prognosis for Hodgkin lymphoma. Involved field lymph node irradiation after chemotherapy is more commonly used than extended field therapy that included the lymphatic chain above or below the diaphragm. Treatment consists of chemotherapy followed by 2000 to 3000 cGy delivered through AP-PA fields or IMRT fields using a megavoltage unit. Chemotherapy may also be indicated for more advanced cases.

BREAST CANCER

Using two tangential fields to the chest wall or intact breast, megavoltage radiation delivers 5000 cGy in 5 weeks (Fig. 30.25). An electron boost to the site of initial lumpectomy adds an additional 1000 cGy. Irradiation of the axillary, supraclavicular, and internal mammary nodes to a dose of 5000 cGy is indicated for patients with a large primary tumor or node-positive disease. IMRT may also be used for the treatment of breast cancer. The breast is one location that respiratory gating may be utilized. A patient's breathing is monitored, and patients are instructed to hold their breath to limit internal organ motion while treatment commences. Respiratory gating limits the dose to the heart in patients with left-sided breast cancer.

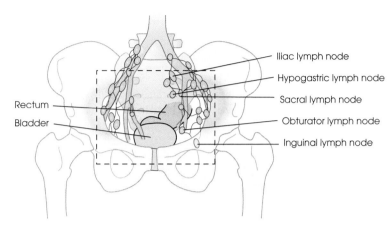

Fig. 30.24 Field used for irradiation of primary tumor and adjacent lymph nodes.

Fig. 30.25 (A) Cross section of thorax showing field arrangements to irradiate the intact breast tangentially while sparing the lung (*lines A* and *B*). (B) Port image of tangential breast field. Note sparing of lung tissue.

Accelerated partial-breast irradiation (APBI) is a breast conservation method being studied as an alternative to whole breast irradiation. This treatment option may be offered to a subset of women who are older than 50 years of age with tumors of less than 3 cm located in the outer quadrant of the breast. The patient must have negative surgical margins and no lymph nodes involved. *Accelerated* is the term used because the treatment is delivered in 1 week with twice-a-day treatments using external beam or brachytherapy. The two commonly used brachytherapy applicators are MammoSite and strut adjusted volume implant applicator (SAVI). Both applicators are placed in the lumpectomy site. The MammoSite applicator is a balloon catheter that is placed in the lumpectomy cavity. The SAVI has individual catheters in the shape of an eggbeater and is placed in the cavity created by the lumpectomy. The applicator used is hooked up to the HDR unit for treatment delivery. A total dose of 3400 cGy is delivered in the 1-week period. Chemotherapy, hormonal therapy, or both are also commonly used to treat breast cancer.

LARYNGEAL CANCER

Cancer of the larynx is best treated with megavoltage radiation. Tumors that are confined to the true vocal cord, with normal cord mobility, have a 90% 5-year cure rate; in addition, the voice remains useful. The method of treatment is usually accomplished by using small 2- × 2-inch (5- × 5-cm) opposing lateral wedged fields and delivering a dose of 6300 to 6500 cGy over a 6-week period.

SKIN CANCER

Carcinomas of the skin are usually squamous cell or basal cell lesions that may be treated with superficial radiation or surgery. Cure rates tend to be 80% to 90%, and basal cell lesions less than ⅜ inch (1 cm) in diameter have a cure rate of almost 100%. The method of treatment is usually a single-field approach with attention given to shielding the uninvolved skin and delivering 4000 to 5000 cGy in a 3- to 4-week period.

MEDULLOBLASTOMA

Children with medulloblastoma are usually referred to the radiation oncology department after a biopsy and shunt procedure. The tumor is radiosensitive, and patients who have had treatment of the entire cerebrospinal axis have a 5-year cure rate of greater than 60%. The therapeutic approach tends to be complicated because the entire brain is irradiated with 3600 cGy, the spinal cord receives a dose of 2340 to 3600 cGy, and the cerebellum receives an additional dose of radiation to bring the total up to 5500 cGy (Fig. 30.26). This irradiation is usually accomplished with parallel opposed fields to the cranial vault and an extended single field to the spinal cord. The boost dose of 2000 cGy to the posterior fossa may be given with IMRT to provide better dose optimization to the target and less dose to critical structures. A megavoltage unit is used, with extreme care given to the areas of abutting fields. Medulloblastoma is one area that has been treated with proton therapy.

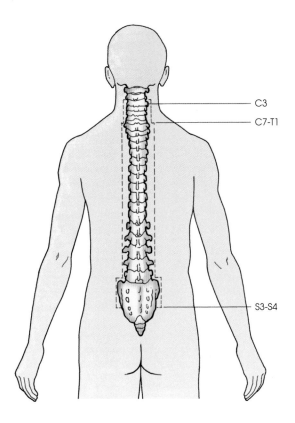

Fig. 30.26 Spinal treatment portal for medulloblastoma.

Future Trends

Radiation therapy has entered the electronic age with increased technologic advancement in the areas of dosimetry, simulation, and treatment. Most institutions use computer-interfaced accelerators with treatment verification software packages to ensure accurate treatment. Paperless treatment charting and filmless departments are the standard design of a facility. VMAT and IMRT are standard treatment techniques used in most facilities to treat various tumor types. Developments will continue to occur in the use of IGRT. Refinements in the application of linac cone-beam CT and other modalities, such as PET, to verify target, isocenter, and patient position before treatment will occur more routinely. Advancements and implementation of respiratory gating will permit better delineation of three-dimensional conformal target volumes, lessen the chance of a geographic miss of the target volume, and further minimize the dose to normal structures. The use of gating may permit higher doses to be prescribed and result in greater control and cure rates. The use of SBRT may expand for use in the treatment of other cancer sites within the body.

Conclusion

From a questionable beginning, radiation therapy has emerged as one of the primary modalities used in the treatment of malignant disease. Radiation therapy departments are currently examining and treating approximately 75% of all patients with a new diagnosis of cancer. Radiation oncologists and radiation therapists are integral members of the health care team that discusses and selects the appropriate treatment regimens for all cancer patients.

As the factors that initiate cellular change, growth, and spread become better understood, the radiation treatments for cancer are expected to become even more effective. The irradiation techniques presently used may change dramatically based on this new information. In addition, new, more sophisticated radiation-producing equipment is currently under design and may lead to the reevaluation of presently accepted therapeutic techniques and dose levels. Finally, new chemotherapeutic agents are being produced that, when used by themselves or with other drugs, may enhance tumor sensitivity when used in conjunction with irradiation.

Definition of Terms

absorbed dose Amount of ionizing radiation absorbed per unit of mass of irradiated material.

accelerator (particle) Device that accelerates charged subatomic particles to great energies. These particles or rays may be used for direct medical irradiation and basic physical research. Medical units include linear accelerators, betatrons, and cyclotrons.

asymmetric jaws Four independent x-ray collimators that are used to define the radiation treatment field.

attenuation Removal of energy from a beam of ionizing radiation when it traverses matter, accomplished by disposition of energy in matter and by deflection of energy out of the beam.

betatron Electron accelerator that uses magnetic induction to accelerate electrons in circular path; also capable of producing photons.

biopsy Removal of a small piece of tissue for examination under the microscope.

brachytherapy Placement of radioactive nuclide or nuclides in or on a neoplasm to deliver a cancericidal dose.

cancer Term commonly applied to malignant disease; abnormal growth of cells; *neoplasm* (new growth) or *-oma* (tumor).

cancericidal dose Dose of radiation that results in the death of cancer cells.

carcinogen Any cancer-producing substance or material, such as nicotine, radiation, or ingested uranium.

carcinoma Cancer that arises from epithelial tissue—either glandular or squamous epithelium.

cerrobend block Beam-shaping device made of a lead alloy that attenuates the x-ray beam, preventing exposure of normal tissue.

chromosome Unit of genetic information that guides cytoplasmic activities of the cell and transmits hereditary information.

cobalt-60 Radioisotope with half-life of 5.26 years, average gamma ray energy of 1.25 MeV (range 1.17 to 1.33 MeV), and ability to spare skin with buildup depth in tissue of 0.5 cm.

collimator Diaphragm or system of diaphragms made of radiation-absorbing material that defines dimension and direction of beam.

conformal radiation Treatment designed to deliver radiation to the exact target volume as seen on any plane (e.g., transverse, sagittal, vertex views); requires a three-dimensional treatment planning system.

contour Reproduction of an external body shape, typically in the transverse plane at the level of the central axis of the beam; facilitates planning of radiation treatment. Other planes of interest may also be obtained.

cure Usually a 5-year period after completion of treatment during which time the patient exhibits no evidence of disease.

decay or disintegration Transformation of radioactive nucleus, resulting in emission of radiation.

differentiation Acquisition of cellular function and structure that differ from that of the original cell type.

direct effect Radiation that interacts with an organic molecule such as DNA, RNA, or a protein molecule. This interaction may inactivate the cell.

dosimetry Measurement of radiation dose in an absorbing medium.

epithelial tissue Cells that line the surfaces of serous and mucous membranes, including the skin.

etiology Study of causes of diseases.

external-beam treatment Delivery of radiation to a patient from a unit such as a linear accelerator in which the radiation enters the patient from the external surface of the body.

field Geometric area defined by collimator or radiotherapy unit at skin surface.

fractionation Division of total planned dose into numerous smaller doses to be given over a longer period. Consideration must be given to biologic effectiveness of smaller doses.

gamma ray Electromagnetic radiation that originates from radioactive nucleus and causes ionization in matter; identical in properties to x-ray.

gray (Gy) International unit for the quantity of radiation received by the patient; previously rad; 1 cGy = 1 rad.

grenz rays X-rays generated at 20 kVp or less.

half-life Time (specific for each radioactive substance) required for radioactive material to decay to half its initial activity; types are biologic and physical.

half-value layer Thickness of attenuating material inserted in beam to reduce beam intensity to half of the original intensity.

high-dose-rate brachytherapy Use of a high-activity radionuclide placed within the body for the treatment of cancer. Delivers more than 1200 cGy per hour.

image-guided radiation therapy (IGRT) Use of images to verify treatment isocenter, target, and patient positioning before initiating radiation treatment.

independent jaws X-ray collimator with four individual blades that can be moved independently of one another (see *asymmetric jaws*).

indirect effect Interaction of radiation with water molecules within the cell; results in the formation of free radicals OH, H, and HO_2, which can damage the cell.

intensity-modulated radiation therapy (IMRT) Modification of beam intensity to deliver nonuniform exposure across radiation field.

ionization Process in which one or more electrons are added to or removed from atoms, creating ions; can be caused by high temperatures, electrical discharges, or nuclear radiations.

ionizing radiation Energy emitted and transferred through matter that results in the removal of orbital electrons (e.g., x-rays or gamma rays).

isocentric Refers to rotation around a fixed point.

isodose line curve Curve or line drawn to connect points of identical amounts of radiation in a given field.

isotope Atoms that have the same atomic number but different mass numbers.

lesion Morbid change in tissue; mass of abnormal cells.

linear accelerator (linac) Device for accelerating charged particles, such as electrons, to produce high-energy electron or photon beams.

linear energy transfer (LET) Rate at which energy is deposited as it travels through matter.

low-dose-rate brachytherapy Use of a low-activity radionuclide placed within the body for treatment of cancer. Dose is slowly delivered, 40 to 500 cGy per hour, to a small volume of tissue over a period of days.

malignancy Cancerous tumor or lesion.

medical dosimetrist Person responsible for calculation of proper radiation treatment dose who assists the radiation oncologist in designing individual treatment plans.

medical physicist Specialist in the study of the laws of ionizing radiation and their interactions with matter.

metastasis Transmission of cells or groups of cells from primary tumor to sites elsewhere in body.

multileaf collimator (MLC) Individual collimator rods within the treatment head of the linear accelerator that can slide inward to shape radiation field.

oncologist Physician specializing in the study of tumors.

oncology Study of tumors.

palliation To relieve symptoms; not for cure.

passively scattered particle therapy Involves the use of special devices to spread the proton beam out laterally and distally.

pathologist Specialist in the study of the microscopic nature of disease.

pencil beam scanning Method of proton beam delivery. The positively charged thin proton beamlet is directed by two magnets to deliver the beam in an alternating scanning fashion to paint the tumor with dose.

prophylactic surgery Preventive surgical treatment.

radiation oncologist Physician who specializes in the use of ionizing radiation in treatment of disease.

radiation oncology Medical specialty involving the treatment of cancerous lesions using ionizing radiation.

radiation therapist Person trained to assist and take directions from the radiation oncologist in the use of ionizing radiation for treatment of disease.

radiation therapy Older term used to define the medical specialty involving treatment with ionizing radiation.

radioactive Pertaining to atoms of elements that undergo spontaneous transformation, resulting in emission of radiation.

radiocurable Susceptibility of neoplastic cells to cure (destruction) by ionizing radiation.

radiosensitivity Responsiveness of cells to radiation.

radium (Ra) Radionuclide (atomic number 88, atomic weight 226, half-life 1622 years) used clinically for radiation therapy. In conjunction with its subsequent transformations, radium emits alpha and beta particles and gamma rays. In encapsulated form, it is used for various intracavitary radiation therapy applications (e.g., for cervical cancer).

reactor Cubicle in which isotopes are artificially produced.

relative biologic effectiveness (RBE) Compares radiation beams with different LETs and their ability to produce a specific biologic response. Dose in gray from 250 kVp beam of x-rays/dose from another type of radiation to produce the same effect.

simulator Diagnostic x-ray machine that has the same geometric and physical characteristics as a radiation therapy treatment unit.

skin sparing In megavoltage beam therapy, reduced skin injury per centigray (cGy) exposure because electron equilibrium occurs below skin; occurs $\frac{1}{4}$ to 2 inches (0.6 to 5 cm) deep, depending on energy.

spread out Bragg peak Individual Bragg peaks are spread across the various depths of the tumor, providing a more useful beam.

stereotactic radiation therapy Use of small focused radiation beams to treat small extracranial or intracranial lesions; delivered with conventional fractionation or in two to five treatments instead of a single treatment as in stereotactic radiosurgery. Rigid immobilization of involving patient is required.

stereotactic radiosurgery Use of multiple, narrow, highly focused radiation beams to deliver a large dose in a single treatment to a small intracranial lesion. The patient is immobilized with a fixed stereotactic head frame.

surgical bed Area of excision and adjacent tissues manipulated during surgery.

systemic Throughout the human body.

teletherapy Radiation therapy technique for which the source of radiation is at some distance from the patient.

treatment field Anatomic area outlined for treatment (e.g., AP or RL pelvis).

tumor/target volume Portion of anatomy that includes tumor and adjacent areas of invasion.

undifferentiation Lack of resemblance of cells to cells of origin.

wedge filter Wedge-shaped beam attenuating device used to absorb beam preferentially to alter the shape of the isodose curve.

Selected bibliography

Accuray: Available at: www.accuray.com. (Accessed 6 June 2009).

American Cancer Society: *Cancer facts and figures 2017*, Atlanta, 2013, American Cancer Society.

Berson AM, et al: Clinical experience using respiratory gated radiation therapy: comparison of free-breathing and breath-hold techniques, *Int J Radiat Oncol Biol Phys* 60:419, 2004.

Boyer AL: The physics of intensity-modulated radiation therapy, *Phys Today* 55:38, 2002.

BrainLab: Available at: www.BrainLab.com. (Accessed 6 June 2009).

Brenner DJ: Dose, volume, and tumor-control predictions in radiotherapy, *Int J Radiat Oncol Biol Phys* 26:171, 1993.

Chan OS, et al: The superiority of hybrid-volumetric arc therapy (VMAT) technique over double arcs VMAT and 3D-conformal technique in the treatment of locally advanced non-small cell lung cancer—a planning study, *Radiother Oncol* 101:298, 2011.

Chang JY, et al: Image-guided radiation therapy for non-small cell lung cancer, *J Thorac Oncol* 3:177, 2008.

Chang SD, et al: An analysis of the accuracy of the cyberknife: a robotic frameless stereotactic radiosurgical system, *Neurosurgery* 52:140, 2003.

Cheng J, et al: Comparison of intensity modulation radiation therapy treatment techniques for nasopharyngeal carcinoma, *Int J Radiat Oncol Biol Phys* 96:126, 2001.

Chirag S, et al: The American brachytherapy society consensus statement for accelerated partial breast irradiation, *Brachytherapy* 12:267, 2013.

Chuong MA, et al: Stereotactic body radiation therapy for locally advanced and borderline resectable pancreatic cancer is effective and well tolerated, *Int J Radiat Oncol Biol Phys* 86:516, 2013.

Coleman A: Treatment procedures. In Washington CM, Leaver DT, editors: *Principles and practices of radiation therapy*, ed 3, St Louis, 2010, Mosby.

Damien C, et al: Intensity modulated proton and photon therapy for early prostate cancer with or without transperineal injection of a polyethylene glycol spacer: a treatment planning comparison study, *Int J Radiat Oncol Biol Phys* 84:e311, 2012.

Das IJ, et al: Intensity-modulated radiation therapy dose prescription, recording and delivery: patterns of variability among institutions and treatment planning systems, *J Natl Cancer Inst* 100:300, 2008.

Dawson LA, Jaffray DA: Advances in image-guided radiation therapy, *J Clin Oncol* 25:938, 2007.

Dieterich SP, Pawlicki TP: CyberKnife image-guided delivery and quality assurance, *Int J Radiat Oncol Biol Phys* 71:126, 2008.

Dische S: Radiotherapy in the nineties: increase in cure, decrease in morbidity, *Acta Oncol* 31:501, 1992.

Elekta: Available at: http://www.elekta.com/healthcare_international_gamma_knife_surgery.php. (Accessed 6 June 2009).

Furlow B: Three-dimensional conformal radiation therapy, *Radiat Therapist* 12(131):2003.

Gierga DP, et al: The correlation between internal and external markers for abdominal tumors: implications for respiratory gating, *Int J Radiat Oncol Biol Phys* 61:2005, 1551.

Gillin MT: Special procedures. In Washington CM, Leaver DT, editors: *Principles and practices of radiation therapy*, ed 3, St Louis, 2010, Mosby.

Goetein M, et al: Treating cancer with protons, *Phys Today* 55:45, 2002.

Grabowski CM, et al: Factors predictive of completion of treatment and survival after palliative radiation therapy, *Radiology* 184:329, 1992.

Greenlee RT, et al: Cancer statistics, *CA Cancer J Clin* 51(15):2001, 2001.

Hovington JA, et al: Treatment of stage I and II non-small cell lung cancer, *Chest* 143(Suppl):e2788, 2013.

Jaffray DA, et al: Flat-panel cone-beam computed tomography for image-guided radiation therapy, *Int J Radiat Oncol Biol Phys* 53:1337, 2002.

Jessup JM, et al: Diagnosing colorectal carcinoma: clinical and molecular approaches, *CA Cancer J Clin* 47:70, 1997.

Khan F: Proton beam therapy. In *The physics of radiation therapy*, ed 4, Philadelphia, 2010, Lippincott Williams, Wilkins.

Landis SH, et al: Cancer statistics, *CA Cancer J Clin* 48(6):1998, 1998.

Leaver D: Intensity modulated radiation therapy: part 2, *Radiat Therapist* 12(17):2003.

Leaver D, et al: Simulation procedures. In Washington CM, Leaver DT, editors: *Principles and practices of radiation therapy*, ed 3, St Louis, 2010, Mosby.

Lipa LA, Mesina CF: Virtual simulation in conjunction with 3-D conformal therapy, *Radiat Therapist* 2:99, 1995.

Marks JE, Armbruster JS: Accreditation of radiation oncology in the US, *Int J Radiat Oncol Biol Phys* 24:863, 1992.

Mell LK, et al: A survey of intensity-modulated radiation therapy use in the United States, *Cancer* 98:204, 2003.

McDermott P, Orton C: Special modalities in radiation therapy. In *The physics & technology of radiation therapy*, Madison, WI, 2010, Medical physics.

Mohan R, Grosshans D: Proton therapy–present and future, *Adv Drug Deliv Rev* 109:26–44, 2017.

Mohan R, et al: Empowering intensity modulated proton therapy through physics & technology: an overview, *Int J Radiat Oncol Biol Phys* 99:304, 2017.

Morgan HM: Quality assurance of computer controlled radiotherapy treatments, *Br J Radiol* 65:409, 1992.

National Association of Proton Therapy: Available at http://www.proton-therapy.org/map.htm.

National Cancer Institute: *Genetic testing for breast cancer risk: it's your choice*, Washington, DC, 1997, National Cancer Institute.

National Cancer Institute: Radiation therapy for cancer: questions and answers. Available at: http://www.cancer.gov/cancertopics/factsheet/Therapy/radiation. (Accessed 9 July 2009).

Navarria P, et al: Volumetric modulated arc therapy with flattening filter free beams for stereotactic body radiation therapy in patients with medically inoperable early stage non-small cell lung cancer, *Radiother Oncol* 107:414, 2013.

Order SE: Training in systemic radiation therapy, *Int J Radiat Oncol Biol Phys* 24:895, 1992.

Otto K: Volumetric modulated arc therapy: IMRT in a single gantry arc, *Med Phys* 35:310, 2008.

Palma D, et al: Volumetric modulated arc therapy for delivery of prostate radiotherapy: comparison with intensity-modulated radiotherapy and three-dimensional conformal radiotherapy, *Int J Radiat Oncol Biol Phys* 72:996, 2008.

Palma D, et al: New developments in arc radiation therapy: a review, *Cancer Treat Rev* 36:393, 2010.

Palmer M: Particle therapy. In Washington CM, Leaver DT, editors: *Principles and practices of radiation therapy*, ed 4, St Louis, 2016, Mosby.

Perez CA: Quest for excellence: ultimate goal of the radiation oncologist: astro gold medal address, *Int J Radiat Oncol Biol Phys* 26(567):1993, 1992.

Prado K, Prado C: Dose distributions. In Washington CM, Leaver DT, editors: *Principles and practices of radiation therapy*, ed 3, St Louis, 2010, Mosby.

Qi XS, et al: Assessment of interfraction patient setup for head and neck cancer intensity modulated radiation therapy using multiple computed tomography based image guidance, *Int J Radiat Oncol Biol Phys* 86:432, 2013.

Ramsey CR, et al: A technique for adaptive image-guided helical tomotherapy for lung cancer, *Int J Radiat Oncol Biol Phys* 64:1237, 2006.

Rietzel E, et al: Four-dimensional image-based treatment planning: target volume segmentation and dose calculation in the presence of respiratory motion, *Int J Radiat Oncol Biol Phys* 61:2005, 1535.

Roberge SL: Virtual reality: radiation therapy treatment planning of tomorrow, *Radiat Therapist* 2:113, 1996.

Shimizu S, et al: Preliminary analysis for integration of spot-scanning proton beam therapy and real-time imaging and gating, *Phys Med* 30:555, 2014.

Sillanpaa J, et al: Integrating respiratory gating into a megavoltage cone-beam CT system, *Int J Radiat Oncol Biol Phys* 60:197, 2004.

Simone CH, II, et al: Stereotactic body radiation therapy for lung cancer, *Chest* 143:2013, 1784.

TomoTherapy: Available at: www.tomotherapy.com. (Accessed 15 June 2009).

Vlachaki MT, et al: IMRT versus conventional 3D CRT on prostate and normal tissue dosimetry using an endorectal balloon for prostate localization, *Med Dosim* 30:69, 2005.

Wagner LK: Absorbed dose in imaging: why measure it?, *Radiology* 178:622, 1991.

Washington CM, Leaver DT, editors: *Principles and practice of radiation therapy*, ed 4, St Louis, 2016, Mosby.

Weber DC, et al: Intensity modulated proton and photon therapy for early stage prostate cancer with or without transperineal injection of a polyethylene glycol spacer: a treatment planning comparison study, *Int J Radiat Oncol Biol Phys* 84:e311, 2012.

Wilkinson B, et al: Evaluation of current consensus statement recommendations for accelerated partial breast irradiation: a pooled analysis of William Beaumont Hospital and American Society of Breast Surgeons MammoSite registry trial data, *Int J Radiat Oncol Biol Phys* 85:1179, 2013.

Yamada Y, et al: A review of image-guided intensity modulated radiotherapy for spinal tumors, *Neurosurgery* 61:226, 2007.

Yashar CM, et al: Initial clinical experience the (SAVI) breast brachytherapy device for accelerated partial-breast irradiation (APBI): first 100 patients with more than 1 year of follow-up, *Int J Radiat Oncol Biol Phys* 80:765, 2011.

INDEX

Page numbers followed by "*f*" indicate figures, "*t*" indicate
tables, and "*b*" indicate boxes. Boldface numbers indicate
the volume.

Index

Index

Index

Index

Index

Index

Index

Sharpen your *radiographic positioning and image analysis skills* with these essential resources.

Mosby's Digital Positioning Consult — Online Course

Learn how to produce the most accurate images possible with this digital diagnostic image critique product that uses questions, answers, and rationales to help you improve your ability to recognize acceptable versus unacceptable images.

- **More than 1,200 online questions** test the critical thinking skills you need for recognizing positioning and technical errors.

- **More than 600 self-study questions** provide the opportunity to expand your knowledge on your own.

- **Questions presented in multiple-response formats** encourage you to exercise the clinical reasoning required to succeed on image critique testing.

- **Targeted content** equips you to identify appropriate technical, procedural, and pathologic factors, and employ corrective actions if necessary.

- **The latest ARRT guidelines** are reflected throughout to prepare you for certification and clinical practice.

2019 • **ISBN: 978-0-323-64136-4**

Also Available

Merrill's Pocket Guide to Radiography, 14th Edition

Get quick access to bulleted, step-by-step explanations of how to position the patient and body part for approximately 170 commonly requested radiographic projections, including mobile, mammography, and neonatal procedures.

2019
ISBN: 978-0-323-59703-6

Mosby's Comprehensive Review of Radiography: The Complete Study Guide and Career Planner, 7th Edition

Prepare for success on the ARRT certification exam with this complete, outline-style review of the major subject areas covered on the exam that also features more than 2,400 multiple-choice format review questions.

2017
ISBN: 978-0-323-35423-3

ELSEVIER

Visit myevolve.us/MDPC to get your copy today!

18-NHPem-0859 TM/CH 10/18

Egas Moniz
(1874-1955)

Schüller
(1874-1957)

Lysholm
(1891-1947)

Albers-Schönberg
(1865-1921)

Béclère, H.
(1880-1937)

Fuchs
(1895-1962)

Waters
(1888-1961)